Coronary Laser Angioplasty

GENERAL SERIES EDITOR
Ronald E. Vlietstra, MD
Department of Medicine (Cardiology)
The Watson Clinic
Lakeland, Florida

OTHER VOLUMES IN THE SERIES
David R. Holmes, Jr., and Kirk N. Garratt, *Atherectomy*

FORTHCOMING VOLUMES
Steven E. Nissen, *Intravascular and Myocardial Imaging*
Robert S. Schwartz, *Coronary Restenosis*

SERIES IN INTERVENTIONAL CARDIOLOGY

∙ ∙

Coronary Laser Angioplasty

EDITED BY

FRANK LITVACK, M.D.

Co-Director
Cardiovascular Intervention Center
Cedars-Sinai Medical Center;
Assistant Professor of Medicine
UCLA School of Medicine
Los Angeles, California

BOSTON

Blackwell Scientific Publications
Oxford   London   Edinburgh
Melbourne   Paris   Berlin   Vienna

Blackwell Scientific Publications

EDITORIAL OFFICES:
Three Cambridge Center, Cambridge, Massachusetts 02142, USA
Osney Mead, Oxford OX2 0EL, England
25 John Street, London, WC1N 2BL, England
23 Ainslie Place, Edinburgh, EH3 6AJ, Scotland
54 University Street, Carlton, Victoria 3053, Australia

OTHER EDITORIAL OFFICES:
Arnette SA, 2 rue Casimir-Delavigne, 75006 Paris, France
Blackwell-Wissenschaft, Meinekestrasse 4, D-1000 Berlin 15, Germany
Blackwell MZV, Feldgasse 13, A-1238 Wien, Austria

DISTRIBUTORS:
USA
Blackwell Scientific Publications
Three Cambridge Center
Cambridge, Massachusetts 02142
(Orders: Telephone: 800-759-6102)

Canada
Times Mirror Professional Publishing Ltd
5240 Finch Avenue E
Scarborough, Ontario M1S 5A2
(Orders: Telephone: 416-298-1588)

Australia
Blackwell Scientific Publications (Australia) Pty Ltd
54 University Street
Carlton, Victoria 3053
(Orders: Telephone: 03-347-0300)

Outside North America and Australia
Blackwell Scientific Publications, Ltd.
c/o Marston Book Services, Ltd.
P.O. Box 87, Oxford OX2 0DT, England
(Orders: Telephone: 011-44-865-791155)

Typeset by Pine Tree Composition
Printed and bound by The Maple-Vail Book Manufacturing Group
Designed by Joyce C. Weston

© 1992 by Blackwell Scientific Publications
Printed in the United States of America
91 92 93 94 5 4 3 2 1

All rights reserved. No part of this book may be reproduced in any form or by any electronic or mechanical means, including information storage and retrieval systems, without permission in writing from the publisher, except by a reviewer who may quote brief passages in a review.

Library of Congress Cataloging in Publication Data

Coronary laser angioplasty / edited by Frank Litvack.
     p.   cm. — (Series in interventional cardiology)
  Includes bibliographical references and index.
  ISBN 0-86542-189-7
    1. Coronary heart disease—Laser surgery.   I. Litvack, Frank.
II. Series.
    [DNLM: 1. Angioplasty, Laser. 2. Angioplasty, Laser—methods.
  3. Coronary Disease—surgery.   WG 300 C8254]
RD598.35.L37C67   1992
617.4'12059—dc20
DNLM/DLC
for Library of Congress   91-17213
                                                      CIP

To my wife, Shelley; my son, William Asher; and my parents, Erika and Jack Litvack.

Contents

Contributors ix
Foreword xiii
Preface xv

1. The Physical and Biological Basis for Laser Angioplasty 1
   Warren S. Grundfest, Jacob Segalowitz, and James Laudenslager

2. Laser-Tissue Interaction 18
   Sabino R. Torre and Timothy A. Sanborn

3. Catheters for Laser Angioplasty—Design Considerations 43
   Tsvi Goldenberg, William B. Anderson and Lynn M. Shimada

4. Technique and Patient Selection for Excimer Laser Coronary Angioplasty 72
   Neil Eigler

5. Results of Excimer Laser Coronary Angioplasty 85
   Neil Eigler

6. Percutaneous Transluminal Coronary Excimer Laser Atherectomy—The German Experience 98
   Karl R. Karsch and Manfred Mauser

7. Excimer Laser Coronary Angioplasty—Illustrative Cases and Applications 127
   Stephen L. Cook and Frank Litvack

8. Other Pulsed Lasers for Angioplasty Including Solid State Lasers 172
   Timothy J. Garrand and Lawrence I. Deckelbaum

9. Laser Balloon Angioplasty: Evolving Technology 192
   J. Richard Spears

10. Laser Safety and Regulatory Issues: FDA Perspective 222
    Lynne A. Reamer and Richard P. Felten

11. Restenosis: From Pathogenesis to Prevention 241
    James S. Forrester, Bojan Cercek, Behrooz Sharifi, Peter Barath, Michael Fishbein, and James Fagin

Index 269

Contributors

William B. Anderson, BS
Senior Engineer
Catheter Development
Advanced Interventional Systems, Inc. (AIS)
Irvine, California

Peter Barath, MD, PhD
Research Scientist
Department of Cardiology
Cedars-Sinai Medical Center
Los Angeles, California

Bojan Cercek, MD
Associate Cardiologist
Cedars-Sinai Medical Center
Los Angeles, California

Stephen L. Cook, MD
Attending Cardiologist
Department of Cardiology
Alvarado Hospital Medical Center
San Diego, California

Lawrence I. Deckelbaum, MD
Associate Professor of Medicine
Department of Internal Medicine (Cardiology)
Yale University School of Medicine
New Haven, Connecticut
Director, Cardiac Catheterization Laboratory
West Haven Veterans Administration Medical Center
West Haven, Connecticut

Neil Eigler, MD
Co-Director, Cardiovascular Intervention Center
Cedars-Sinai Medical Center
Los Angeles, California

James Fagin, MD
Medical Director
Weight Control and Endocrinology
Cedars-Sinai Medical Center
Los Angeles, California

Richard P. Felten
Center for Devices and Radiological Health
Office of Science and Technology
Division of Life Sciences
Radiation Biology Branch
Food and Drug Administration
Rockville, Maryland

Michael Fishbein, MD
Associate, Pathology and Laboratory Medicine
Cedars-Sinai Medical Center
Los Angeles, California

James S. Forrester, MD
George Burns and Gracie Allen Professor of Cardiovascular Research
Cedars-Sinai Medical Center
Los Angeles, California

Timothy J. Garrand, MD
Department of Internal Medicine (Cardiology)
Yale University School of Medicine
New Haven, Connecticut
West Haven Veterans Administration Medical Center
West Haven, Connecticut

Tsvi Goldenberg, PhD
Director of Catheter Development
Advanced Interventional Systems, Inc. (AIS)
Irvine, California

Warren S. Grundfest, MD
Assistant Director of Surgery
Director, Laser Surgery and Technology Development
Cedars-Sinai Medical Center
Assistant Clinical Professor of Surgery
UCLA School of Medicine
Los Angeles, California

Karl R. Karsch, MD
Professor of Medicine/Cardiology
University of Tubingen
Tubingen, Germany

James Laudenslager, PhD
Vice President, Laser Development
Advanced Interventional Systems, Inc. (AIS)
Irvine, California

Frank Litvack, MD
Co-Director
Cardiovascular Intervention Center
Cedars-Sinai Medical Center
Assistant Professor of Medicine
UCLA School of Medicine
Los Angeles, California

Manfred Mauser, MD
Professor of Medicine/Cardiology
University of Tubingen
Tubingen, Germany

Lynne A. Reamer
Center for Devices and Radiological Health
Office of Device Evaluation
Division of Cardiovascular Devices
Surgical, Therapeutic and Diagnostic Devices Branch
Food and Drug Administration
Rockville, Maryland

Timothy A. Sanborn, MD
Associate Professor of Medicine
Director, Interventional Cardiology Research and Laser Angioplasty Program
Arthur Ross Scholar in Cardiovascular Medicine
Division of Cardiology
Mount Sinai Medical Center and the New York Cardiac Center
New York, New York

Contributors xi

Jacob Segalowitz, MD
Clinical Instructor of Surgery
UCLA School of Medicine
Associate in Cardiovascular
  Laser Surgery
Department of Surgery
Cedars-Sinai Medical Center
Los Angeles, California

Behrooz Sharifi, MD, PhD
Research Scientist
Department of Cardiology
Cedars-Sinai Medical Center
Los Angeles, California

Lynn M. Shimada, MS
Senior Engineer
Catheter Development
Advanced Interventional Systems, Inc. (AIS)
Irvine, California

J. Richard Spears, MD
Department of Medicine
Division of Cardiology
Harper Hospital/Wayne State
  University
Detroit, Michigan

Sabino R. Torre, MD
Interventional Research Fellow
Division of Cardiology
Mount Sinai Medical Center
New York, New York

Foreword

THIS is the second in a series of monographs devoted to emerging cardiovascular technologies. Each volume addresses technical issues, clinical application, comparative utility versus alternative devices, and includes insights as to what changes might be expected in the near future. The series is timely in that a wide variety of devices are under investigation, and their relative strengths and weaknesses are poorly understood by most of us.

The volume editors have been selected not only for being leaders in their field, but also for their capacity to give a balanced perspective. We believe that authoritative and sober presentations may help counter the "hyped" and unrealistic expectations that can be fostered by limited or inaccurate information.

Dr. Litvack and his contributors have the necessary experience to fully appreciate the strengths and weaknesses of the exciting new laser catheter technology. Their comprehensive technical and clinical text helps demystify the laser approach. Importantly, the authors also help the clinical reader interpret some of the technical and regulatory factors involved in device development—issues that often seem to frustrate the prompt incorporation of useful devices into clinical practice.

Blackwell Scientific Publications is enthusiastically supporting this effort with the result that further contributions on other exciting technology issues will soon be published. Much remains to be discussed.

RONALD E. VLIETSTRA
Series Editor

Preface

IT was not without some trepidation that I accepted the kind offer to edit this volume when first approached by Ronald Vlietstra and Blackwell Scientific Publications. Although I was impressed by the caliber of the series on Interventional Cardiology, I was also respectful of the difficulties in producing a text on such an adolescent and dynamic subject as Coronary Laser Angioplasty.

A book, which necessarily is published many months or even a year or so following its writing, competes on uneven ground with the many journals and periodicals now available. Further, live courses, congresses, and demonstrations now serve as the primary media of communication for most interventional cardiologists. One may justly inquire, Is there any role for any book about such a subject nowadays? Upon reflection, I answered in the affirmative and began the task of outlining the contributions. What we have endeavored to present is a comprehensive but not exhaustive view of the subject. Neither have we attempted to cover every obsolete device ever conceived or tested nor to speculate on future (and sometimes futuristic) technologies currently in the seminal or earlier phase.

I requested Grundfest, Sanborn, Goldenberg, and their colleagues to present the basics of laser science, laser tissue interactions, and fiberoptic theory, upon which all useful research thus far performed has been based and upon which future developments will be predicated. Failure to examine basic principles and to incorporate these principles into clinical projects in the past has resulted in research that generated media hype but has served no patients well and blemished the entire field of laser angioplasty in the eyes of some. The scientific principles presented in these chapters, although certain to be expanded and modified in the future, should remain useful to investigators and clinicians in the years to come.

Excimer laser angioplasty with the 308 nanometer device has, to date, dominated our clinical experience with ablative lasers and is therefore covered in the greatest detail. There are major differences between the three excimer laser angioplasty systems (Technolase, Spectranetics, and Advanced Interventional Systems) thus far used clinically. These differences rest both in laser and delivery system design. Clinical results of any one system may not necessarily be extrapolated to another. All three systems are discussed but no effort has been made to provide comparative analysis. Such an attempt would be precocious as all systems are undergoing rapid evolution. Furthermore, direct comparisons necessarily evoke commercial instincts—something we have attempted to avoid in this text.

The Advanced Interventional Systems, Inc., excimer devices have received the most attention in this work, and the reasons are twofold. First, this is the system that has been most widely tested and that has thus far provided the broadest clinical experience. Second, this is the system that I and my Cedars-Sinai colleagues have been investigating for several years. I believe it my responsibility to disclose that Grundfest, Forrester, and I were involved with the founding of this company several years ago and remain to this day shareholders. Without the 12–15 million dollars this company has invested in research and development, excimer laser coronary angioplasty would never have happened. The technology was not available, even in preclinical form, in the early 1980s. Despite this potential conflict of interest, we have made every effort to present our data honestly and without embellishment.

Deckelbaum and Garrand have contributed a chapter on other pulsed lasers potentially useful for coronary angioplasty. No good clinical data is yet available on these devices, and we await some serious clinical trials. Spears has presented his most interesting work with the laser balloon angioplasty system he has developed. This "nonablative" laser angioplasty system is finding a role in the treatment of complications encountered during balloon angioplasty.

Reamer and Felten have provided a chapter on laser safety and regulatory issues. This chapter is designed to aid physicians and hospital administrators who may consider setting up or running a laser program. It should also assist device developers at better understanding the broad regulatory issues. Since the government and specifically the Food and Drug Administration play such an important role in device development, I felt they should be heard from.

Forrester and colleagues have provided a broad overview on our great nemesis—restenosis. At the time of this writing detailed restenosis data following excimer angioplasty is just being analyzed (see Chapter 5). We must, however, have no illusions. Available data leads us to believe that this technology, at least as applied today, has had no impact on reducing restenosis rates in general. The chapter on restenosis is presented to provide scientific facts and theory upon which researchers and clinicians may draw in the future. When one accounts for the critical (and often overlooked) parameters of vessel diameter and lesion length it is clear that none of the plaque-removing, shaving, or ablative devices has had any real positive effect on restenosis. Each of the new device developers has searched their data for a subgroup within a subgroup that could provide some positive results. The net results, with respect to reduction of restenosis, have been unimpressive despite some claims to the contrary. We have much yet to learn.

FRANK LITVACK, M.D.
Los Angeles, January, 1991

Notice
The indications and dosages of all drugs in this book have been recommended in the medical literature and conform to the practices of the general medical community. The medications described do not necessarily have specific approval by the Food and Drug Administration for use in the diseases and dosages for which they are recommended. The package insert for each drug should be consulted for use and dosage as approved by the FDA. Because standards for usage change, it is advisable to keep abreast of revised recommendations, particularly those concerning new drugs.

Coronary Laser Angioplasty

CHAPTER **1**

The Physical and Biological Basis for Laser Angioplasty

WARREN S. GRUNDFEST
JACOB SEGALOWITZ
JAMES LAUDENSLAGER

T H E goals of this chapter are threefold: first, to discuss the basic physics of lasers, light generation, and light propagation; second, to examine the laser-tissue interaction in terms of its component parts including the type of laser, tissue composition, and energy-delivery parameters of the laser light; and third, to explore some engineering aspects of the design of laser angioplasty systems.

The idea for a "laser" was first conceived by Albert Einstein in 1905. The term "laser" is an acronym developed from the description of the device in which *l*ight *a*mplification by *s*timulated *e*mission of *r*adiation occurs. The laser device can generate an intense, monochromatic, directional, polarized, coherent beam of light. Each of these terms describes some of the unique features of laser light. Laser light can be generated at enormous intensities (gigawatts) in one color, in a beam that propagates in one direction with minimal divergence of the light. Light generated from nonlaser sources is incoherent; the various wavelengths that compose it interfere with each other or cancel each other out as the light propagates in all directions. White light diminishes in intensity as the square of the distance between the source and the observer. Laser light is usually of one wavelength and the waves of light travel synchronously in time and in electromagnetic phase with one another; therefore, there is minimal interference in a laser beam. Thus, this organized, structured beam of light propagates with minimal dispersion at high intensities.

Lasers produce intense monochromatic radiation, which can be delivered to a small area of tissue with great precision through fiber optics. This energy may be absorbed, reflected, scattered, transmitted, diffracted, refracted, or absorbed and reemitted as fluorescence. Once absorbed, the energy may be converted to heat, may break chemical bonds, may form a plasma, or may be reemitted as fluorescence. Each of these outcomes produces different biological effects on the tissue. Thus, the choice of laser depends upon the desired application, the tissue encountered, and the biologic constraints placed on the laser-delivery system.

The first working laser was demonstrated by Maiman in 1959 using a ruby crystal as the lasing medium (1). Throughout the 1960s a variety of lasers was developed based on using gases, solids, and liquids as the lasing medium. Maiman's ruby laser was soon followed by a helium neon laser, demonstrated by Javan (2) in 1961, and several other lasers developed between 1961 and 1970, including the argon ion, carbon dioxide, and metal vapor lasers. Combinations of lasers and the ability to generate laser light from organic dye molecules expanded the range of laser wavelengths. In the 20-year period between 1970 and 1990 the development of solid-state crystalline lasers based on doped yttriumaluminumgarnet and excimer lasers based on combinations of halogen and noble gases further extended the range of wavelengths available for biological applications (3–5).

The first laser applied for medical applications was the ruby laser, which emitted a pulsed intense beam of red light. This laser's application was limited largely to ophthalmologic procedures. In its initial configuration the intense laser pulse was difficult to control and often produced unpredictable results. In 1964 the carbon dioxide laser was used to cut and coagulate tissue. This was the first laser that reached broad medical application. However, the CO_2 laser emits light in the far infrared region of the spectrum. For more than 20 years, no fiber-optic-delivery system was available, and therefore, complex articulated arms and handpieces (a series of lenses, mirrors, and tubes) were devised to deliver the energy to the operative site. This cumbersome delivery system, the need for specialized training, and the expense of the devices limited medical application.

The Physical and Biological Basis for Laser Angioplasty   3

The advent of argon ion and Nd:YAG lasers was touted as a revolution in laser surgery since both could be delivered through fiber optics. However, initial models of these "new" lasers had several drawbacks: they were expensive, difficult to maintain, and required water cooling and high-voltage electrical outlets. More importantly, from the standpoint of hospital economics, the devices were continually modified and "upgraded" as the technology improved. Additional costs were incurred as physicians realized the need for appropriate safety measures, ancillary devices, and additional tools. Typically, each medical application of laser technology has required 7–10 years of developmental research. Since the first attempts at laser angioplasty using continuous-wave argon lasers took place in 1984, it is not surprising that a reliable clinical system was not developed until 1989.

Initial versions of laser devices, particularly for angioplasty, were often crude and ineffective. Despite the experimental nature of these initial systems, they were touted as miracle cures and purchased to attract patients. This unfortunate circumstance led to a negative impression of laser technology, in particular for laser angioplasty. Lasers were employed with little or no understanding of their effects on vascular tissue. Delivery of laser energy was accomplished through crude single fiber-optic systems without the benefit of guidance mechanisms. The preliminary results of laser angioplasty reported in the literature (6–8) were often used to compare laser systems to other more mature technologies (balloon angioplasty). Unfortunately, this apples-to-oranges comparison was inappropriate since not all lasers produce the same effects on tissue. Laser angioplasty can be compared to other forms of vascular recanalization only after the laser system has been optimized to produce the best result. As with any engineering project, defining the "optimal" system requires a thorough understanding of the parameters that govern its operation. Further, optimization, particularly in systems as complex as lasers, is an iterative process. The ideal laser angioplasty system does not yet exist.

Currently, a broad range of laser systems is under investigation. As more sophisticated technologies reach clinical trials, the older and more primitive continuous-wave systems appear less likely to have any clinical role in laser angioplasty. Therefore, the physician is faced with increasingly complex choices when considering purchase and clinical application of laser angioplasty. To make this choice, the physician must understand both the fundamental physical properties that define and constrain the laser angioplasty system and the current clinical results. The physician must examine the various laser angioplasty systems available and select that system that appears to be optimal. Each laser has specific operating parameters that govern its emission of light. The effect of this light on tissue is controlled by the absorption, scattering, and transmission of the particular light by the tissue. Both the mode in which the laser light is delivered and the tissue with which it interacts play a major role in determining the outcome of the interaction. To predict the outcome of the interaction of laser light with tissue the operating parameters of the laser, the delivery system employed, and the tissue being irradiated must be described. The concept of a "generic" laser that is useful for multiple applications is misleading and deceptive. Laser light can be used for lithotripsy, coagulation, tissue ablation, and drug activation. However, each of these processes requires its own set of parameters. Laser angioplasty also requires its own set of parameters for optimal therapeutic effectiveness and safety.

Basic Physics of Lasers and Light

Fundamentally, lasers are energy-conversion machines that transmute electrical, chemical, or light energy into intense beams of light of one color. A laser has several basic components (Fig. 1.1). These include the lasing medium that fills the laser cavity, and an energy source. At one end of the laser cavity is a totally reflecting mirror, and at the other end is a partially reflecting mirror. Various methods are used to excite the lasing medium within the cavity. Energy can be pumped into the cavity by means of a flashlamp or electrical discharge to excite or stimulate the atoms. In some lasers the combination of an electrical discharge and a chemical reaction produces a new chemical species. The chemical reaction provides the energy to excite the atoms. To produce laser light there must be more excited than unexcited atoms in the laser chamber. This condition is termed a "population inversion." When the excited atoms relax (lose energy), they spontaneously release one photon or packet of light. The spontaneously released photon can strike either an excited or an unexcited atom. If it strikes an unexcited atom it can be absorbed, leading to excitation of that particular atom. However, if it strikes an excited atom a stimulated release of two photons can occur. Thus, one excited atom generates one photon, which can strike a second excited atom to generate two photons. Each of these photons can strike more excited atoms, leading to an exponential increase in the re-

The Physical and Biological Basis for Laser Angioplasty 5

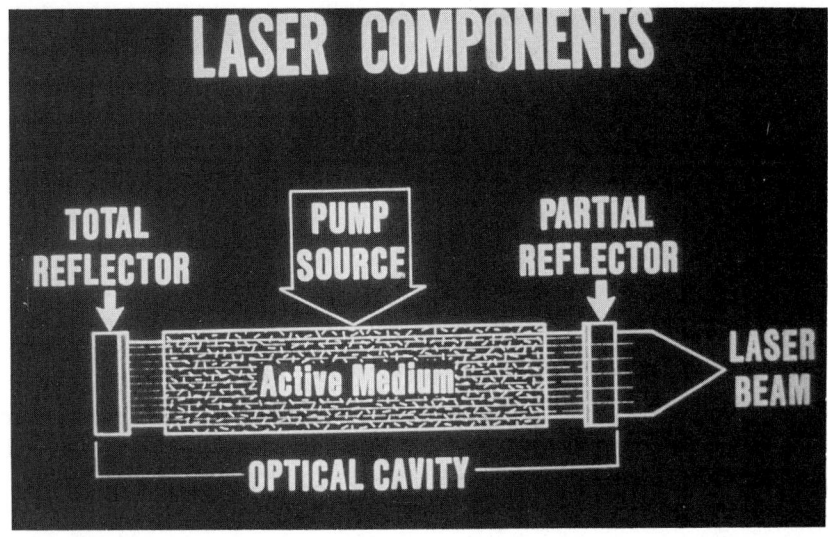

Figure 1.1. The basic laser components consist of an energy or "pump" source that excites atoms of the active medium. The active medium is held between two mirrors, a total reflector and a partial reflector. The laser beam is emitted through the partial reflector.

lease of light, from one to two to four to eight, etc. For this process to proceed there must be more excited atoms than unexcited atoms. When the number of excited atoms exceeds the number of unexcited atoms a population inversion occurs. To maintain lasing action the lasing material must be continually excited to produce the population inversion. This amplification step is critical to laser action. The specifics of the process vary from one lasing material to another. However, the process of amplification is common to all lasers.

This process of amplification is relatively inefficient and converts only 1 to 10 percent of the input energy to light output. Thus, a laser with a 10-watt output may require 10,000 watts of electrical energy for operation. This inefficiency can have a major impact on the engineering aspects and size of clinical lasers. The more inefficient the device the greater the size and the need for large electrical inputs (three-phase 220-volt power) and water cooling.

The wavelength of emitted light is a function of the lasing medium within the laser cavity. Solids, liquids, and gases can be used as the lasing medium. The wavelength of emitted light is determined by the electronic structure of the lasing medium. Light is emitted in the infrared region of the spectrum when a population inversion is established between a ground state and a higher-level vibrational rotational energy level. To produce light in the visible or ultraviolet region of the spectrum, excitation of the lasing medium must produce a population inversion between two electronic energy levels. Thus the emitted light is dependent upon the molecular structure of the lasing medium and its excited states.

The Interaction of Light with Matter

Several processes are required to describe the interaction of light with matter. Absorption, transmission, reflection, refraction, diffraction, and several types of scattering can occur simultaneously as light interacts with matter. Absorption of light by an irradiated material increases the energy content of the material. All atoms and molecules have characteristic energy levels and can exist in different energy states. These atoms or molecules contain rotational, vibrational, and translational energy that is characteristic of the temperature of their own environment. In addition, atoms and molecules also have various electronic states. In these electronic states the electrons orbiting around the nucleus can be raised to higher or excited energy levels by the absorption of a photon of radiation. These excited species can also gain or lose energy levels as a result of molecular collisions. When light is absorbed it characteristically increases the translational energy level, which increases molecular motion. This mechanism of light absorption results in heating of the material. Alternatively, if the absorbed photon has sufficient energy to cause electronic excitation, an excited electronic intermediate can be generated. These electronic intermediates can lead to chemical rearrangements, or the energy can be converted from an electronic excited state to a vibrational rotational state. Once in the vibrational rotational state the increased energy appears as heat. For typical laser applications the absorption of laser light results in conversion of light to heat. However, if light absorption leads to electronic excitation, chemical bond breaking and subsequent alteration of material can occur.

When the light path crosses an interface between two optically clear materials with differing refractive indices, a portion of the light beam is reflected at the interface and the rest of the light beam undergoes a change in direction as it passes through the second material. The refractive index is the velocity at which light travels through the transmitting medium as compared to the velocity of light in a vacuum. For a given set of materials such as an air-glass or a glass-water interface, the portion of reflected light and the portion of transmitted light are a function of wavelength and the angle at which the light beam travels through the interface. Light traveling perpendicularly from air into a glass target loses approximately 4 percent of its intensity due to reflection. Thus, from one lens with two surfaces a light beam may be diminished by an 8 percent loss of energy. These factors become critical in the design of a complex laser delivery system where multiple lenses, mirrors, and fiber optics are required to deliver light to the target. Thus, the output of the laser must be sufficient to overcome the losses in the delivery system and still achieve a therapeutic effect.

In general, the absorption of light increases the temperature of the absorbing medium. The mathematical formula that describes the relationship between the absorption and transmission of monochromatic light by a homogeneous material is the Beer-Lambert equation: $I = I_o(-ax)$, where I is the intensity of light transmitted through the medium of length x with an attenuation coefficient of a, and I_o is the intensity of the light beam as it is incident on the interface. The ratio of I/I_o is the transmittance through the medium. A ratio of 1 describes a material that is totally transparent with no absorption. The above formula describes the attenuation of light as an exponential process with the proportion of light absorbed per unit length as a constant. This law holds only for ideal conditions; however, tissue is not ideal. In addition to absorption, scattering plays a major role in the distribution of light within the tissue.

In contrast to absorption, scattering of a beam of light does not always cause an increase in the energy content of the medium and a corresponding rise in temperature. There are several different types of scattering. If light is scattered by particles smaller than the wavelength of the incident light, the beam is dispersed away from the path of the light beam. This type of scattering is known as Rayleigh scattering and is commonly seen in shorter wavelengths, particularly in the ultraviolet. Rayleigh scattering is symmetrical in both forward and backward directions. If the scattering particles are larger in size than the wavelength of light, for example, for green light, 0.4 microns in diameter, the scattering is called Mie scattering. Unlike Rayleigh scattering, Mie scattering is predominantly in the forward direction and depends upon the size and shape of the particles as well as the wavelength of light. Rayleigh scattering predominates when the particles in the light-transmitting medium are small, while Mie scattering predominates when the particles are much larger than the wavelength of the light. Dust particles or smoke permits visualization of a laser beam through a combination of Mie scattering and diffraction. The effects of scattering and variation in tissue absorption of laser energy must be considered when choosing the optimal wavelengths for laser angioplasty.

A variation of the process of reflection and refraction is used to guide light through fiber optics. In a fiber-optic wave guide, once the light enters the material, total internal reflection occurs. In this situation two transparent materials are used. One material serves as a core, which is surrounded by a cladding composed of the second material. By appropriately choosing the index of refraction of the materials total reflection occurs at the core-cladding interface.

The above descriptions of absorption, reflection, and scattering are designed to describe relatively ideal phenomena. However, the processes that occur in tissue are not ideal and are therefore difficult to model mathematically. The description of these processes is further complicated by the enormous energy densities used during the ablation of tissue. Tissue is not an ideal material, and the atheromatous process generates highly heterogeneous tissue. Thus, multiple scattering phenomena with wide variations in absorption and transmission can occur within a very short segment of tissue. Thus, predicting the interaction of light with atheroma becomes an extremely complex, difficult task. Further complicating the issue is the phenomena of nonlinear absorption. These nonlinear processes occur when high peak-power pulses of light are used to ablate tissue and may produce unexpected results (tissue breakdown, shock wave formation, and chemical rearrangements).

Given the complexity of describing the interaction of laser light with biological materials, mathematical modeling of these processes often results in inadequate conclusions. The additional complexities introduced by nonlinear processes require that observational methods be used to optimize laser selection for laser angioplasty. Further complicating the analysis of the interaction of laser light with tissue is the presence of a fiber-optic delivery system and the constraints imposed by the biological system. The presence of blood and the heterogeneity of the arterial wall must be taken into account when selecting the energy source for laser angioplasty.

For each specific application, such as laser angioplasty, there exists an optimal set of energy-delivery parameters. This set of parameters must be clearly defined and reproducible from procedure to procedure. These parameters include the energy delivered per unit time at the target, the area of the target irradiated, the time of irradiation, and if a pulsed laser is used, the duration of the laser pulse and the number of pulses per second. When pulsed lasers are employed, knowledge of the pulse duration becomes critical to controlling the laser's biological effects. These pulse durations can range from a few milliseconds to a few picoseconds (10^{-12} seconds). For any laser the average power is the energy delivered per unit of time. For pulsed lasers the peak power is the energy of a single pulse divided by its pulse width. The pulse width of the laser is determined by the laser's electronics and the lasing medium and is measured using photodiodes and an oscilloscope. Two lasers operating at an average power of 5 watts will have distinctly different effects on the tissue if one is operating in the continuous-wave mode and the other operates in a pulsed mode (9,10). Unfortunately, the literature lacks clarity when describing laser power. Descriptions of average power without statements of the laser spot size or pulse characteristics are inadequate for characterization of the biological effects.

The following example illustrates the difference between average power and peak power. If a pulsed laser emits light with an energy of 100 millijoules at 100 pulses per second with a pulse duration of 10 nanoseconds and this energy is delivered to a 1 cm^2 spot, the average power density is 100 millijoules $\times$ 100 pulses per second per cm^2 or 10 watts per cm^2 in average power terms. However, the peak power is calculated as 100 millijoules divided by 10×10^{-9} seconds/cm^2 or 10 megawatts per cm^2. In this example the peak power is enormous while the average power is much lower. The peak power has a dramatic influence on the biological effect. At energy levels of a megawatt or above, nonlinear effects begin to occur. Generation of photoplasmas and excited states also requires high peak powers.

For pulsed lasers the term "energy fluence" is used to describe the irradiance level of the tissue. Energy fluence is the energy per pulse divided by the area under irradiation and is expressed in joules/cm^2 or millijoules/mm^2. For a continuous-wave laser the energy fluence equals the laser output power in watts multiplied by the exposure time in seconds divided by the irradiated area. Thus, tissue effects are usually related to the energy per unit area delivered to the tissue. These effects, including heating, vaporization, ablation (layer-by-layer removal of tissue), and fragmentation, are a function of the wavelength of light, the energy density at which the light is delivered, and the properties of the tissue. Because of its ability to deliver highly concentrated monochromatic light, the laser provides a unique source of energy for biological applications. The combination of pulsed delivery and spatial confinement of energy (due to intense absorption and resultant minimal depth of penetration) provides a unique method of energy delivery for laser angioplasty. The short pulse duration limits the time available for heat transfer to occur during irradiation, and the spatial confinement produced by the use of ultraviolet light limits the area irradiated. Understanding this process requires a brief description of the mechanisms of laser action.

Laser/Tissue Ablation Mechanisms

The following sections describe the four basic physical processes that result from the absorption of laser light by tissue. Energy that is not absorbed can be scattered or transmitted through the tissue and produce effects remote from the site of energy application. The extent of scattering depends upon the organization structure and particulate size within a given tissue, the depth of penetration of a particular wavelength within the tissue, and the presence of molecules that strongly absorb the light (chromophores). Energy delivered in short intense pulses can generate a photoplasma. Alternatively, rapid deposition of energy can lead to almost instantaneous conversion of solid or liquid to the gas phase. From either process explosive ejection of material occurs and is accompanied by acoustic transients or shock waves. These shock waves can disrupt the tissue.

Thermal Processes

The first and most common mechanism results when continuous-wave or pulsed infrared lasers are used to irradiate tissue (11). The absorbed photons are converted to heat, which increases the molecular motion of the molecules. As sufficient energy is pumped into the tissue water begins to vaporize and proteins denature. If water is the absorbing chromophore the tissue undergoes rapid dehydration as the water is converted to steam. The resulting shock wave from the conversion of water to steam can be quite pronounced. As energy delivery continues, heating of the surrounding tissues occurs as light is scattered through the dehydrated tissue. Protein coagulation can be prominent, particularly in the infrared wavelengths. The fundamental process, the conversion of light to heat, occurs with all continuous-wave lasers and at pulse durations greater than 50 microseconds, regardless of the wavelengths chosen and the energy delivery parameters. As heat increases, thermal conduction and diffusion cause temperature rises in the surrounding tissue. To minimize the lateral spread of energy it is necessary to select a pulsed laser with a pulse duration shorter than the average thermal conduction time of the tissue.

When laser irradiation occurs from continuous-wave, infrared, or visible sources, the light is converted to heat. Continued deposition of energy raises the tissue temperature. As the tissue is heated from 43°–50° C, the collagen helices uncoil, resulting in reversible tissue denaturation. If the heating is not prolonged, cooling may occur and the coils may actually fuse together. This annealing process is the basis for laser welding and laser tissue fusion experiments. Efforts to control this process are complicated by the enormous number of variables involved. The clinical application of laser welding has been slow to evolve due to the inability to predict the outcome of the process (12). As the temperature of the tissue increases beyond 60° C, irreversible protein denaturation occurs. If exposure to this level of heat is short, the cells are injured; prolonged heating results in cell death. As temperatures exceed 80° C the underlying structural elements of the tissue—collagen, elastin, and proteoglycans—begin to degrade. At 100° C, water within the tissue boils, leading to a potentially explosive release of steam. When temperatures exceed 150° C, pyrolysis of the tissue is observed. At temperatures above 200° C the tissue begins to carbonize. Only the carbon particles are left behind as the rest of the organic material is oxidized. With continuous-wave lasers, attempts to ablate calcified tissue can result in temperatures in excess of 500° C.

When laser energy is converted to heat in the tissues, thermal diffusion begins. Diffusion of heat through the tissue depends on the thermal properties of the irradiated material. Vascular tissue tends to have thermal diffusion constants in a range of 1–10 microseconds. Pulses longer than several microseconds allow thermal energy to diffuse over 10–100 microns in a few milliseconds. Pulses in the millisecond range are sufficiently long to allow heat generated to diffuse between 100 and 1000 microns away from the zone of irradiation. The thermal relaxation (cooling) phenomenon is influenced by 1) the thermal coefficient of the tissue, 2) the properties of the surrounding tissue or fluids, and 3) the temperature differential between the irradiated and nonirradiated tissue (13).

Photochemical Processes

A second method of tissue ablation results from irradiation of tissue with short- (nanosecond) pulse-duration ultraviolet laser energy. Ultraviolet photons contain sufficient energy per pulse to break molecular bonds. This electronic process is more efficient than thermal processes because the laser energy is employed directly in bond breaking without a thermal intermediate. The primary chromophore (energy-absorbing material) is protein or lipid, not water. Thus, pulsed ultraviolet light can lead to direct electronic bond breaking of organic material and does not require vaporization of water. As large molecules are converted to small molecules, they are ejected from the surface of the material, removing much of the energy used to break the chemical bonds (14). Since the pulse duration is less than 500 nanoseconds, there is little time for radiative or conductive heat transfer to the adjacent tissue. Thus, the input energy is not deposited in the adjacent tissue. For the process to be effective, the tissue must be a strong absorber of the laser wavelength. Atherosclerotic tissue, although highly heterogeneous, is composed primarily of water and organic compounds with a few inorganic salts. The atherosclerotic proteins and lipids strongly absorb ultraviolet light and serve as the primary chromophore. While the exact nature of this mechanism remains the subject of intense debate, ablation produced by pulsed ultraviolet light at levels above threshold is precise, controllable, and predictable. On a theoretical basis, therefore, pulsed ultraviolet light would appear to be the optimal energy source for laser angioplasty (15).

Photochemical change can occur as a result of direct excitation of electronic bonds by the laser energy and is one of the proposed mechanisms of action of pulsed ultraviolet lasers. Electronic excitation by laser is not 100 percent efficient; therefore, heat is also generated during this process. The physical chemistry of pulsed tissue ablation is as yet not well defined. Two potential mechanisms appear to operate. At shorter wavelengths, tissue components, proteins, and lipids absorb photons and become electronically excited. This "photoexcitation" leads to rupture of molecular bonds and formation of molecular fragments. These molecular fragments then undergo a process known as "photochemical desorption" and are ejected from the irradiated surface in less than 200 nanoseconds. The ejected fragments carry with them much of the energy that was initially deposited within the tissue to generate the fragments. This electronic excitation occurs before conversion to heat or thermal diffusion occurs. A second possible mechanism to explain this phenomenon is very-high-speed, localized absorption, which leads to formation of a very small area of vaporized photoproducts. These products expand rapidly away from the tissue surface, again carrying away the incident energy. By either mechanism the result is the removal of tissue with minimal thermal damage to adjacent structures.

Photoacoustic Processes

The deposition of large numbers of photons in a short period of time produces a very intense local electric field. This sudden rise in electrical energy produces a plasma. These plasmas can be produced through a variety of mechanisms, the most common of which is dielectric breakdown, in which large numbers of electrons are released as the conductivity of the material is altered due to the intense electric field. This energy is then transferred in a very localized fashion to the surrounding tissue, producing a small area of vaporized material. The sudden expansion of the vaporized material generates an intense shock wave. As the shock wave expands radially outward, tissue disruption and ejection of material may result. This mechanism is employed in the treatment of thickened posterior capsule membranes, which occur after cataract operations. Typically, two infrared beams of subthreshold energies are focused to the spot on the posterior capsule of the lens where membrane disruption is desired. While each beam is insufficient to destroy the tissue, the two beams together produce a photoplasma that disrupts the tissue (16).

This photoacoustic shock wave mechanism is not readily adaptable to fiber-optic transmission. The high peak powers and short pulse durations employed tend to destroy the fiber optics as well as the tissue. In addition, this mechanism does not work well in heterogeneous tissue, and its application to atherosclerotic tissue therefore produces variable results.

These three ablation mechanisms, photothermal, photoacoustic, and photochemical, occur at distinctly different energy and power densities and wavelengths. Thus, the desired outcome can be achieved by selecting the appropriate wavelength and energy-delivery parameters. Unless the appropriate parameters are selected, the desired result may not be achieved. For pulsed ultraviolet ablation of tissue through a photochemical mechanism, there must be sufficient energy deposited to break molecular bonds. This occurs above a certain threshold level that is a unique combination of both the laser wavelength and the tissue under irradiation. If the light irradiating the tissue is at subthreshold levels, insufficient chemical intermediates are formed for the photochemical processes to occur and the light is converted to heat. If too much energy is employed, dielectric breakdown occurs and a photoacoustic mechanism predominates. Thus, the same laser, if operated in a different mode, can produce considerably different tissue effects even though the wavelength is the same.

Fluorescent Phenomena

Fluorescence occurs when photons of light are absorbed by tissue and reemitted at a longer wavelength. This rapidly occurring process (nanoseconds or less) is strongly affected by the electronic bond structure and the chemical composition of the irradiated matter. Fluorescence can be used to detect and monitor specific compounds that occur naturally or that have been added to the system. A particular wavelength fluorescence must be distinguished from the baseline autofluorescence that occurs in tissue. This can be done using various filters after identifying the specific wavelengths of the emitted (fluorescent) light. To date this work has primarily focused on photodetection of hematoporphyrin derivatives, tetracycline, and carotenoids.

Laser-induced fluorescence results when a portion of the laser light is absorbed and reradiated. Given the high intensity and monochromaticity of the laser beam, the reradiated light can be of sufficient intensity to permit detection and analysis. The returning fluorescent light pattern can act as a fingerprint for identification of certain compounds. Analysis of the fluorescent pattern is now under study as a means of differentiating normal from atherosclerotic tissue (17,18). This would permit target-specific laser angioplasty. Preliminary results are encouraging; however, the laser-induced fluorescence is so sensitive to chemical changes that irradiated or ablated tissue may give different signals than normal or atherosclerotic tissue (Fig. 1.2).

The Physical and Biological Basis for Laser Angioplasty 15

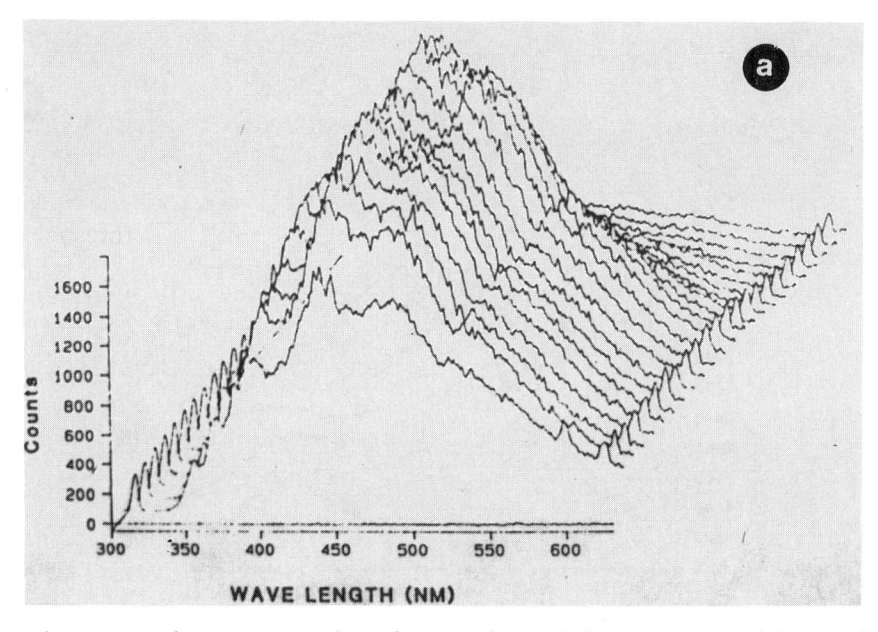

Figure 1.2. This sequence of graphs was obtained during excimer ablation of human aorta using a multifiber catheter. Ablation was performed at 45 mJ/mm^2. The spectroscopic signals were obtained using the ablation catheter for collection and transmission of the fluorescence signal. The graph represents ablation of normal *(A)* and atherosclerotic *(B)* tissue. The X axis represents the wavelength of the fluorescence light, the Y axis shows the intensity (count), and the Z axis represents number of pulses. Normal vascular tissue has a relatively well-defined peak at 400–450 nanometers while atherosclerotic tissue has a broader signal with a second peak occurring at 500–550 nanometers. A comparison of *(A)* and *(B)* shows the difference in spectra.

The Physical Basis for Observed Phenomena

Initial attempts to use continuous-wave lasers for laser angioplasty demonstrated the futility of this approach. The light emitted from a carbon dioxide laser at 10.6 microns is in the far infrared. This radiation is absorbed primarily by water with a relatively short depth of penetration (approximately 100 microns). This wavelength is unacceptable for several reasons. First, no fiber-optic transmission system exists for this wavelength. Second, the primary chromophore or light-absorbing material is water, which results in conversion of water to steam. Third, this wavelength is relatively ineffective in ablating calcified material.

The argon ion laser was also proposed as a source for laser angio-

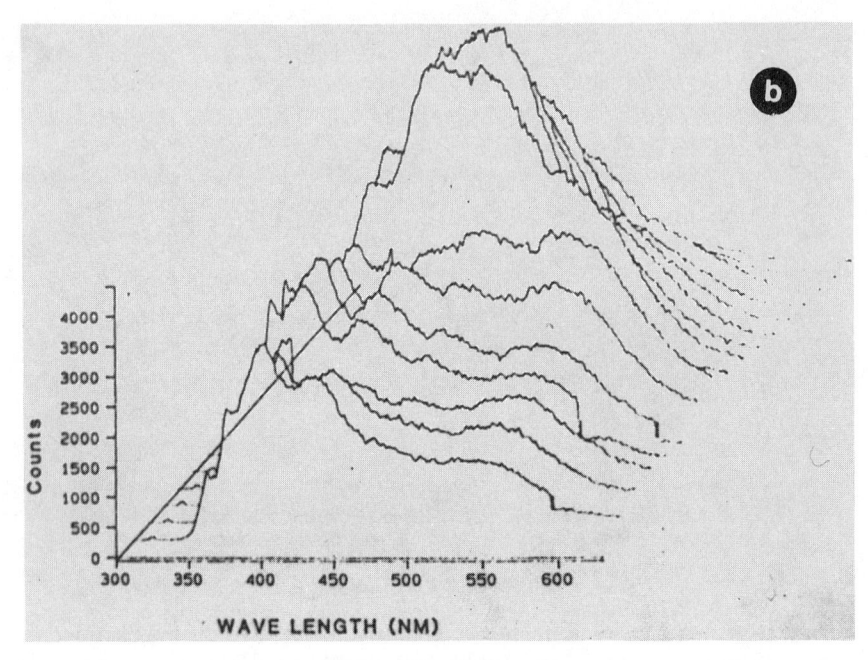

Figure 1.2. Continued

plasty. This source produces light at 514 and 488 nm. While this wavelength can be transmitted through fiber optics, its effects on biologic tissue are highly dependent upon the presence of absorbing chromophores such as blood or carotenoid pigments. Tests revealed that this laser ablates tissue with considerable thermal injury to adjacent tissue even when delivered in a chopped-beam mode and is relatively ineffective in ablation of calcified tissue.

The Nd:YAG laser can operate in a variety of modes. Light is emitted at 1064 nm in the infrared and penetrates tissue to a depth of ½ cm or more. This large depth of penetration coupled with the variability of ablation based on the presence or absence of chromophores makes this laser a poor choice for laser angioplasty.

The CO_2, argon ion, and Nd:YAG lasers represent the traditional continuous-wave lasers employed in surgical applications of lasers. For the reasons listed above, none of these devices are appropriate for laser angioplasty. Attempts to optimize these devices were doomed to fail due to the nature of the ablation mechanism of continuous-wave lasers. All of these lasers produce their ablative effects through the conversion of

The Physical and Biological Basis for Laser Angioplasty 17

light to heat. Although the chromophores may be different, ablation with each of these lasers generates large volumes of steam (water converted to its vapor phase) with subsequent thermal denaturation of surrounding tissues. Attempts to limit the thermal injury to tissue, including the use of optical shields with fixed spot sizes from multifiber catheters, the use of lenses and irrigation systems to limit thermal injury, and the development of "hot tips" to radially distribute the thermal injury, were unable to produce precisely controlled, predictable ablation.

Based on early observations that continuous-wave lasers produce significant thermal damage during ablation of atherosclerotic material, our group began to investigate the possibility of pulsed ultraviolet laser ablation of tissue in 1983. Thus we began our search for a laser source that emitted light directly in the ultraviolet and could be transmitted through fiber optics (19).

A variety of pulsed lasers are currently being investigated for use in laser angioplasty. These lasers span the wavelength range from 2.9 microns to 248 nm. Given current fiber-optics technology and the need for precisely controllable ablation with minimal damage to adjacent tissue, we believe there is an optimal set of wavelengths, energy delivery parameters, and fiber optics for a laser angioplasty system. The subsequent paragraphs describe our experimental observations at each of these pulsed wavelengths (19–21).

The erbium:YAG laser emits light at 2.94 microns in the mid-infrared region of the spectrum. Two forms of operation are possible with this laser: a long-pulse mode with approximately 200-microsecond pulse trains, and a Q-switched mode with 70–100-nanosecond individual pulses. In the long-pulse mode the laser emits a burst of pulses, each approximately 100 picoseconds to 1 nanosecond in duration, with approximately 1 to 2 nanoseconds between each pulse. The complexity of this pulse structure makes a precise determination of peak powers difficult. This wavelength is primarily absorbed by water with very short depths of penetration. This suggests that it might be an ideal candidate for laser angioplasty. Unfortunately, despite an intense search, no viable fiber-optic transmission system is available for this wavelength. A variety of fiber-optic materials are under consideration for use as transmission systems. The most promising of these are a zirconium-fluoride fiber optic or a sapphire fiber optic. Unfortunately, both of these materials are extremely brittle, relatively inflexible, and difficult to produce at this time (Plate I).

The holmium:YAG laser, emitting at 2.1 microns, can be transmitted through low-OH silica fiber optics. Like the erbium:YAG laser its output can be obtained in two modes: a long-pulse and a Q-switched version. The primary chromophore absorbing this wavelength is water but the absorption depth is quite large. This results in correspondingly large ablation thresholds at approximately 3000 millijoules/mm^2 for soft atherosclerotic tissue to 10,000 millijoules/mm^2 for calcified tissue. These high pulse energies produce enormous shock waves during tissue ablation. Since the mechanism is conversion of water to steam with correspondent generation of heat, this wavelength also causes significant thermal damage and dissection to the adjacent tissue. The enormous tissue stresses generated by the acoustic shock waves and the adjacent thermal injury produced by conversion of water to steam make this laser a less than optimal choice for laser angioplasty (Plate II). Attempts to shift the wavelength closer toward the water absorption peak at 1.93 microns by addition of thulium to the laser rod and birefringent filters to selectively turn the laser from 2.01 microns to 1.96 microns do decrease the ablation threshold to approximately 300 millijoules/mm^2. With the decrease in depth of penetration the process is more controllable. Unfortunately, the laser repetition rate at this wavelength is currently limited to 4 Hz (pulses per second). Even with the decreased depth of penetration and lowered threshold, tissue ablation proceeds with significant shock-wave and thermal damage to tissue since the primary chromophore is water. Thus, while 1.93 or 1.96 microns appears to produce less damage during tissue ablation, the attendant shock waves are still pronounced.

A variety of pulsed lasers operating in the visual portion of the spectrum have been investigated for laser angioplasty, and some have reached clinical trials. Unfortunately, none of the wavelengths between 600 and 400 nm produces consistent ablation of atherosclerotic tissue. Attempts to use 504 nm or 480 nm dye lasers for laser angioplasty were unsuccessful despite early reports in the literature of their ability to ablate atherosclerotic plaque. These reports were based on the ability of these lasers to ablate pigmented atheroma (yellow or red). However, most atheroma is glossy white or translucent (22). These lasers operate at pulse durations of 1–10 microseconds. Energies used for tissue ablation produced a photoplasma and subsequent shock wave. Often the photoplasma was produced at the blood-tissue interface, resulting in the transmission of a jackhammerlike shock wave into the tissue. This produced a blast crater and was relatively unpredictable. These wavelengths are poorly absorbed by collagen, elastin, and noncolored lipids. Thus, it is a poor wavelength choice for laser angioplasty.

Several pulsed ultraviolet wavelengths have been investigated for application to laser angioplasty. The longer wavelengths, 355 nm from a frequency-tripled Nd:YAG laser and 351 nm from a xenon-fluoride excimer laser, can be transmitted easily through fiber optics. However, the energy per photon is less than 3.4 electron volts, which makes direct bond breaking less probable with these wavelengths (most organic bonds require 3.6 EV or higher for excitation). Both laboratory experience and clinical investigation have demonstrated that the ablation thresholds at these wavelengths are on the order of 60–70 millijoules/mm^2. Ablation is often accompanied by some thermal injury and the depth of penetration is approximately 250–500 microns per pulse. These wavelengths, therefore, appear to be suboptimal for laser angioplasty.

At 308 nm each photon has 3.8 EV; thus, this wavelength is the longest that might produce direct photochemical excitation on a one-photon-per-one-bond basis. Transmission of this wavelength through fiber optics requires pulse stretching of the laser. Research by Litvack et al. (23) has demonstrated that over the range of 10–500 nanoseconds, energy density is the key parameter in determining ablation thresholds. In contrast, fiber-optic damage occurs as peak powers are increased (as pulse duration is decreased). Thus, a long pulse (200 nanoseconds) of 100 millijoules can be easily transmitted through a multifiber catheter, while a short pulse (60 nanoseconds or less) at the same energy invariably leads to fiber destruction within a few pulses. Stretching the pulse decreases the shock wave during ablation since the ejection of material and escape of gases occur over a longer time period. However, as the pulse duration increases, poor beam quality and high repetition rates may lead to thermal injury of the tissue. Optimal pulse durations for ablation of tissue with minimal thermal damage and shock wave appear to be between 200–350 nanoseconds.

Three hundred eight–nm light is strongly absorbed by most vascular and atherosclerotic tissue. Depth of penetration ranges from 10 microns for blood to 30 microns for lipoid atheroma. As calcification increases the energy threshold rises for ablation. At 308 nm, ablation thresholds for noncalcified tissue are between 18–25 millijoules/mm^2. For moderately calcified atheroma, the threshold rises to 35 millijoules/mm^2, and for densely calcified tissue such as calcified heart valves, the ablation threshold can exceed 60 millijoules/mm^2. In densely calcified tissues dead space from the cladding of the fiber optics may often limit the ability to advance the fiber. In clinical practice this is a potentially serious problem. To avoid this problem, careful attention must be paid to the fiber-optic design of the delivery system.

Ablation at 308 nm proceeds with minimal transfer of heat into the adjacent tissue. High-speed filming and histologic and thermographic studies have all demonstrated that tissue adjacent to areas ablated by an excimer laser suffer minimal, if any, thermal trauma. When properly operating, that is, with uniform beam quality and minimal variation of energy from pulse to pulse, ablation occurs uniformly across the area irradiated by the laser beam. If the beam is irregular, an irregular crater will form. If the delivery system injects energy into the tissue at subthreshold levels, this energy is converted to heat. Thus, the challenge for system engineers is to produce a relatively uniform energy output across the surface of the catheter while maintaining flexibility and trackability of the angioplasty system. This complex engineering problem requires multiple iterative design sequences.

At energies necessary to ablate plaque, wavelengths shorter than 308 nm are currently difficult to transmit through fiber optics. Although the threshold at these wavelengths is lower than the threshold of ablation at 308 nm, transmission losses within the fiber optics and fiber damage are so substantial that a practical system using short-wavelength UV pulses is impractical at this time. However, ablation at these shorter wavelengths is highly precise and controllable. Ablation of calcified tissue proceeds more readily at these shorter wavelengths.

Excimer Lasers

Excimer lasers are a family of gas lasers in which the lasing action is produced by a chemical reaction. The chemical reaction is induced by transmitting a high-voltage electrical discharge through a gas mixture. The gas mixture is primarily composed of an inert gas such as helium or neon into which a few percent of another inert gas such as argon, xenon, or krypton and trace amounts (0.1–0.5%) of a halogen such as hydrogen chloride or fluorine are added. The excimer gas laser emits pulsed light directly in the ultraviolet region of the spectrum. These lasers operate only in the pulsed mode. The word "excimer" is derived from the initial description of these lasers as emitting from an excited-state dimer molecule, although this characterization proved to be a simplification of the actual physical process.

A variety of engineering considerations is critical to excimer laser design. Each combination of gases produces light at a different wavelength and requires variation in the electronics and discharge circuits to produce an optimal laser. Excimers can be formed from mixtures of xenon and fluorine (XeF) emitting at 351 nm, xenon and chlorine (XeCl) emitting at 308 nm, krypton and flourine (KrF) emitting at 248 nm, and argon and fluorine (ArF) emitting at 193 nm. Excimer lasers have a variety of advantages for medical applications. Since they emit in the ultraviolet, penetration depth is short and absorption is strong. The ArF laser has the strongest absorption but is presently difficult to transmit through silica-based fiber optics. The KrF laser is poorly transmitted through fiber optics at present. The XeF laser emits at 351 nm and can be transmitted through fiber optics but at this wavelength it is much less effective in ablation of calcified material than the 308 nm light from the XeCl laser. An additional complexity is introduced through the use of fluorine-based systems, which are more difficult to handle in the medical environment than hydrogen chloride–based systems. The XeCl excimer appears to have the optimal combination of pulsed ultraviolet emission; intense tissue absorption; ablation of calcified material; precise, predictable ablation; and delivery through fiber optics.

The XeCl excimer can be made to operate in the so-called "long-pulse" mode. Typically commercially available excimers for industrial applications operate between 7–25 nanoseconds. For ablation of biologic tissue approximately 30–50 millijoules/mm^2 of energy fluence per pulse are required. The power produced by such a pulse in units of energy per time is enormous and is calculated in the megawatt range. These high peak-power pulses destroy the fiber optics with corresponding loss of transmission of the laser light. When short-pulse laser designs are used for clinical applications they do not have sufficient reliability and predictability to produce optimal results. Recent results reported by Karsch et al. using a XeCl excimer laser with 60 or 110 nanosecond pulse durations showed significant loss of energy transmission during the procedure. However, the XeCl excimer can be operated at 200–300 nanoseconds pulse, producing an order of magnitude reduction in the peak power. This stretching of the pulse permits reliable fiber-optic transmission.

Critical to the development of clinical systems for excimer laser angioplasty is the iterative design process. Experiments by Laudenslager, Kinley, and Goldenberg have demonstrated that the transmission of pulsed ultraviolet light through fiber optics is a function of peak power, spatial and temporal uniformity of the beam, and the construction of the fiber optics themselves (Fig. 1.3). Use of a long-pulse excimer is not sufficient to achieve fiber-optic transmission. The laser must have a relatively uniform beam profile with an output of sufficient size to power large-diameter (3 mm or greater) fiber-optic arrays. If the laser is underpowered, energy will be insufficient to ablate harder plaques with large-diameter catheters. When only small catheters can be employed the laser must be used primarily as an adjunctive hole-drilling device.

Thus the choice of laser depends on the requirements of the particular application. Our laboratory investigations have defined the optimal laser system given current fiber-optic technology. The laser, a 308-nanometer excimer laser, is designed to emit pulsed ultraviolet light at a pulse duration of 225 nanoseconds at energy levels of 250–300 millijoules/pulse. These requirements permit uniform transmission of

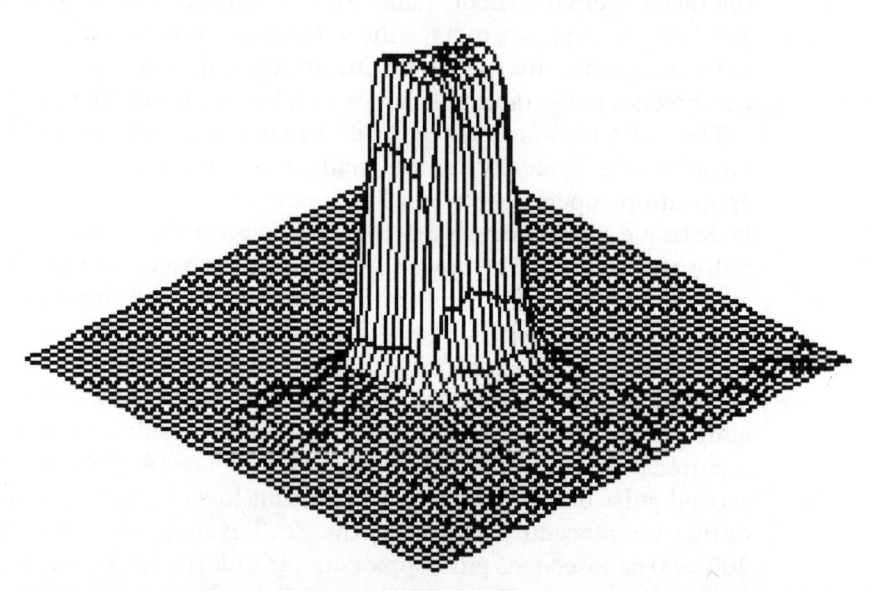

Figure 1.3. Three-dimensional spatial energy profile from a DYMER 200+ laser at the focus out of the coupler before input to a multiple fiber optic catheter. Note the uniform "top hat" energy distribution, which ensures uniform energy filling of each fiber optic in the catheter.

the laser pulse through a multifiber concentric over-the-wire catheter. The catheters are designed to deliver 50–70 millijoules/mm^2 in contact with the tissue. Given the losses in the system from both fiber optics and coupler, an energy pulse from the laser must be sufficient to deliver this fluence through the catheter. The high energy output of the laser accounts for these energy losses, which occur in the optical train and optical coupler, and losses that occur during transmission through the fiber optics.

The magnetically switched "pulse-stretched" excimer provides laser pulses at 225 nanoseconds. Typical commercial excimer lasers emit pulses of 7–40 nanoseconds duration. At these short pulse durations, the peak power of the individual pulse destroys the fiber optics. Thus, the clinical system requires a stretched pulse that permits reliable transmission of the pulses through the fiber optics. The improvement in fiber optic transmission occurs because the peak powers of the clinical system are an order of magnitude less than those of available commercial excimer lasers. Our research demonstrated that both pulse duration and beam quality were required for reliable fiber-optic transmission. Therefore, the clinical unit was designed specifically to meet these requirements (23).

The design, construction, and testing of laser angioplasty systems must consider the requirements at each level of development: the laser, the optical system, the angioplasty catheters, and the guidance system. Integration of these individual components into a working system requires close cooperation between laser physicists, engineers, medical researchers, and clinicians. The translation of the prototype system requires close cooperation between the developers and the clinical trial investigators. The learning process continues well after the initial clinical prototypes are developed. As clinicians acquire this new technology for laser angioplasty, it is critical that they learn from the experience of the initial investigators (24).

References

1. Maiman TH. Stimulated optical radiation in ruby. *Nature* 1960;187: 493–494.
2. Javan A, Bennett WR Jr, Herroit DQ. Population inversion and continuous optical laser oscillation in a gaseous discharge containing a He-Ne mixture. *Phys Rev Lett* 1961;6:106–110.

3. Burham R, Harris NW, Djeu N. Xenon fluoride laser excitation by transverse electric discharge. *Appl Phys Lett* 1976;28:86–87.
4. Wang CP, Mirels H, Sutton DG, et al. Fast-discharge-initiated XeF laser. *Appl Phys Lett* 1976;28:236–238.
5. Laudenslager JB, Pacala TJ, Wittig C. Electric discharge pumped nitrogen ion laser. *Appl Phys Lett* 1976;29:580–582.
6. Forrester JS, Litvack F, Grundfest WS. Laser angioplasty and cardiovascular disease. *Am J Cardiol* 1986;57:990–992.
7. Ginsburg R, Wexler L, Mitchell RS, et al. Percutaneous transluminal laser angioplasty for treatment of peripheral vascular disease: clinical experience with 16 patients. *Radiology* 1985;156:619–624.
8. Sanborn TA, Faxon DP, Haudenschild CC, et al. Experimental angioplasty: circumferential distribution of laser thermal energy with a laser probe. *J Am Coll Cardiol* 1985;5:934–938.
9. Grundfest WS, Litvack F, Doyle L, et al. Comparison of in vitro and in vivo thermal effects of argon and excimer lasers for laser angioplasty, abstracted. *Circulation* 1986;74 (suppl 2):204.
10. Litvack F, Doyle L, Grundfest WS, et al. In vivo excimer laser ablation: acute and chronic effects on canine aorta, abstracted. *Circulation* 1986;74 (suppl 2):360.
11. Gorisch W, Boargen KP. Heat-induced contraction of blood vessels. *Lasers Surg Med* 1982;2:1–13.
12. Anderson RR, Parrish JA. Selective photothermolysis: precise microsurgery by selective absorption of pulsed radiation. *Science* 1983;220:524–527.
13. Hu C, Barnes FS. The thermal-chemical damage in biological material under laser irradiation. *IEEE Trans Biomed Eng* 1970;17:220–231.
14. Srinivasan R. Ablation of polymers and biological tissues by ultraviolet lasers. *Science* 1986;234:559–565.
15. Grundfest WS, Litvack F, Morgenstern L, et al. Effect of excimer laser irradiation on human atherosclerotic aorta: amelioration of laser-induced thermal damage. *IEEE-CLEO Tech Dig* 1984; 248–249.
16. Prince MR, Deutsch TF, Mathews-Roth MM, et al. Preferential light absorption in atheromas in vitro: implications for laser angioplasty. *J Clin Invest* 1986;78:295–302.
17. Cothren RM, Hayes GB, Cramer JR, et al. A multifiber catheter with an optical shield for laser angiosurgery. *Lasers Life Sci* 1987;1:1–12.
18. Sartori MP, Bossaller C, Weilbacher D, et al. Detection of atherosclerotic plaques and characterization of arterial wall structure by laser-induced fluorescence, abstracted. *Circulation* 1986;74 (suppl 2):7.
19. Grundfest WS, Litvack F, Forrester JS, et al. Laser ablation of human

atherosclerotic plaque without adjacent tissue injury. *J Am Coll Cardiol* 1985;5(4):929–933.
20. Grundfest WS, Litvack F, Goldenberg T, et al. Pulsed ultraviolet lasers and the potential for safe laser angioplasty. *Am J Surg* 1985;150:220–226.
21. Grundfest WS, Litvack F, Hickey A, et al. The current status of angioscopy and laser angioplasty. *J Vasc Surg* 1985;5(4):666–673.
22. Forrester JS, Litvack F, Grundfest WS, et al. A perspective of coronary disease seen through the arteries of living man. *Circulation* 1987;75:505–513.
23. Litvack F, Grundfest WS, Goldenbert T, et al. Pulsed laser angioplasty: wavelength power and energy dependencies relevant to clinical application. *Lasers Surg Med* 1988;8(1):60–65.
24. Litvack F, Grundfest WS, Segalowitz J, et al. Interventional cardiovascular therapy by laser and thermal angioplasty. *Circulation* 1990;81(3)(suppl IV):109–116.

CHAPTER 2

Laser-Tissue Interaction

SABINO R. TORRE
TIMOTHY A. SANBORN

FOLLOWING the development of the first practical laser by Theodore Maiman in 1960 (1), the laser quickly gained widespread acceptance as a useful device in the fields of medicine and surgery (2). Percutaneous recanalization of coronary occlusions utilizing laser irradiation delivered through flexible optical fibers was first described by Choy et al. (3,4). Since 1981, dramatic developments in laser systems and fiber-optic catheters have occurred, solely for the purpose of laser angioplasty.

Although many different lasers are in various stages of experimental and clinical development, the utility of any particular laser for percutaneous angioplasty is closely linked to its ability to safely deliver high-power laser irradiation through percutaneous fiber-optic catheters. Once the laser irradiation has reached the target tissue, the subsequent outcome of laser ablation depends upon several related laser and tissue factors. The objectives of this chapter are to review laser-tissue interaction, both acute and chronic, as functions of the type of laser and components of the irradiated tissue.

Laser Fundamentals

To understand the true nature of laser-tissue interaction, it is necessary to review certain fundamental principles of laser irradiation. These include: 1) continuous-wave (CW) vs. pulsed lasers, 2) laser energy dosage, and 3) tissue optics.

Continuous-Wave vs. Pulsed Lasers

Lasers are generally categorized by their laser source, unique wavelength, and mode of operation (Table 2.1). Most biomedical applications of laser irradiation have utilized continuous-wave energy delivery. The energy profile of a CW laser is characterized by power delivery that is constant over time (Fig. 2.1). Most such CW lasers employed for biomedical purposes are constructed to yield outputs under 100 watts. A CW laser may be used in two ways: continuous or periodically interrupted. The latter has been referred to as an intermittent or "chopped" mode. A CW laser used in an intermittent or chopped mode must be differentiated from a true pulsed laser. Intermittent or chopped delivery differs from CW delivery only with respect to emission-free intervals; power output during intervals of laser emission is identical for both modes. This is in marked contrast to true pulsed lasers. Pulsed lasers include emission-free intervals similar to the chopped mode. Unlike chopped lasers, pulsed lasers use a variety of techniques (i.e., mode-

Table 2.1. Laser Sources

LASER	WAVELENGTH (NM)	OPERATING MODE
Excimer	193 (ArF)	Pulsed
	248 (KrF)	
	308 (XeCl)	
	351 (XeF)	
Argon ion	488	CW
	514.5	
Ruby	694	CW
Alexandrite	700–820	Pulsed
Neodynium:YAG	1064	CW/pulsed
Holmium	2100	Pulsed
Erbium	2940	Pulsed
Carbon dioxide	10,600	CW/pulsed

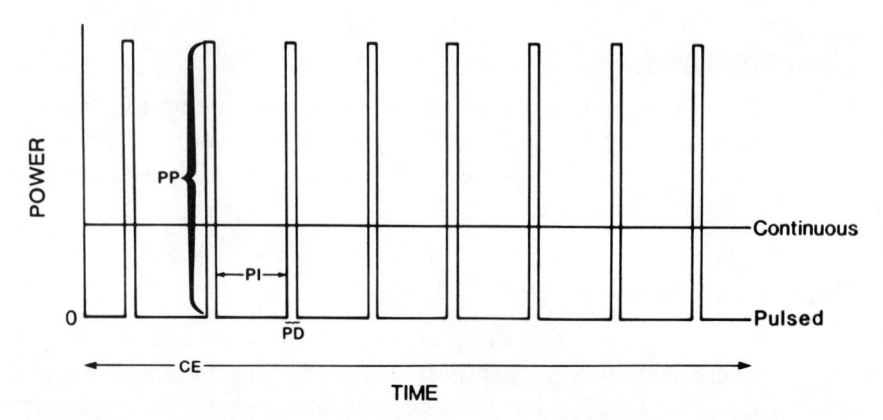

Figure 2.1. Laser energy profile. Continuous-wave (CW) lasers deliver constant power over time. Pulsed lasers deliver energy in discrete bursts. The pulse duration (PD) of each burst is typically in nanoseconds or microseconds. The duration of the pulse interval (PI) depends upon the repetition rate. Peak power (PP) is typically in the mega- or kilowatt range. CE = cumulative exposure. (Isner JM, Clarke RH, eds. Cardiovascular laser therapy. New York: Raven Press Ltd., 1989. Reproduced with permission of J M Isner and Raven Press, Ltd.)

locking or Q-switching) that allow energy storage within the laser cavity; as a result, each emission is characterized by a peak power substantially greater than the continuous power output of a CW laser. Because of these differences, CW lasers (argon, Nd:YAG, and carbon dioxide) produce intense heating of the irradiated tissue, resulting in significant thermal injury (5), while pulsed-wave lasers (excimer and holmium) emit very short, high-energy pulses that can ablate irradiated tissue without thermal injury. The rapid delivery of short pulses of high-peak-power laser irradiation by the pulsed-wave lasers permits thermal relaxation of tissue between subsequent pulses. Thus, no thermal accumulation occurs between laser pulses (6, 7).

Laser Energy Dosage

To further understand tissue response to laser irradiation, several optical variables must be specified. These are 1) the energy delivered per unit time, 2) the spot size of the area irradiated, and 3) the total time of irradiation, and if pulsed laser is used, the duration of the laser pulse. Collectively, these variables provide the total laser energy dosage delivered to the target tissue. There are two types of laser light power designations when a pulsed laser is used, average power and peak power. Average power is the energy delivered per unit of time, whereas peak power is the energy contained in a single laser pulse divided by its pulse width. The average power delivered by a pulsed laser is the total energy delivered per unit of time, which equals the number of pulses per second from the laser multiplied by the individual pulse energy. Interestingly, these two forms of average power level, one for a pulsed laser and the other for a CW laser, usually produce distinctly different effects on tissue even when the total energy dosage and wavelength are the same.

Designating average power without knowing the other characteristics of the laser, especially if it is used in a pulsed manner, is insufficient for understanding the procedure. In all cases, the power per unit area, referred to as "energy fluence," is one of the most important characteristics for understanding laser-tissue interaction. For a CW laser, the energy fluence is given by the laser output in watts multiplied by the exposure time in seconds divided by the area irradiated; this is expressed as watts per square centimeter. For a pulsed laser, the energy fluence is the energy per pulse divided by the beam spot area; this is expressed as joules per square centimeter.

Tissue Optics

Once these parameters of the laser light are measured, the next important effect is absorption and scattering of the light energy, which typically is wavelength-dependent. If the laser irradiation is reflected there will be little effect; if the laser irradiation is absorbed at the tissue surface, only the cells irradiated may be affected. However, if the light scatters and penetrates deeply into the tissue, the effects of this energy may occur at some site distant from the point of irradiation. The laser wavelengths currently used for laser angioplasty vary from 308 nm to 10.6 μm. These laser wavelengths are from the ultraviolet, the visible, and the far-infrared portions of the electromagnetic spectrum. Within these wavelength ranges, the ratio of absorption to scattering varies substantially (Fig. 2.2). Absorption predominates over scattering at wavelengths of less than 150 nm or greater than 2000 nm (i.e., carbon dioxide); absorption and scattering are about equally important between 250 nm and 350 nm (i.e., XeCl) and also between 1200 nm and 2000 nm; and scattering predominates over absorption at wavelengths between 350 nm and 1200 nm (i.e., Nd:YAG).

In addition to wavelength, the structural components of the target tis-

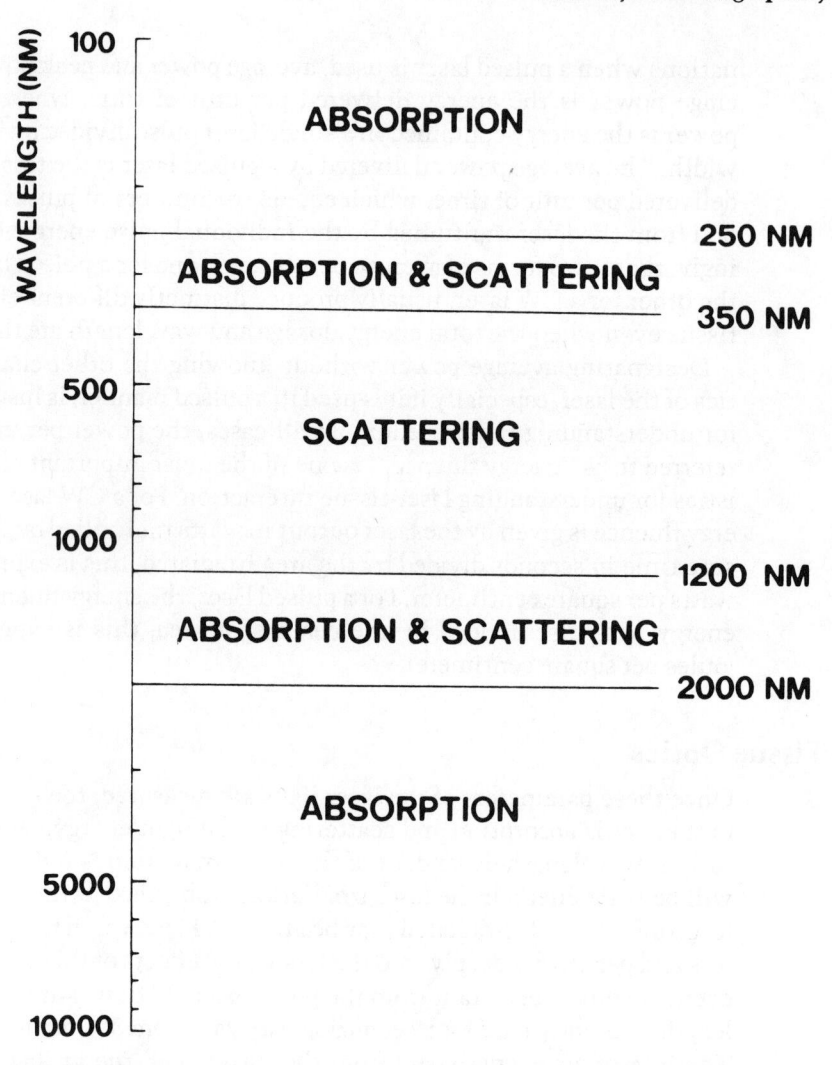

Figure 2.2. Approximates wavelength bands where absorption dominates scattering, scattering dominates absorption, and absorption and scattering are about equal. (Abela GS, ed. Lasers in cardiovascular medicine and surgery. Boston: Kluwer Academic Publishers, 1990. Reproduced with permission of M. J. C. van Gemert and Kluwer Academic Publishers).

sue may strongly influence the absorption of laser irradiation. Normal cardiovascular tissue is primarily composed of water, various structural proteins, and lipids. In contrast, atherosclerotic vessels have a much higher content of lipid and a small amount of calcium contained within complex atheromatous plaques. Thus, the ideal laser source for the ablation of atherosclerotic plaque should promote intense absorption of laser irradiation by atheromatous tissue and minimal absorption of laser irradiation by water. Interestingly, a plot of the absorption coefficient of water as a function of laser wavelength (Fig. 2.3) demonstrates that ultraviolet laser irradiation is poorly absorbed by water. On the other hand, a plot of the absorption coefficient of atheroma as a function of laser wavelength (Fig. 2.4) demonstrates that ultraviolet laser irradia-

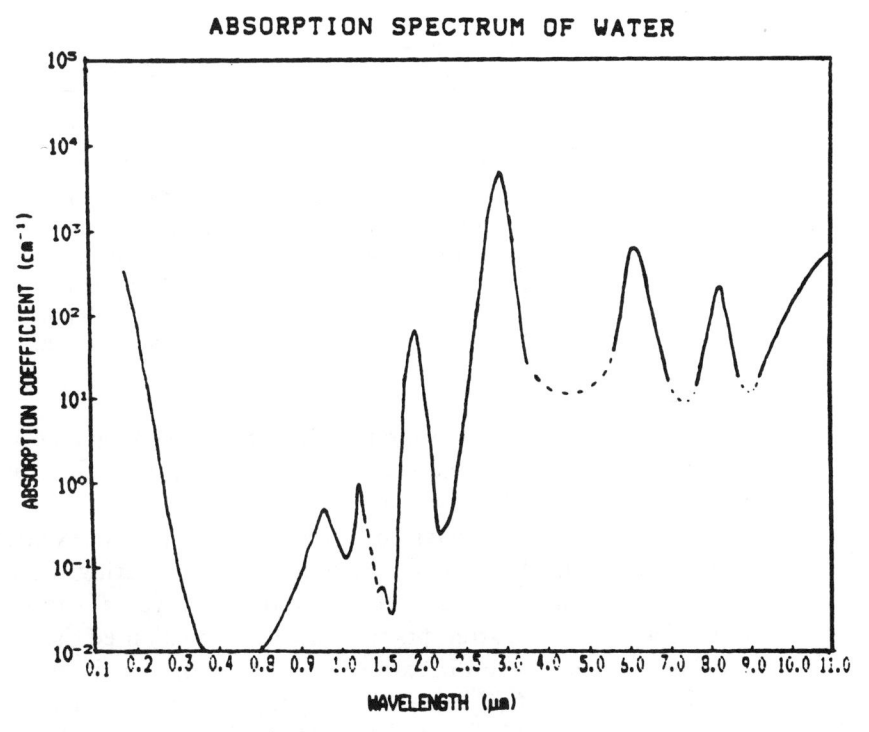

Figure 2.3. Absorption coefficient of water as a function of wavelength. Note that absorption of laser irradiation by water is minimal in the ultraviolet range (400 nm). (J Soc Photoptic Instrum Eng 1986;605:32–36. Reproduced with permission of R. F. Bonner and the Society of Photoptic Instruments and Engineering.)

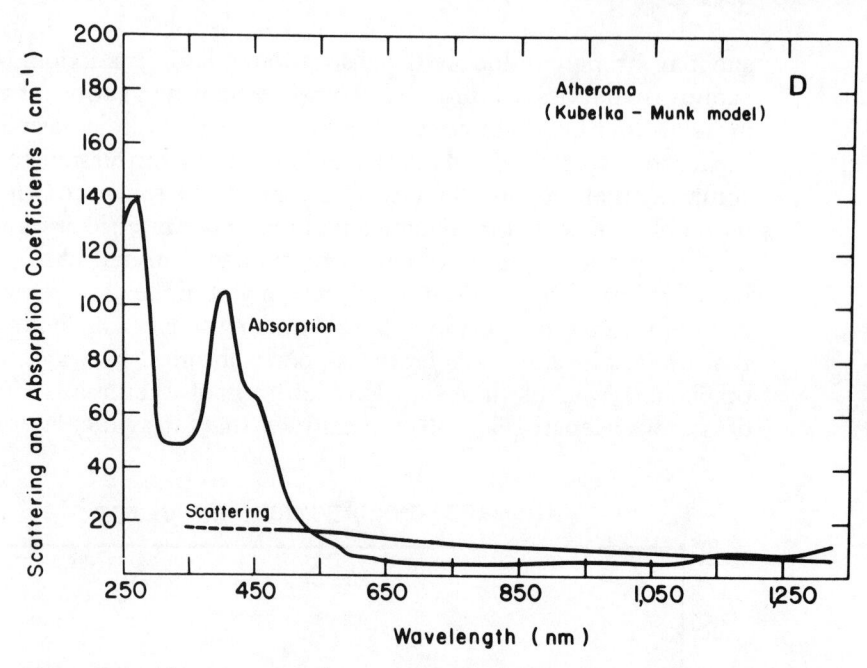

Figure 2.4. Absorption coefficient of typical atheroma (1.5 mm thick) as a function of wavelength from ultraviolet to infrared. Note the absorption peaks corresponding to known tissue chromophores (hemoglobin at 550–570 nm, aromatic amino acids and DNA at 250–290 nm, and the extra absorbance for atheroma at 400–450 nm). (J Clin Invest 1986;78:295–392. Reproduced with permission of M. R. Prince and the Journal of Clinical Investigation).

tion is highly absorbed by atheroma. Therefore, ultraviolet laser sources appear to be the logical choice for ablation of atherosclerotic plaque without vaporization of water and subsequent injury to adjacent tissue.

The small amount of calcium contained within complex atherosclerotic plaques may become a serious impediment during the laser angioplasty procedure. Because calcific deposits are typically refractory to CW laser irradiation, attempts to ablate heavily calcified tissues with a CW laser typically result in extensive charring. In fact, the resistance of calcific deposits to CW laser ablation may at times predispose to thermal perforation as the laser fiber "seeks" the path of least resistance through the noncalcified plaque or normal wall (8,9). In a series of elegant experiments, Tobis et al. (10) observed that if an arterial obstruction is composed of thrombus or soft atheroma, the hot-tip CW laser

Laser-Tissue Interaction 33

probe can burn through the tissue relatively easily. However, when the obstruction is a hard, fibrocalcific plaque, the probe may be deflected and burn through the intimal plaque, advance between the plaque and the media, and either reenter the lumen distally or perforate externally.

Three mechanisms of absorption of laser light have been proposed: 1) photothermal, 2) photochemical, and 3) photoplasmic (Fig. 2.5). The most common mechanism for CW and pulsed lasers in the visible and infrared spectrum is the conversion of the absorbed photons into heat or thermal motion of the molecules that compose various tissues. Once heat is deposited into an irradiated area, there is thermal conduction by the tissue to its surrounding area. To minimize the lateral spread of this heat conduction, a pulsed laser with a pulse duration shorter than the characteristic thermal relaxation time of the tissue is used. As the ab-

ABSORPTION OF LASER ENERGY

PHOTOCHEMICAL
- THERMAL DEGRADATION
- DIRECT BOND BREAKING
↓
CONVERSION OF LONG CHAINED MOLECULES TO SMALLER FRAGMENTS
↓
RAPID VAPORIZATION
↓
TISSUE ABLATION

PHOTOTHERMAL
↓
CONVERSION OF ENERGY TO HEAT
↓
TEMPERATURE RISE OF TISSUE
↓
CELL NECROSIS
↓
WATER VAPORIZATION
↓
TISSUE VAPORIZATION

PHOTOPLASMA
↓
HIGH POWER DENSITY
↓
HIGH ELECTRIC FIELD
↓
DIELECTRIC BREAKDOWN
↓
PLASMA FORMATION
↓
SHOCK WAVE IONIZATION
↓
TISSUE RUPTURE

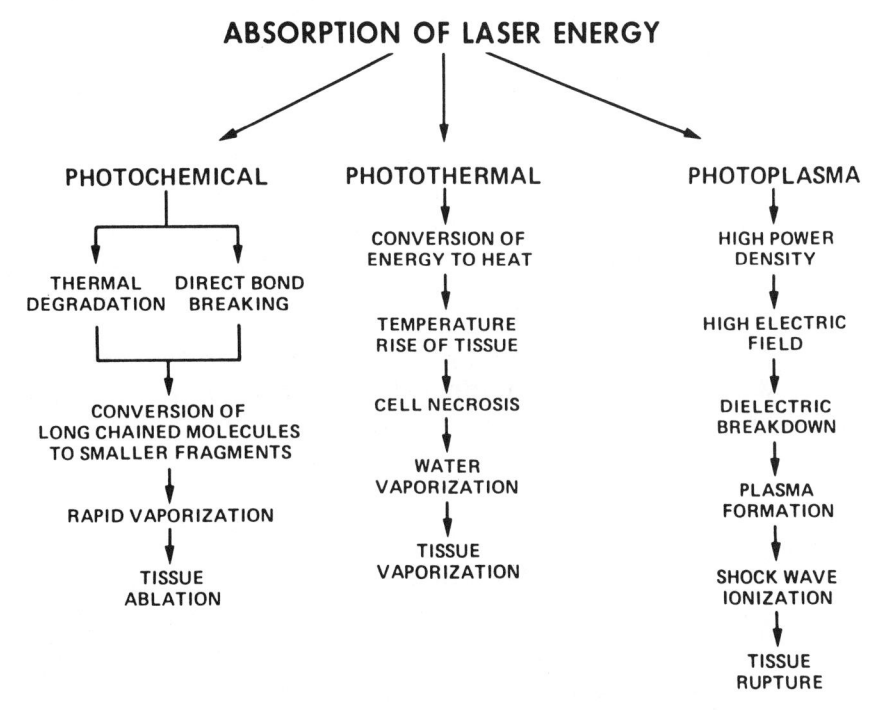

Figure 2.5. Schematic of three mechanisms of energy deposition in tissue following absorption of laser energy. (White RA, Grundfest WS, eds. Lasers in cardiovascular disease. Chicago: Year Book Medical Publishers, 1987. Reproduced with permission of J. B. Laudenslager and Year Book Medical Publishers.)

sorbed laser energy is converted into heat, the temperature of the tissue rises, causing cell necrosis. The temperature of the tissue continues to rise until it reaches the level where water vaporization occurs. This thermal absorption process occurs with both CW and pulsed laser sources when the pulse duration is greater than the thermal relaxation time for the tissue or the energy per pulse is below the ablation threshold.

The other two absorption mechanisms in medical applications are predominantly produced by high peak-power laser sources. The second mechanism only pertains to short-pulse ultraviolet wavelengths and is called photochemical ablation. If the energy of an ultraviolet photon is absorbed by a molecule, molecular bonds can rupture directly, causing a change of a large molecule into smaller fragment molecules, which then leave the substrate in a rapid expansion. This is a very efficient tissue ablation mechanism and produces clean incisions with minimal thermal heat retention in the nonirradiated tissue when short-pulsed ultraviolet laser sources are used (10–200 nsec). This process requires strong absorption of the laser wavelength by the tissue in the ultraviolet, and for pulsed ultraviolet sources, multiphoton processes may occur along with single-photon absorption for the photochemical bond-breaking mechanism. The third mechanism is somewhat independent of laser wavelength and is referred to as the photoplasma mechanism. This process can occur in materials normally transparent to the laser wavelength at low power levels. Very high peak-power laser radiation produces a very intense local electric field, causing dielectric breakdown of material and heating of liberated electrons, which avalanche to produce a local plasma. The sudden expansion of vaporized material produces a shock wave, causing localized rupture of the tissue.

Acute Effects of Laser Irradiation

The current understanding of the acute effects of laser irradiation is derived from numerous in-vitro and in-vivo experiments utilizing both normal and atherosclerotic cardiovascular tissue. In this section, several different aspects of the acute laser-tissue interaction are discussed: 1) macroscopic and histologic analysis, 2) debris and byproduct formation, 3) thrombogenicity, and 4) vasoactivity. In addition, we will make distinctions between CW and pulsed lasers whenever possible.

Laser-Tissue Interaction 35

Macroscopic and Histologic Analysis

Pathologic examination of cardiovascular tissues irradiated with CW lasers, regardless of whether such lasers are used in continuous or chopped mode, has consistently disclosed two distinctive light microscopic findings in the perimeter of the laser crater: a superficial zone of charring or carbonization, and a subjacent zone of polymorphous lacunae or vacuolization (Fig. 2.6;5,11–13). These findings have come to be recognized as the histologic hallmarks of thermal injury. Very often, such thermal injury is manifested as grossly apparent charring that is easily recognizable by nonmagnified visual inspection. On occasion, however, extensive histologic signs of thermal injury may be absent on gross examination, yet be deep and extensive when examined by light microscopy. The magnitude of charring observed by light microscopy is

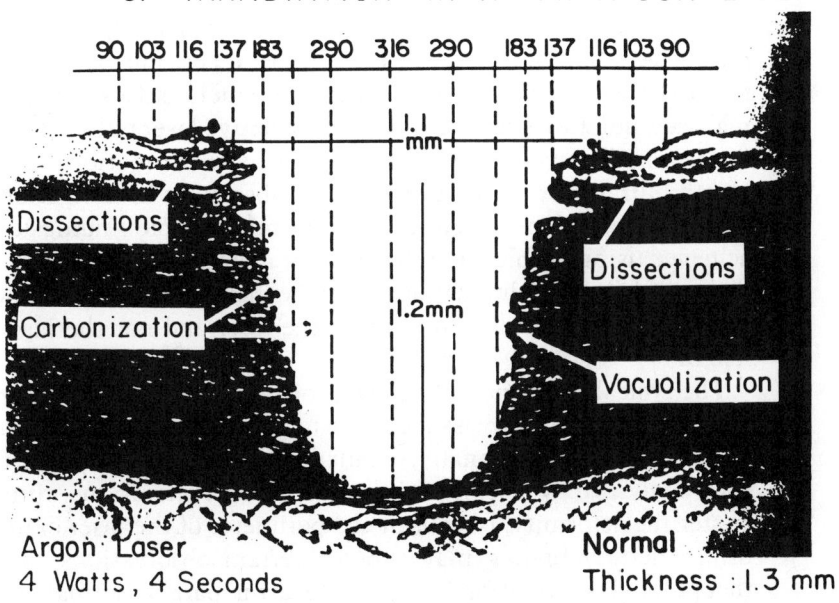

Figure 2.6. Hematoxylin-eosin–stained section of nonatherosclerotic aorta irradiated with 4W argon ion laser for 4 sec via a 300-μm optical fiber, 700-μm spot size in air. (Circulation 1987;76:1353–1363. Reproduced with permission of A. J. Welch and the American Heart Association.)

variable: it may range from a discontinuous linear alteration at the perimeter of the ablation site to a slightly thicker zone of injury.

The subjacent zone of vacuoles underlying the superficially charred zone has been described as the zone of "acoustic injury" or "polymorphous lacunae." The latter term is adequately descriptive without implying specific mechanisms. The best evidence that plasma-mediated "acoustic" transients play a role in laser ablation, for example, involves experiments carried out using pulsed-laser ablation (14,15), and histologic analyses of tissues irradiated in such experiments have never disclosed "acoustic injury."

Studies performed by Srinivasan and Mayne-Banton in 1982 (16) demonstrated that far ultraviolet radiation (193 nm) emitted by an excimer laser could be used to inscribe exceptionally clean and precisely etched cuts devoid of thermal injury in synthetic organic polymers, human hair, cartilage, and corneal tissue. Similar findings have been made in cardiovascular tissues, including myocardium, calcified aortic valves, and atherosclerotic plaque (Fig. 2.7;7,17). As mentioned above, the underlying mechanism of plaque ablation is the rapid delivery of short, high-peak-energy pulses by using a pulse repetition rate that allows thermal relaxation of tissue between subsequent pulses. Thus, no thermal accumulation occurs between the ablative laser pulses (6,7). While it was initially suggested that these results were a function of the wavelength (ultraviolet) of light employed, subsequent investigations demonstrated that identical gross and light microscopic findings could be achieved using visible and infrared laser radiation (10,18). The absence of thermal injury is thus a function of the thermal relaxation time of the substrate and the pulse duration of the laser and not the laser wavelength.

The typical gross and light microscopic studies of pulsed laser irradiation of cardiovascular tissues consistently demonstrate the absence of thermal injury. Occasionally, detailed light microscopic and ultrastructural analysis may disclose subtle morphologic alterations, similar to a blisterlike deformity, of cells at the perimeter of the laser crater. This ultrastructural finding may support certain observations suggesting that pulsed laser ablation involves, at least in part, a thermal process in which thermal injury is minimized by pulsed energy delivery (19).

The distinction between chopped and pulsed energy delivery, as well as considerations regarding pulse duration and repetition rate, are directly relevant to the elimination of laser-induced thermal injury. Experiments by Hayes and Wolbarsht (20) and Anderson and Parrish (21)

Laser-Tissue Interaction 37

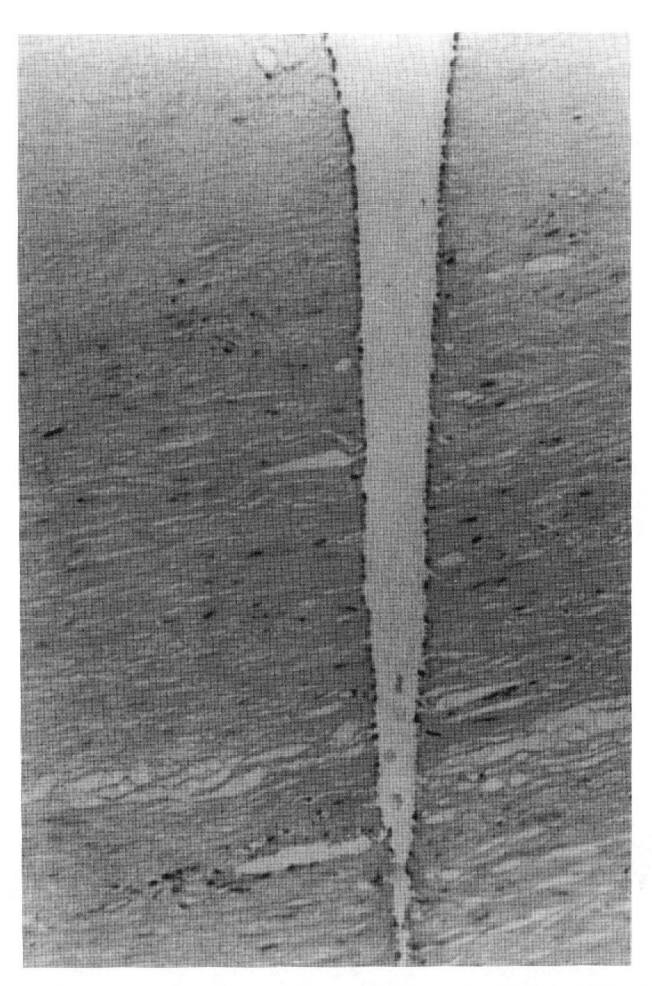

Figure 2.7. Atherosclerotic aortic segment displays the effect of 90 pulses at 35 mJ per pulse with 10-nanosecond pulse duration from a pulsed XeCl (308 nm) excimer laser. Beam dimensions at impact point were 1.2 mm by 0.4 mm after focusing with 600 mm lens. Laser ablation produced a scalpellike incision with smooth regular walls and minimal, if any, evidence of thermal injury. Depth of penetration 1.8 mm, width 0.4 mm. No carbon particles are seen and fiber architecture is undisturbed. Hematoxylin-eosin stain; magnification × 40. (Am J Surg 1985;150:220–226. Reproduced with permission of W. S. Grundfest et al. and the American Journal of Surgery.)

have suggested that thermal injury can be avoided when exposure time for each pulse is shorter than the thermal relaxation time of the irradiated tissue. If the pulse duration and cumulative exposure are sufficiently brief, and if the interval between consecutive pulses is sufficiently long, then the heat generated by each pulse may be sufficiently dissipated before delivery of the subsequent pulse. Consequently, thermal injury of tissue outside the path of the laser beam can be avoided. It has been suggested that CW laser irradiation delivered in the "chopped" mode may diminish the magnitude of thermal injury (22). Results identical to those using true pulsed lasers, however, cannot be duplicated with chopped delivery, because further compromise of the relatively low power output by addition of emission-free intervals ultimately requires an increase in the repetition rate or protracted cumulative exposure to ablate the target tissue (18). Either or both of these "solutions" ultimately overwhelm the thermal relaxation time of the target tissue, causing thermal injury. Interestingly, pulsed lasers may cause charring when used in an unfocused manner, that is, when the target tissue is irradiated proximal or distal to the focal spot (6). Such nonfocused use of the pulsed laser beam results in a lower energy density at the irradiated surface. The longer exposure time required to vaporize a given volume of tissue in this manner may ultimately overwhelm the heat-dissipating capabilities of the tissue adjacent to the target site.

Debris and By-Product Formation

One of the earliest concerns raised about laser angioplasty was the formation of debris and distal vessel embolization. During the initial feasibility studies of laser recanalization in a live circulation using CW argon ion and Nd:YAG lasers in an atherosclerotic rabbit model, no distal embolization was noted by angiography of the treated vessel (23). These data, however, were not sufficient to detect small, particulate debris.

Debris generation using different laser systems has been systematically evaluated by Provosti et al. (24). Studies were performed comparing a pulsed XeCl (308 nm) excimer laser and a CW argon (488 nm) laser. Both systems were used to irradiate atherosclerotic plaque, with the beam perpendicular to the plaque, until the plaque was perforated. Particle number and size were measured using a flow cytometer. Particle density and size were generated five to ten times more with excimer laser irradiation than with CW argon irradiation. It is presumed that shock waves generated by the pulsed excimer system have a greater potential for forming larger debris particles.

In-vitro experiments were then designed to evaluate debris products formed by laser degradation and vaporization of cardiovascular tissues and blood elements. Isner et al. (8) evaluated photoproducts liberated by argon laser irradiation of atherosclerotic plaque, myocardium, and calcific aortic valves. This was done using gas chromatography, mass spectroscopy, and absorbance spectroscopy. The gaseous products were those of pyrolized proteins such as light-chain hydrocarbon fragments, carbon monoxide, and water vapor. These photoproducts indicated that a thermal degradation process was occurring in the cardiovascular tissue.

Subsequently, gas chromatography was utilized to identify gaseous photoproducts liberated during pulsed excimer laser (ArF, 193 nm; XeF, 351 nm) irradiation of myocardium and atherosclerotic coronary arterial segments (25). In every case, the gas chromatographic spectrum of the photoproducts released was indistinguishable from those observed during CW laser irradiation. Identification of these specific photoproducts as a result of pulsed excimer laser photoablation further supports the hypothesis that the process of excimer laser tissue ablation is similar to that of continuous-wave laser irradiation. Pulsed laser ablation may be interpreted to represent the results of a thermal process in which thermal diffusion has been optimized.

Thrombogenicity

There have been several studies of the relative thrombogenicity of continuous-wave thermal irradiation versus pulsed excimer laser irradiation. Prevosti et al. (26) irradiated 15 rabbit atherosclerotic aortic segments in vitro with both a pulsed XeCl (308 nm) excimer laser and a catalytic hot-tip catheter and used scanning electron microscopic morphometry to determine the percentage of surface area covered with adherent platelets and platelet thrombi. They demonstrated less platelet accumulation and thrombus formation following thermal ablation of plaque when compared to either the control segments or those aortic segments irradiated with the pulsed excimer laser. They hypothesized that thermal ablation causing denaturation of surface proteins may be responsible for the reduction in platelet adherence.

Subsequently, Ragimov et al. (27) irradiated 99 peripheral canine vessel segments with the following lasers: 1) CW Nd:YAG (1060 nm) laser;

2) CW argon ion (480 and 514 nm) laser; 3) pulsed XeCl (308 nm) excimer laser; and 4) a CW Nd:YAG (1060 nm) laser-heated metal probe. The irradiated arterial segments were then exposed to platelet-enriched plasma in an in-vitro circulation system and adherent platelets were counted by scanning electron microscopy over 20 randomly selected fields. These experiments demonstrated a high thrombogenicity for laser-irradiated arterial segments; however, no significant difference was observed in the relative thrombogenicity of the four laser systems used. The authors concluded that irrespective of the laser utilized the laser angioplasty should be accompanied by a number of thrombosis-preventive adjuvant measures.

Since these two studies were performed in vitro rather than in vivo and platelet deposition was semiqualitative rather than quantitative, Sanborn et al. (28) conducted a study of the relative thrombogenicity of pulsed excimer and CW thermal laser angioplasty in vivo in normal swine coronary arteries using angiographic, histologic, and quantitative indium-111–labeled platelet analysis. In this study, all three coronary arteries in seven normal pigs were randomly treated with either excimer or thermal laser angioplasty. The coronary arteries had already been perfused in vivo for 24 hours with autologous platelets labeled with indium-111. In addition to gross and light microscopic inspection of the arterial segments for platelet accumulation and thrombus formation, platelet deposition was calculated from the blood platelet count and indium-111 counts on the arterial wall and in blood, as previously described (29). This study demonstrated that there was a greater incidence of both angiographic complications (thrombosis, perforation) and mural or occlusive thrombus formation after thermal laser angioplasty. In addition, quantitative indium-111 platelet deposition was significantly increased after thermal laser angioplasty compared with excimer-treated or control segments. Thus, excimer laser angioplasty resulted in less thrombosis and platelet accumulation than did thermal laser angioplasty.

Vasoactivity

Light-induced relaxation of vascular smooth muscle was observed more than 30 years ago by Furchgott et al. (30,31), who used a monochromator to study the effects of selected wavelengths from 240 to 675 nm generated by a xenon arc lamp. Interestingly, maximum relaxation was observed in the ultraviolet portion of the spectrum. Subsequently, Steg et al. (32) demonstrated that CW argon (457–514 nm) laser irradiation of isolated segments of rabbit aorta at powers exceeding 1.0 watts consistently produces contraction of vascular smooth muscle. Simultaneous recordings of tissue-temperature profiles indicated that such increases in vascular tone were consistently accompanied by a significant rise in tissue temperature. In these same experiments, however, CW laser irradiation at lower powers (less than 0.1 watts) was unaccompanied by a significant increase in temperature and consistently produced vascular smooth muscle relaxation.

Recently, Steg et al. (33) were the first to study the effects of pulsed ultraviolet laser irradiation on vascular smooth muscle reactivity. Although pulsed ultraviolet lasers typically produce high-intensity laser light, such irradiance is nevertheless unaccompanied by significant tissue heating (7,34). The investigators irradiated 250 rings of rabbit thoracic aorta while simultaneously measuring tissue-temperature profiles and the tension generated by the vascular rings. They demonstrated that pulsed laser irradiation did not cause contraction of vascular smooth muscle but instead induces a relaxation response. Simultaneously recorded tissue-temperature profiles disclosed that during pulsed laser irradiation, tissue temperature rise did not exceed 5°C. Thus, it appears that the observed relaxation of vascular smooth muscle represents the net result of photoillumination, unaccompanied by significant tissue heating.

Chronic Effects of Laser Irradiation

Few studies have examined the chronic effects of laser irradiation. The work completed thus far has been limited to studies of the short-term healing responses following laser irradiation in several animal models. In this section, the discussion focuses on two different aspects of the chronic laser-tissue interaction: 1) macroscopic and histologic analysis, and 2) restenosis.

Macroscopic and Histologic Analysis

Gerrity et al. (35) were the first to examine the cellular response of normal and atherosclerotic aortic intima after in vivo laser irradiation with a CW carbon dioxide laser in hyperlipidemic swine. At energy levels greater than 5 joules, laser burns appeared as craters less than 1 mm in depth and 2 mm in diameter. Two days following exposure, the craters were filled with platelet-fibrin thrombi and surrounded by a ring of densely packed leukocytes at the edge of the normal endothelium. Two weeks after laser irradiation, the depressed crater surface was mostly reendothelialized with small, closely packed endothelial cells. The subjacent thrombus contained numerous phagocytic cells with inclusions of fibrin, erythrocytes, and membranous debris. Proliferative invaginations containing smooth muscle cells, mitotic figures, and collagen extended into the pit from the lateral aspects. Eight weeks after laser irradiation, the laser craters were still depressed and therefore less occlusive than adjacent lesion areas. In addition, a fibrous cap had formed over the remaining necrotic area (Fig. 2.8). These observations demonstrated the rapid healing, including reendothelialization and intimal fibrous scarring, with minimal damage to surrounding tissue following laser irradiation.

In a similar series of experiments, Abela et al. (36) evaluated the healing response of both normal and atherosclerotic arteries to in-vivo CW argon laser irradiation. In monkeys studied at 1 hour and 4 days, light and electron microscopy of laser-treated sites demonstrated craters filled with a coagulum of blood and cellular debris with only a few adherent platelets. Healing occurred with only a minimal inflammatory response and involved both fibroblasts and smooth muscle cells. Reendothelialization was seen in all animals killed between 7 and 14 days after laser irradiation and was complete by 30 to 60 days.

A study by Sanborn et al. (37) compared laser thermal angioplasty and balloon recanalization effects in an atherosclerotic rabbit model. In that study, angiographic and histologic consequences of laser thermal and balloon angioplasty were examined and compared both immediately and at 4 weeks following the procedure. Nineteen arteries were randomly treated. Nine arteries were treated with either 1.5- or 2.0-mm laser thermal probes using 6 or 8 watts, respectively, for 5 sec over a 2-cm-long arterial segment. Balloon angioplasty was performed in ten stenotic lesions using a 2.5-mm balloon catheter inflated three times each for 30 sec. Histologic examination 4 weeks after the procedure revealed less fibrocellular proliferation after laser thermal angioplasty, whereas vessels treated with balloon angioplasty demonstrated evidence of prior fracture and dissection of the vessel wall with more fibrocellular proliferative response.

The healing process following pulsed laser irradiation has not been extensively studied. Higginson et al. (38) reported on the chronic effects

Laser-Tissue Interaction 43

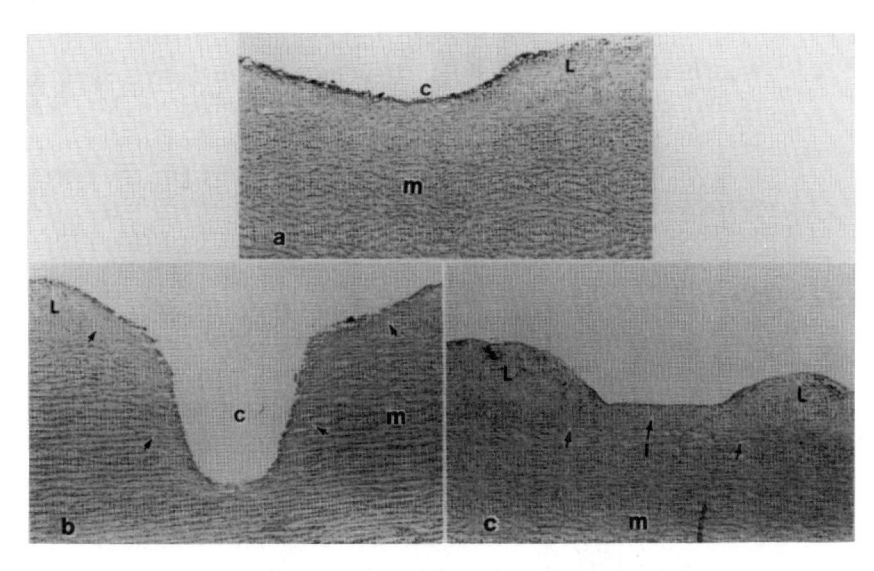

Figure 2.8. [a] Light micrograph of section through laser burn crater *(c)* at 3 joules in a mildly atherosclerotic swine aorta. Burn depth roughly coincides with depth of lesion *(L)* but does not extend into the media *(m)*. [b] In contrast, a 15-joule burn in the same vessel resulting in a crater *(c)* extending deep into the media *(m)* well beyond the lesioned intima *(L)*. Considerable tissue damage is present lateral to the pit, particularly on the intimal aspect *(arrows)*. [c] Light micrograph of section through 5-joule burn in atherosclerotic lesion after 8 weeks of recirculation to demonstrate healing of low-energy burn. Crater is reendothelialized, and slightly thickened intima *(I)* below crater is much thinner than that of the lesioned intima *(L)* on the lateral aspects. Internal elastic lamina *(arrows)* and media *(m)* are intact. No necrotic core is present in this crater, and the intimal area *(I)* is composed of a fibromuscular cap. Hematoxylin-eosin stain; magnification × 54. (J Thorac Cardiovasc Surg 1983;85:409–421. Reproduced with permission of R. G. Gerrity and the Journal of Thoracic and Cardiovascular Surgery.)

of laser irradiation using a pulsed XeCl (308 nm) excimer laser in an atherosclerotic swine model. Both argon and excimer laser irradiation were applied to the infrarenal abdominal aorta in anesthetized swine via an anterior aortotomy. After laser irradiation, the incisions were sutured and the animals were allowed to recover. Treated sites were examined at 48 hours, 3 weeks, and 9 weeks. Early response seen by histology involved the formation of a thrombotic plug at the base of the crater. As expected, thermal necrosis was seen in only those sites irradiated with CW argon laser energy. At 3 weeks, reconstitution of the vascular surface was seen for both argon and excimer craters. At 9 weeks, all arteries were healed by a fibrocellular tissue reaction and covered with an endothelial cell layer. Also, as previously described (36,37), the intimal thickness at the crater site following laser irradiation was significantly reduced from the original thickness, as measured on the lateral aspects of the craters.

Restenosis

Although conventional balloon angioplasty has gained wide acceptance in the treatment of atherosclerotic coronary artery disease, restenosis continues to be the "Achilles' heel" of this procedure. Unfortunately, there have been few studies of the effects of laser angioplasty or laser-assisted angioplasty on restenosis. Sanborn et al. (37) examined the angiographic luminal diameters immediately and 4 weeks after both balloon angioplasty and laser thermal angioplasty in an atherosclerotic rabbit model. The immediate enlargement of the angiographic luminal diameters was similar for both procedures: from 1.0 to 1.9 mm for laser thermal angioplasty vs. 1.0 to 2.0 mm for balloon angioplasty. However, 4 weeks later the vessels treated with laser thermal angioplasty had less restenosis (22% vs. 100%), defined as a 20 percent greater reduction in luminal diameter, and a significantly larger mean luminal diameter (1.6 vs. 1.0 mm) than those treated with conventional balloon angioplasty. Morphometric analysis of histologic cross-sections of these arterial segments confirmed a significantly larger lumen after laser thermal angioplasty compared with balloon angioplasty (1.24 vs. 0.64 mm^2).

Pulsed lasers, such as the excimer, are capable of precise tissue ablation without evidence of thermal injury. In contrast to CW lasers, pulsed lasers appear to be less thrombogenic and have the unique ability to cause vasodilatation. These unique properties may portend a reduced incidence of restenosis following pulsed laser angioplasty. At this writing, the authors are not aware of any systematic studies of the effects of pulsed laser irradiation on restenosis. No conclusions may be drawn regarding the effects of pulsed laser angioplasty on restenosis until such studies are completed.

Summary

Several laser systems have been shown to vaporize atheromatous plaque in vitro and in vivo. There appear to be certain advantages and disadvantages to all these systems. CW lasers such as the argon, Nd:YAG, and carbon dioxide debulk plaque essentially by thermal degradation following the conversion of light energy into heat within the plaque. The argon and Nd:YAG lasers are readily transmitted via standard optical fibers. The disadvantage of these systems is the spread of thermal damage to adjacent tissues. Pulsed lasers provide energy that results in little thermal damage to the adjacent tissue. While providing for more precise cutting, pulsed lasers were previously limited by destruction of the fiber optics used to transmit these high-peak-power pulses. This problem, however, has been largely overcome by using long pulse durations, as in the case of the XeCl (308 nm) excimer laser. Debris production appears to be small; however, a larger and greater number of particles are produced by pulsed laser irradiation. Although there is something of a controversy regarding the issue of thrombogenicity, it appears that CW lasers may be more thrombogenic than pulsed lasers. Finally, CW laser irradiation characteristically causes vasospasm, while the pulsed lasers have the unique ability to cause photorelaxation of vascular smooth muscle and vasodilatation.

The healing process following laser irradiation of both normal and atherosclerotic arteries with either CW or pulsed lasers appears to occur in a similar fashion. This process occurs within a few hours after irradiation as the crater fills with a platelet-fibrin plug. Fibrocellular infiltration of the crater is seen soon after laser irradiation. By 7 days an endothelial lining is present, and by 30–60 days the endothelial surface has covered the entire crater surface. The healing process following laser angioplasty appears to be a benign event. Although more randomized studies are needed, it appears that laser irradiation during laser angioplasty has the potential to reduce the high rate of restenosis seen with conventional balloon angioplasty. These data support the advancement of the laser as a clinical tool for interventional cardiovascular procedures.

References

1. Maiman TH. Stimulated optical radiation in ruby. *Nature* 1960;187:493–494.
2. McGuff PE, Bushnell D, Soroff HS, Deterling RA. Studies of the surgical applications of laser. *Surg Forum* 1963;14:143–152.
3. Choy DSJ, Stertzer Z, Rotterdam HZ, et al. Transluminal laser catheter angioplasty. *Am J Cardiol* 1982;50:1206–1208.

4. Choy DSJ, Stertzer Z, Rotterdam HZ, et al. Laser coronary angioplasty: experience with nine cadaver hearts. *Am J Cardiol* 1982;50:1209–1211.
5. Welch AJ, Bradley AB, Torres JH, et al. Laser probe ablation of normal and atherosclerotic human aorta: a first thermographic and histologic analysis. *Circulation* 1987;76:1353–1363.
6. Isner JM, Donaldson RF, Dechelbaum LI, et al. The excimer laser: gross, light microscopic and ultrastructural analysis of potential advantages for use in laser therapy of cardiovascular disease. *J Am Coll Cardiol* 1985;6:1102–1109.
7. Grundfest WS, Litvack IF, Goldenberg T, et al. Pulsed ultraviolet lasers and the potential for safe laser angioplasty. *Am J Surg* 1985;150:220–226.
8. Isner JM, Donaldson RF, Funai JT, et al. Factors contributing to perforations from laser angioplasty. *Circulation* 1985;72:II–191.
9. Abela GS, Seeger JM, Barbieri E, et al. Laser angioplasty with angioscopic guidance in humans. *J Am Coll Cardiol* 1986;8:184–187.
10. Tobis J, Smolin M, Mallery J, et al. Laser-assisted thermal angioplasty in human peripheral artery occlusions: mechanism of recanalization. *J Am Coll Cardiol* 1989;13:1547–1554.
11. Abela GS, Normann S, Cohen D, Feldman RL, Geiser EA, Conti CR. Effects of carbon dioxide, Nd:YAG, and argon laser radiation on coronary atheromatous plaques. *Am J Cardiol* 1982;50:1199–1204.
12. Isner JM, Clarke RH, Donaldson RF, Aharon AS. Identification of photoproducts liberated by in vitro laser irradiation of atherosclerotic plaque, calcified cardiac valves and myocardium. *Am J Cardiol* 1985;55:1192–1198.
13. Deckelbaum LI, Isner JM, Donaldson RF, Laliberte SM, Clarke RH, Salem DN. Use of pulsed energy delivery to minimize tissue injury resulting from carbon dioxide laser irradiation of cardiovascular tissues. *J Am Coll Cardiol* 1986;7:898–902.
14. Teng P, Nishioka NS, Anderson RR, Deutsch TF. Acoustic studies of the role of immersion in plasma-mediated laser ablation. *IEEE J Quant Elec* 1987;23:1845–1856.
15. Clarke RH, Isner JM, Gauthier T, et al. Spectroscopic characterization of cardiovascular tissue. *Lasers Surg Med* 1988;8:45–51.
16. Srinivasan R, Mayne-Banton V. Self-developing photoetching of poly(ethylenephtalate) laser radiation. *Appl Phys Lett* 1982;41:576–578.
17. Linkser R, Srinivasan R, Wayne JJ, Alonso DR. Far ultraviolet laser ablation of atherosclerotic lesions. *Lasers Surg Med* 1984;4:201–208.
18. Decklebaum LI, Isner JM, Donaldson RF, et al. Reduction of laser-in-

duced pathologic tissue injury using pulsed energy delivery. *Am J Cardiol* 1985;56:662–666.
19. Keys T. Theory of photoablation and its implication for phototherapy. *J Phys Chem* 1985;89:4194–4195.
20. Hayes JR, Wolbarsht M. A thermal model for retinal damage induced by pulsed lasers. *Aerospace Med* 1968;39:474–485.
21. Anderson RR, Parrish JA. Selective photothermolysis: precise microsurgery by selective absorption of pulsed radiation. *Science* 1983;220:524–526.
22. Gammon RW, Fox KR, Coster AA. Energy threshold for argon laser ablation of arterial plaque. *Applied Optics* 1987;26:3164–3167.
23. Abela GS, Normann SJ, Cohen DM, et al. Laser recanalization of occluded atherosclerotic arteries: an in-vivo and in-vitro study. *Circulation* 1985;71:403–411.
24. Prevosti LG, Cook JA, Leon MB, Bonner RF. Comparison of particulate debris size from excimer and argon laser irradiation. *Circulation* 1987;76:IV-410.
25. Clarke RH, Isner JM, Donaldson RF, Jones G. Gas chromatographic-light microscopic correlative analysis of excimer laser photoablation of cardiovascular tissues: evidence for a thermal mechanism. *Circ Res* 1987;60:429–435.
26. Prevosti LG, Lawrence JB, Leon MB, et al. Surface thrombogenicity after excimer laser and hot-tip thermal ablation of plaque: morphometric studies using an annular perfusion chamber. *Surg Forum* 1987;38:330–333.
27. Ragimov SE, Belyaev AA, Vertepa IA, et al. Comparison of different lasers in terms of thrombogenicity of the laser-treated vascular wall. *Lasers Surg Med* 1988;8:77–82.
28. Sanborn TA, Alexopoulos D, Marmur JD, et al. Coronary excimer laser angioplasty: reduced complications and indium-111 platelet accumulation compared with thermal laser angioplasty. *J Am Coll Cardiol* 1990;16:502–506.
29. Badimon L, Badimon JJ, Galvez A, Chesbro JH, Fuster V. Influence of arterial damage and wall shear rate on platelet deposition: ex-vivo study in swine model. *Arteriosclerosis* 1986;6:312–320.
30. Furchgott RF, Sleator W, McCaman MW, Elchlepp J. Relaxation of arterial strips by light, and the influence of drugs on this photodynamic effect. *J Pharmacol Exp Ther* 1955;113:22–23.
31. Furchgott RF, Ehrreich SJ, Greenblatt E. The photoactivated relaxation of smooth muscle of rabbit aorta. *J Gen Phys* 1961;44:499–519.
32. Steg PG, Gal D, Rongione AJ, DeJesus ST, Clarke RH, Isner JM. Effect

of argon laser irradiation on rabbit aortic smooth muscle: evidence for endothelium-independent contraction and relaxation. *Cardiovasc Res* 1988;22:747–753.
33. Steg PG, Rongione AJ, Gal D, DeJesus ST, Clarke RH, Isner JM. Pulsed ultraviolet laser irradiation produces endothelium-independent relaxation of vascular smooth muscle. *Circulation* 1989;79:189–197.
34. Isner JM, Clarke RH. The paradox of thermal ablation without thermal injury. *Lasers Med Sci* 1987;2:165–173.
35. Gerrity RG, Loop FG, Golding LAR, Ehrhart LA, Argenyi ZB. Arterial response to laser operation for removal of atherosclerotic plaques. *J Thorac Cardiovasc Surg* 1983;85:409–421.
36. Abela GS, Crea F, Seeger JM, et al. The healing process in normal canine arteries and in atherosclerotic monkey arteries after transluminal laser irradiation. *Am J Cardiol* 1985;56:983–988.
37. Sanborn TA, Haudenschild CC, Garber GR, Ryan TJ, Faxon DP. Angiographic and histologic consequences of laser thermal angioplasty: comparison with balloon angioplasty. *Circulation* 1987;75:1281–1286.
38. Higginson LA, Farrell EM, Walley VM, et al. Arterial response to excimer and argon laser irradiation in the atherosclerotic swine. *Lasers Med Sci* 1989;4:85–92.

CHAPTER **3**

Catheters for Laser Angioplasty—Design Considerations

Tsvi Goldenberg
William B. Anderson
Lynn Shimada

THE fundamental characteristics that determine the success of a laser delivery system are safety and efficacy. A safe delivery system must negotiate the tortuous paths of the peripheral and coronary arteries without causing trauma to the vessel. An efficacious catheter must create a large enough channel to restore blood flow to ischemic tissues. This chapter describes the fundamental issues concerning the development of fiber-optic delivery systems designed to meet the necessary and sometimes conflicting requirements for safety and efficacy. Discussions of the physics of high-energy transmission through optical fibers and catheter design basics are included. Catheter design issues such as device flexibility, steerability, ablation area, atraumatic tip design, and spatial tradeoffs are also addressed.

Physics of Energy Transmission Through Optical Fibers

When light is considered as a plane wave moving through space, the concept of refraction becomes easy to visualize. Refraction is responsible for the light-guiding properties of optical fibers. The speed of light depends on the material it is moving through. Light travels fastest through a vacuum, but when propagating through gases, liquids, and solids, its speed is lower, depending on the properties of the transmissive material. The slowing of the speed of light in a given material is characterized by that material's index of refraction, n. The variable n is the ratio of the speed of light in a vacuum to the speed of light in the transmissive medium. When a light wave approaches a boundary between two materials of different refractive indices, it is deflected. The part of the wave that passes through the interface changes speed (see Fig. 3.1). In the case of Figure 3.1, the secondary material (n_2) has a lower index of refraction than the first, and thus the speed of the light wave increases in the second material.

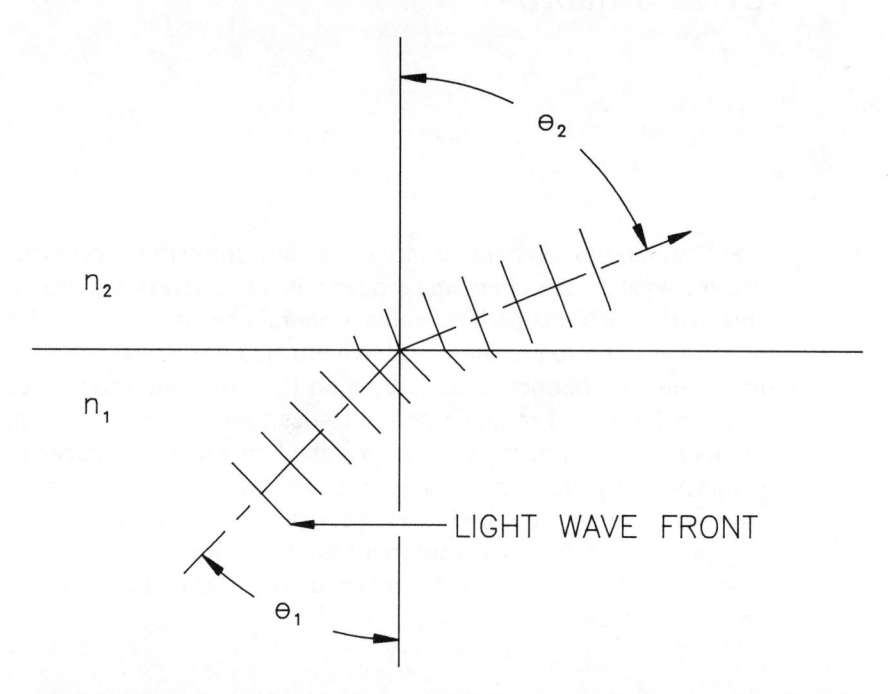

Figure 3.1. Conceptual illustration of light wave refraction at a boundary between two different materials. The arrow denotes the travel direction of the light ray. In addition, the illustration defines the angle of incidence (θ_1) and angle of refraction (θ_2). The indexes of refraction of the boundary materials are also noted (n_1, n_2).

Catheters for Laser Angioplasty—Design Considerations 51

The principle governing the specific relationship between the indices of refraction and the incident and refracted angle is called Snell's Law.

$$n_1 sine\theta_1 = n_2 sine\theta_2$$

Figure 3.1 defines the reference points of angles and gives respective refraction indices. For θ_1 equal to the inverse sine of n_2 over n_1, θ_1 becomes the critical angle. In this case θ_2 is 90° and the light wave is totally reflected.

$$\theta_{critical} = sine^{-1} \frac{n_2}{n_1}$$

Optical fibers use the principle of total reflection to guide light. The type of optical fiber used in delivery systems has a core material (index of refraction n_1) and a cladding material (index of refraction n_2) over the core (see Fig. 3.2).

A light wave that enters the core material of the fiber travels through the core until it strikes the core-cladding interface. If the incident angle of the light wave is greater than or equal to the critical angle (defined by the core and cladding material), it is totally reflected back into the fiber

$\theta_1 < \theta_{CRITICAL}$
$\theta_2 > \theta_{CRITICAL}$

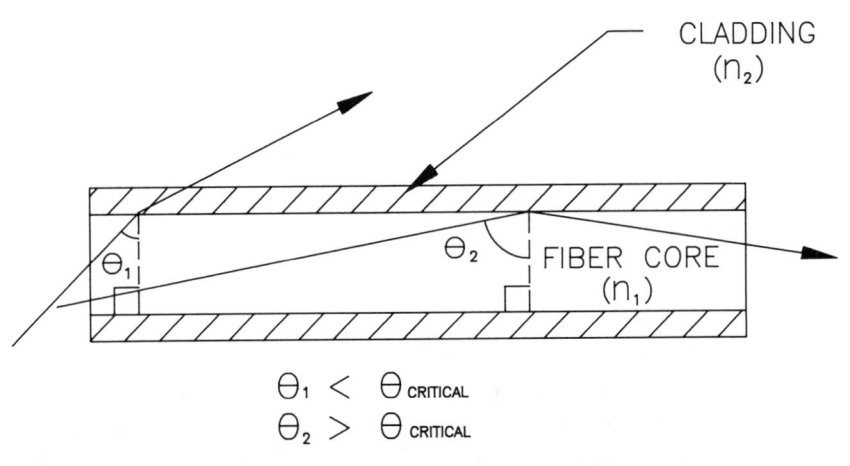

Figure 3.2. Longitudinal cross-section of a multimode fiber showing the core and cladding with their respective refractive indices (n_1, n_2). Entering the fiber core are two rays of light. The ray striking the core-cladding boundary at angle θ_1 has an angle of incidence below the critical angle. The ray subsequently refracts through the boundary and is lost. The ray striking the boundary at angle θ_2 strikes at an angle greater than the critical angle and is totally reflected back into the core.

core at the point of incidence. This process repeats until the light is absorbed by fiber optic loss mechanisms or the light exits the end of the fiber (see Fig. 3.2).

Numerical Aperature

The numerical aperature of an optical fiber is a measure of the fiber's acceptance angle for light. Consider a ray of light traveling in a fiber core, striking the core-cladding interface at an angle greater than the critical angle, and undergoing total reflection each time. At the threshold angle, the light ray does not undergo total internal reflection and the ray refracts into the cladding and is lost. The numerical aperature is the sine of the half angle of the cone of light exiting a fiber (assuming some or all of the light is at or near the critical angle). The numerical aperature also defines the boundaries of the cone of light that are accepted and transmitted by a fiber.

A fiber with a numerical aperature of 0.1, for example, has an output divergence angle of 5°, while an optical fiber with a numerical aperature of 0.5 has an output divergence angle of 20°. Numerical aperature can be defined in terms of the ratio of the index of refraction of the core vs. the index of refraction of the cladding of the fiber:

$$NA = \sqrt{n_1 - n_2}$$

Numerical aperature is also an important factor affecting the amount of bending loss in an optical fiber.

Bending Loss in Optical Fibers

The reflective angle of incidence remains constant for a light ray traveling the length of a fiber that is held in a straight line. If the fiber is bent, however, a light ray that hits the bend hits at an angle slightly different from the angle in the straight section. If a tight bend is imposed upon an optical fiber, a light ray traveling inside it that is almost at critical angle bounces around the bend, progressively adding to the incident angle of reflection until it reaches the critical angle and escapes through the core-cladding boundary. This phenomenon is known as bending loss (see Fig. 3.3). Bending loss can be a problem when an angioplasty system requires operator knowledge of the energy density exiting the distal tip

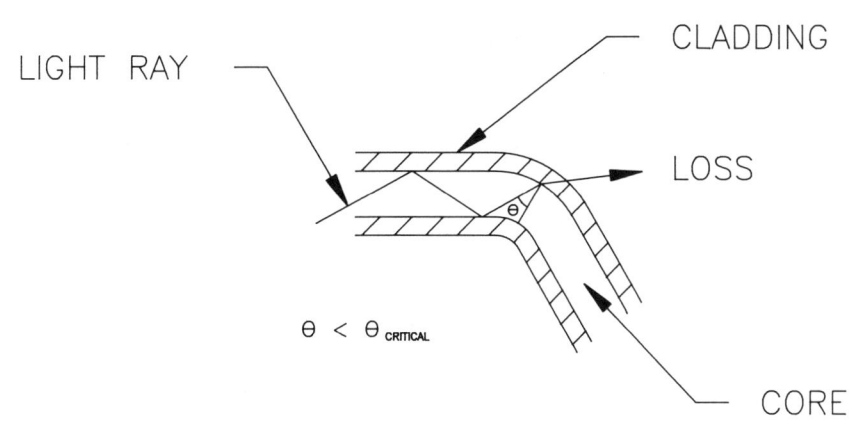

Catheters for Laser Angioplasty—Design Considerations 53

LIGHT RAY

CLADDING

LOSS

θ < θ_{CRITICAL}

CORE

Figure 3.3. Bending loss. The light ray traveling through the core encounters a tight bend and strikes the core-cladding boundary at an angle less than the critical angle. The ray then refracts through the boundary and is lost. Note that this is an extreme case and normally many reflections around a bend would be required to significantly alter the angle of incidence.

of the catheter during a procedure. Suppose a physician sets up the laser catheter at a predetermined energy. The procedure is begun and the laser catheter is inserted through the guiding catheter to reach a lesion in the heart. The laser catheter bends while proceeding through the guiding catheter, and subsequent bending loss of laser energy results. The physician can no longer be sure of the energy setting. It is imperative, therefore, that the energy needed for efficient ablation be measured directly and that no significant bending loss occur during the procedure.

Three ways to minimize bending loss are: 1) choose a fiber with high *NA* (1); 2) minimize the divergence of the light entering the fiber, and 3) use small-core fiber (2). With a higher *NA*, the critical angle of reflection is reduced, allowing more bend in the fiber before the light rays reach the critical angle inside and escape. Minimizing input divergence has a similar effect to raising the *NA* of the fiber. The light rays are at a high angle of incidence (as defined by θ_2, Fig. 3.2) inside the fiber and well above the critical angle threshold for total internal reflection. While a bend in the fiber decreases the angle of incidence of the light ray, the angle may still be above the critical angle and the light ray may be totally reflected.

For a given bend radius, the smaller of two fibers with similar numerical aperatures is less susceptible to bending loss. This can be explained intuitively by considering the fact that the geometry inside a small fiber in a tight bend is the same as the geometry of a large fiber in a large bend. It follows that a small fiber in a large bend is less likely to induce changes in the incidence angle of light traveling through it.

Fiber Coating

The outer coating of an optical fiber protects the core-cladding from mechanical damage and chemical contamination and reduces laser energy leakage into the surrounding environment. Common coating types include silicone, lacquers, urethanes, polyimides, and ultraviolet acrylates (3). Ultraviolet-curable coatings and polyimides have overcome most stability and durability problems (3–6). Important features of fiber coatings include biocompatibility, mechanical strength, resistance to abrasion, bondability to glass substrates and potting adhesives, and the thickness that must be applied to make a strong fiber.

The importance of mechanical strength and abrasion resistance of a coating are obvious. During assembly, shipment, and clinical use, the fibers of a delivery system are subjected to mechanical stress and must remain intact.

The bondability of a coating to the glass cladding substrate is important because silica fiber is extremely susceptible to water contamination. Water particles that contact the silica core or cladding create a weak spot that may fail during mechanical load. A coating that chemically bonds to the glass fiber substrate as it comes out of the melt of the drawing tower is desirable since it ensures that no water contamination occurs along the length of the fiber. It is not sufficient for a coating to be simply impermeable to water because the fibers are often polished in an aqueous environment during assembly. If the coating separates from the glass during polishing, the water can creep back under the coating and weaken the fiber. The same would be true for the polymers used as cladding in hard-clad fibers.

Bondability to potting epoxies is also important because the fibers must inevitably be terminated in a stable fashion at the distal tip of the delivery system. As this is often accomplished by applying a potting epoxy around the ends of the fiber or fibers, it is necessary to have a good bond between the two materials. The amount of coating (thickness) that must be applied to produce a durable fiber is a concern because space is usually limited within a laser delivery system, and thick fiber coating reduces available space for fibers.

Fiber Selection

The ideal optical fiber is durable, has minimal energy loss during transmission, and has a large core-to-cladding ratio to reduce unused cross-sectional surface area. Highly pure silica core fibers are acceptable for most laser angioplasty applications (7,8). Plastic-clad silica (PCS™), Hard-clad silica (HCS™), and glass-clad silica fibers are among the fibers manufactured with a highly pure silica core and a large core-to-cladding ratio (9–11). Glass-clad silica, which provides the best transmission for most laser angioplasty applications, has a relatively low NA (0.2). This is a drawback for catheters that use fibers larger than 100 microns, but the bend loss is not serious for fibers at or below this size. In contrast, PCS and HCS fibers have an NA of 0.37 to 0.47 (9,10), which effectively eliminates bend loss or coronary applications that used fibers in the 100-micron size range.

The purity of the core material is the most important factor affecting the transmission of laser energy through silica fiber. The fiber must contain a substantially pure silica core made synthetically, particularly with ultraviolet (UV) and infrared (IR) applications. Contaminants that strongly degrade transmission are oxides and intermetallics. A desirable core silica for high-energy ultraviolet and infrared transmission would have an intermetallic contaminant level at or below 1 ppm. Reasonable contamination levels of other elements can be seen in Table 3.1. The presence of OH (water) radicals in the core silica creates strong absorption bands in the infrared region of the spectrum, particularly at 1.38, 2.22, and 2.72 micrometers. Infrared applications, therefore, generally require a core silica with a low OH content (less than 5 ppm).

Carbon dioxide laser energy is strongly absorbed by tissue. The availability and low cost of a CO_2 laser system make it a desirable combination to develop. The 10.6-micron wavelength of the carbon dioxide laser, however, is strongly absorbed by both tissue and silica. Development of a fiber suitable for delivery of 10.6-micron radiation from the CO_2 laser is under investigation. To date, however, no cost-effective fiber is commercially available (12–14).

Table 3.1. Silica Glass Composition

ELEMENT		CLEAR FUSED QUARTZ FROM ROCK CRYSTAL COMMERCIAL, OPTOSIL, HOMOSIL	CLEAR SYNTHETIC FUSED SILICA SUPRASIL-W, SUPRASIL
Aluminum	(Al)	10. to 50.	.1
Antimony	(Sb)	.15	.002
Arsenic	(As)	.08	.03
Boron	(B)	0 to 1	0 to .01
Cadmium	(Cd)	0 to .1	.0002
Calcium	(Ca)	.8 to 3.	.1
Chromium	(Cr)	1. to 2.	n.d.
Copper	(Cu)	.07	.004
Gallium	(Ga)	0 to .008	n.d.
Gold	(Au)	.0003	n.d.
Iron	(Fe)	.8	.2
Lithium	(Li)	0 to 2.	0 to .05
Magnesium	(Mg)	.2	0 to .1
Manganese	(Mn)	.01	0 to .01
Phosphorus	(P)	.1	.01 to .1
Potassium	(K)	.8	0 to .001
Silver	(Ag)	n.d.	0 to .05
Sodium	(Na)	1.	.04
Titanium	(Ti)	.8	0 to .1
Uranium	(U)	.0003	n.d.
Zirconium	(Zr)	0 to .1	0 to .001

PARTS PER MILLION (PPM) BY WEIGHT

n.d. = not determined

Other Energy Loss in Optical Fibers

In addition to bending loss, several other types of losses occur in optical fibers during high-energy laser transmission. The extent to which high energy-loss mechanisms are a factor is a function of the peak energy being transmitted (15). Reflective losses account for 4 percent at the input and output of the fiber. Energy losses also occur in the core material where absorption and scattering mechanisms turn laser energy into heat. An example of such a mechanism is called Rayleigh scattering, which is primarily due to microscopic defects in the core material scattering the light. The attenuation coefficient for this phenomena is inversely proportional to the fourth power of the wavelength, making shorter wavelengths more severely attenuated (1).

Nonlinear loss mechanisms are present in the pulsed laser systems due to the high peak-threshold powers being transmitted through the core material of the fiber. The additional losses are a drawback, but pulsed systems have the ability to cut tissue without thermal damage, which is clinically advantageous (16–20). Two nonlinear effects that result in energy loss are Raman and Brillouin scattering (1,21,22). These mechanisms convert laser energy into heat, which reduces output.

Losses within the core (mechanisms other than bending loss) remain fairly constant if the energy launched into the fiber input is constant, and such losses do not present any significant clinical problems. Once the power has been adjusted and set for the laser delivery system, the loss mechanisms should remain stable throughout the clinical procedure.

Nevertheless, energy losses do present a challenge to the delivery-system designer. Enough energy must be transmitted to the end of a 3 to 4-meter piece of optical fiber to remove tissue. In extreme cases, loss mechanisms can result in laser damage to the fiber material. The basic types of laser damage to optical fibers include input surface, output surface, and bulk damage to the fiber core material.

Surface Damage of Fiber Input

To have levels of energy above the ablation threshold exit distal tip of a laser delivery system and overcome optical losses over the length of the delivery system, energy must be launched into the fiber at a very high fluence, which may approach the damage threshold for silica fiber. The input surface of the fiber at the proximal end of the delivery system has to cope with this high energy. When damage occurs to a delivery system, it is usually at the input surface (8,15,23–25). Because the input surface is the part of the catheter exposed to the highest energy density of any part of the delivery system, the preparation of that surface is crucial, particularly with the pulsed laser systems where peak input densities are on the order of megawatts per square centimeter. Mechanical polishing must be done carefully as this process inevitably leaves some contamination from the polishing media buried in the glass surface. Contamination results in an absorption site for laser energy that may lead to cracking or chipping (21,23).

Fiber Output Damage

In continuous-wave (CW) systems, intense heat develops at the distal end of the delivery system. In addition to causing thermal damage to tissue (12,26–28), the heat can also damage the output surfaces of optical fibers (29). Output surface damage has been reduced in CW systems by attaching metal or sapphire tips to the fiber optic for protection (29,30). The sapphire tip is more resilient to thermal shock than the silica fiber and remains intact during the tissue removal procedure. The metal tips are designed to absorb the laser energy and create heat for ablation.

At the output surface of fibers in pulsed systems, optical reflection and other surface effects can create catastrophic stresses (23). If the electric fields or mechanical shock becomes strong enough, the molecules of the silica fiber may be torn apart. The most effective way to eliminate catheter output surface damage in pulsed laser systems is to reduce the energy density exiting the delivery system to just above the ablation threshold for the target lesion. A well-polished output surface is also an important factor in reducing surface damage.

Fiber Core Damage

One cause of fiber core damage is contamination or voids in the core, which occur when the quality of the fiber is not carefully controlled during manufacture (23,31). If the void or the contaminant is large enough, it absorbs enough laser energy to initiate a thermal stress crack (23). Once this crack is exposed to high-density laser energy, it spreads and destroys the fiber. Raman and Brillouin scattering, involving the transformation of energy into heat and sound waves, can also lead to bulk damage if the energy densities are high enough (22).

Self-focusing or self-trapping is an effect that can raise energy densities above the damage threshold of the fiber (22,32). When strong electric fields induced by electromagnetic laser radiation are present in some dielectrics (silica), their index of refraction is altered. The altered index of refraction acts as a focusing lens inside the dielectric. In this way, a laser beam traveling through the fiber becomes continually focused until the energy density exceeds the damage threshold. A common indication of this type of damage is linear destruction along the axis of a fiber (21,22).

Catheters for Laser Angioplasty—Design Considerations 59

Laser Energy Coupling

Angioplasty systems are required to concentrate the large-aperature, low-energy-density beam exiting a laser and to funnel it into the fiber-optic delivery system. This is done to achieve the high-energy densities necessary for plaque removal. The energy density delivered to the optical fiber input surface should be adjustable so the proper energy fluence can be delivered to the distal tip of the system. Energy coupling is generally accomplished by either a convex lens–based apparatus or a tapered fiber that converges with the laser beam to a sharp focal point. Additionally, the energy coupler positions the optical fiber surface precisely in the focused beam. Precise positioning of the input surface ensures consistent energy density delivery and provides for interchanging systems without making adjustments. Fig. 3.4 illustrates a conceptual version of an energy coupler.

The beam exits the laser and is focused by the lens. The fiber input is then moved with precision into and away from the focal spot of the beam to adjust the energy density launched into it. There are many variations of this general scheme. One such variation is the liquid energy

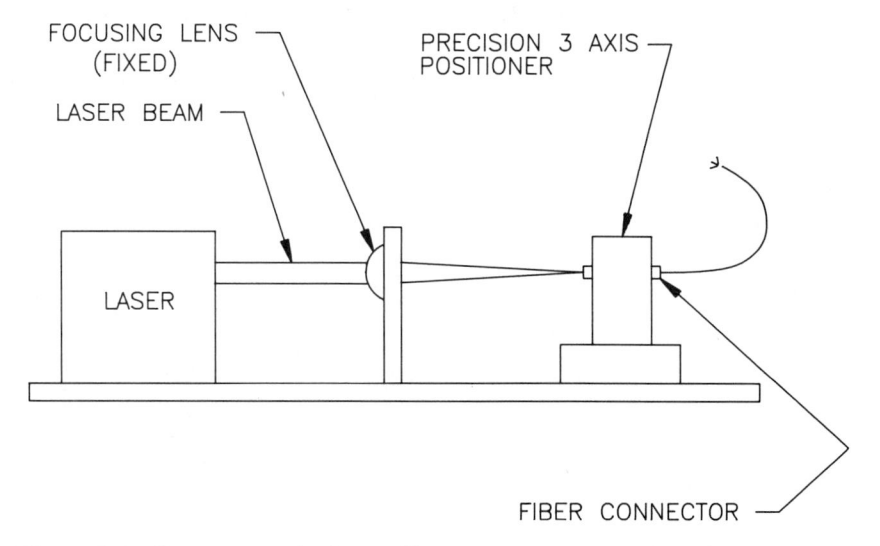

Figure 3.4. Illustration of a basic fiber-optic energy coupler. The two main components are the focusing lens and the three axis positioners. It is important that the laser-focusing lens and the three axis positioners be mounted in a stable mount. The fiber input can then be positioned in the focused laser beam to achieve the desired energy input.

coupler. This type of coupler allows the input surface of the fiber to be immersed in a fluid that matches the index of refraction of the silica fiber. The index-matching fluid reduces the severity of the discontinuity between the air and glass present in a standard coupler.

Catheter Basics

The type of energy that has good tissue removal ability tends to be difficult to transmit through optical fibers, and because of this, the early delivery systems for laser angioplasty consisted of a large single optical fiber packaged in a plastic tube made of a polymer. A large single fiber is easier to couple to a laser because it can be aligned symmetrically to the laser beam axis. Being a large fiber, the entire beam of a laser can be focused with a lens onto the fiber input surface. If the divergence of the focused laser beam is less than the *NA* of the fiber, all of the laser's output can be transmitted through the fiber notwithstanding losses within the fiber (see Fig. 3.5).

One of the first laser angioplasty catheters used clinically consisted of a single 600-micron fiber protected by a polymer sheath. The catheter had epoxy around the circumference of the distal tip to give an atraumatic shape. This system was used in the periphery but was too

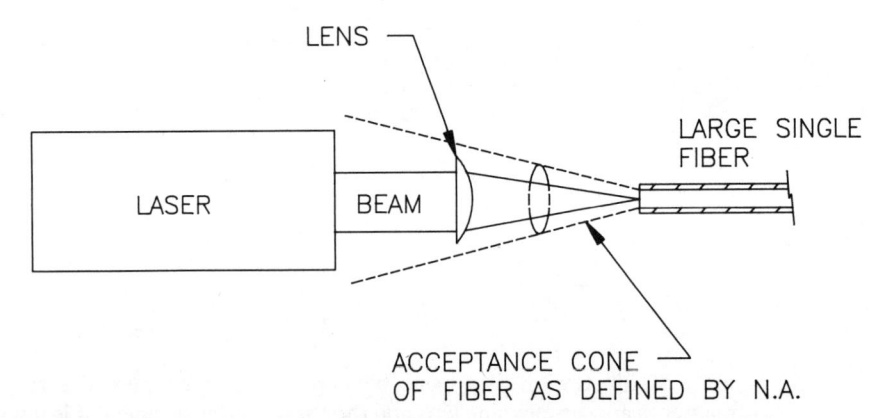

Figure 3.5. Illustration of the input of an entire laser beam into a single large core fiber. Note that the beam convergence matches the fiber acceptance cone divergence.

stiff to negotiate anything but straight vessel occlusions in the mid to distal femoral arteries.

An improvement of the 600-micron catheter is an expanded tip system. Such a peripheral delivery system has the flexibility of a 400-micron fiber but the cutting area of a 600-micron fiber. This can be achieved by attaching onto the distal tip a 4-meter piece of 400-micron fiber that allows the beam inside the 400-micron fiber to expand to 600 microns (see Fig. 3.6).

For an expanded tip system, losses and fiber damage have to be overcome so that enough energy could be launched into the 400-micron input, travel 4 meters to the distal tip of the system, expand to the 600-micron diameter (2.25 times the area of a 400-micron fiber), and still have enough energy density to ablate calcified plaque.

Since fiber stiffness is approximately equal to the diameter of the fiber to the fourth power (33), this system has the cutting area of a 600-micron fiber but is five times more flexible than the system constructed with 600-micron fiber over the full 4-meter length. In addition to increased flexibility, the expanded tip catheter has the advantage of improved cutting efficiency. The distal tip cross-section of an expanded 600-micron system has a high percentage of active cutting area. Pulsed ultraviolet and infrared laser systems are contact cutting systems. The absorption of this type of energy by tissue is strong, and a beam leaving an optical fiber in a blood field or in contact with tissue penetrates a short distance before it is absorbed (16). The size of the hole cut by the

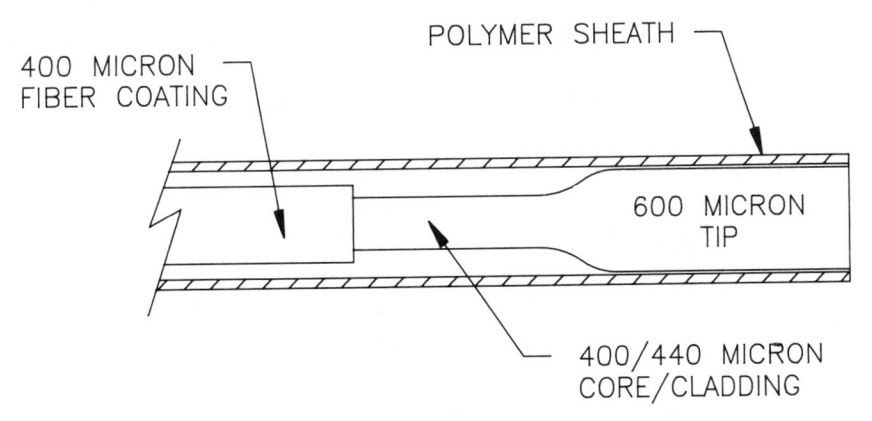

Figure 3.6. Cutaway view of a 600-micron catheter with an expanded tip. Note that the outer diameter (O.D.) of the coating of the 400-micron fiber is less than the O.D. of the cladding of the 600-micron tip.

catheter, therefore, is equal to the size of the core glass at the distal output of the fiber.

The 600-micron expanded tip catheter cuts a 600-micron hole. The area on the catheter located radially outward from the 600-micron core, which does not transmit any energy (i.e., cladding, fiber coating, epoxy for atraumatic tip shaping), is impeding the progress of the catheter as it tries to move through the 600-micron hole it has cut.

The advantage of the expanded 600-micron catheter is that some of the excess outer materials (fiber coating, etc.) are for a 400-micron fiber. The coating diameter of a 400-micron fiber can be less than the cladding diameter of a 600-micron fiber. The protective polymer sheath, therefore, can go over the coating of the 400-micron fiber and the cladding of the 600-micron tip attachment (see Fig. 3.6).

Although the expanded 600-micron catheter is very efficient and somewhat flexible, it has a severe size limitation. The lumen it creates is below 1 mm in diameter, which is large enough to pass a dilatation balloon but not sufficient for peripheral recanalization.

The next logical improvement in producing a coronary catheter is to use a multiple-fiber system. Multiple-fiber design enables a delivery system to have a greater cutting area than a large single fiber and gives the system much greater flexibility. Cutting area is proportional to the square of the fiber diameter; stiffness is proportional to the fourth power of the fiber diameter. If a system is designed for a single 400-micron-diameter fiber, one can use four fibers of 200-micron diameter and have the same cutting area at the distal tip. The flexibility of the four 200-micron fibers, however, is four times greater than that of a single 400-micron fiber.

Coupling multiple-fiber delivery systems to a laser requires a uniform beam profile and consistent energy from the laser. Empty space at the input between the fibers of a multiple-fiber delivery system at the input necessitates a more powerful laser than would be required for a single-fiber catheter with the same active area. Typically, multiple-fiber inputs consist of a circular bundle. A multiple-fiber system operates safely only if similar energy densities exit each fiber. If the energy density from each fiber is not the same, some of the fibers may be below the ablation threshold.

The problem of efficient cutting at the distal tip with multiple-fiber bundles is the empty space between them. Unless the fibers are formed to a hexagonal shape, there is a significant amount of empty space between them, no matter how tightly they are packed.

Catheters for Laser Angioplasty—Design Considerations   63

The clinical significance of this dead space between the fibers of multifiber bundles occurs in the form of displaced, rather than ablated tissue. The portion of the target lesion that lies between the active cutting area of a multiple-fiber catheter is not ablated, yet the catheter advances regardless. Random (transverse) motion of the catheter distal tip during lasing helps correct this situation, but the dead space between and around fibers reduces the performance of the delivery system when a hard calcified lesion is encountered. Nevertheless, the advantages of arranging multiple fibers symmetrically around a guidewire lumen (or any shape, for that matter) far outweigh the disadvantages.

A multiple-fiber system that could be used in peripheral arteries could have seven or more 200-micron fibers arranged concentrically around a guidewire lumen. This system would be able to create a hole approximately 1.5 mm in diameter in lesions that can be crossed with a guidewire. Although the 7 × 200-micron system would be an advance over the expanded 600-micron system, it still would not be flexible enough to be used in coronary arteries.

Combining the best features of the expanded 600-micron system and the 7 × 200 with further improvements results in a safe and effective laser catheter for coronary use. Consider a catheter with 12 100-micron fibers 4 meters long, each fiber expanded to 200 microns at the distal tip. The fibers can be arranged concentrically around a guidewire lumen as in the 7 × 200 system (see Fig. 3.7). This utilizes the beam expansion and cutting efficiency of the expanded 600-micron catheter with the flexible concentrically arranged multiple fibers of the 7 × 200 system. The flexibility of the 12 × 200 is greater than that of a single unexpanded 200-micron fiber but with twelve times the cutting area. The 12 × 200 can create a 1.6 mm channel, which would be sufficient for recanalization by laser alone in a large percentage of coronary cases.

A disadvantage of the 12 × 200 catheter is the areas of nonablation between the 200-micron fibers at the distal tip. Even though the overall ablation efficiency is very good (total core glass area/total distal tip area without the guidewire), the triangular areas between the fibers still tend to hinder advancement of this system through hard calcified lesions.

In response to this inadequacy, a more advanced design is comprised of hundreds of very small fibers (50-micron core or smaller) arranged in a similar manner around a guidewire lumen (see Fig. 3.8). Flexibility is achieved by using very small fibers. A large cutting area is possible because of the number of fibers. In addition, the nonablative areas between the fibers are small and random motion or tapping of the catheter

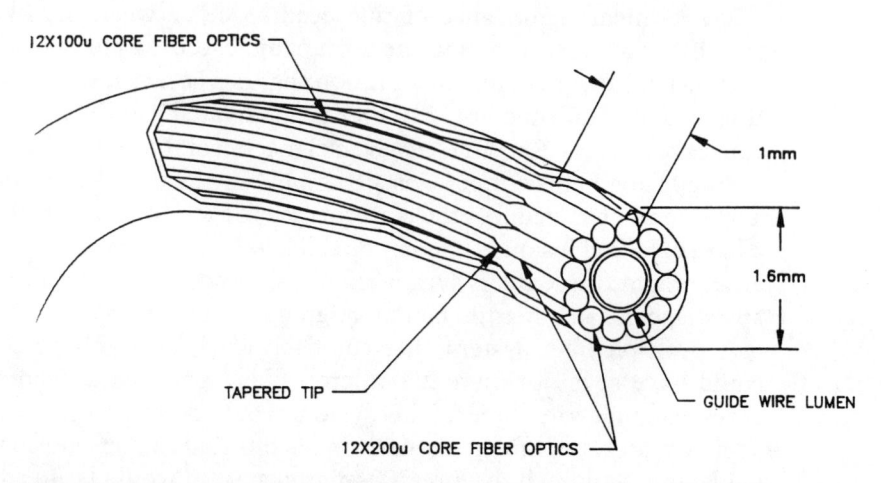

Figure 3.7. Cutaway view of 12 × 200 coronary catheter. Note expanded fiber tips and concentric arrangement around guidewire lumen.

distal tip during ablation tends to overlap the ablative core with the nonablative areas around it. These features combine to give a more uniform circular channel. This design, the multiple-fiber, 50-micron system, is the fiber-optic arrangement used in the current Advanced Interventional Systems, 1.3-mm, 1.6-mm, 2.0-mm, 2.2-mm, and 2.4-mm coronary catheters.

Catheter Guidance

For a delivery system to be safe it must be flexible, but it must also be capable of being guided to and through the target lesion (34,35). There are several modalities in use and under consideration for guiding laser delivery systems.

One approach to recanalize a vessel without over-the-wire guidance can be used to cross a totally occluded vessel (36). A specially designed balloon (37) can be percutaneously introduced and advanced to the occlusion. A 200-micron silica fiber optic is passed through the balloon catheter using fluoroscopic imaging to the distal tip of the balloon where it emerges from the center lumen. Ringer's lactate solution is injected to replace the blood layers between the fiber distal tip and lesion.

Catheters for Laser Angioplasty—Design Considerations 65

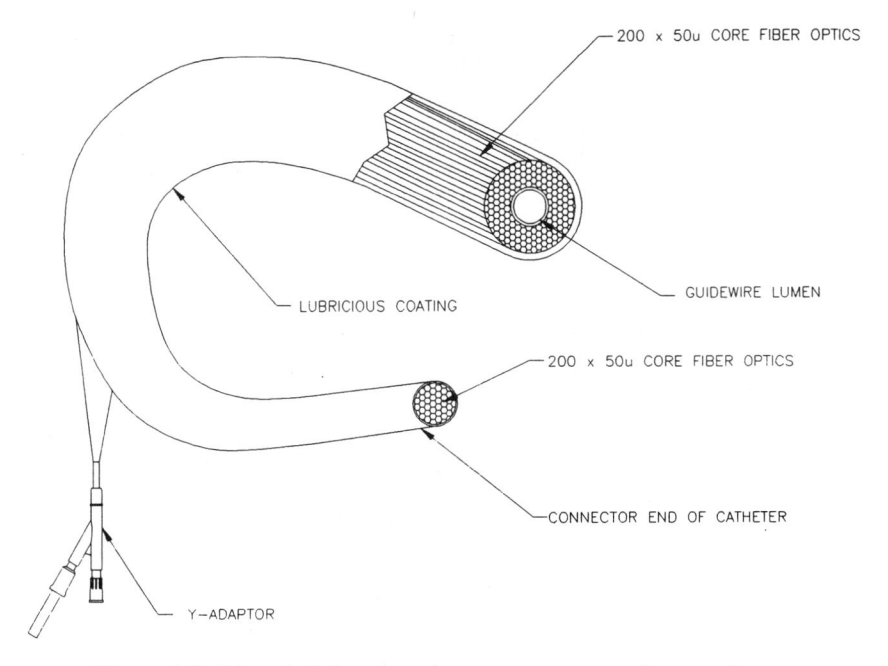

Figure 3.8. Litvack 1.6-mm percutaneous coronary laser catheter.

A continuous-wave argon laser is triggered to deliver 10 watts for 1-, 2-, or 5-second intervals. A funnel-like channel in the lesion is created. The clinician withdraws the optical fiber and passes a conventional guidewire across the lesion, followed by a percutaneous transluminal coronary angioplasty (PTCA) balloon that dilates the lesion. This system represents the catheter developed by GV Medical. A modification of this system could incorporate an excimer or other pulsed laser source.

If the beam is not allowed to expand outside of the laser catheter, the size of the hole cut by the catheter is limited by the inner diameter of the delivery balloon. Either of the two methods above (over-the-wire, balloon-guided) would be dangerous to use on a lesion that was in a bend (38). The centering balloon has the advantage, however, of being able to treat total occlusions.

Another technique for guiding a laser catheter through a lesion is accomplished with spectroscopic feedback (39,40). A low-energy light pulse is sent through the fiber of the delivery system, and the reflected spectrum is analyzed by computer to determine if the reflective material is diseased or healthy tissue. If the spectrum reveals plaque or diseased tissue, the catheter is advanced. If not, the catheter is withdrawn and another attempt made. The ability to deflect the distal tip of the delivery system would be very useful in this application since the catheter would probably follow the same path on successive attempts. Although this technique also works for total occlusions, it has yet to be proven safe and effective. At this time, no system of this design is under commercial development.

A system that uses angioscopic visualization for guidance is another possibility. For this technique to be safe, the system would have to visualize the target lesion while lasing was taking place (34). As with spectroscopic guidance, it would be necessary to have some means of mechanically directing and manipulating the distal tip of the laser catheter. A design concern for this type of complicated system would be the amount of space available for the deflection mechanism, the angioscope, and the fiber for laser transmission. Packaging all of these components in one small, flexible system would be difficult.

A simple and effective method is to put the laser catheter itself over a guidewire. This is the mode of guidance for the currently employed multiple-fiber coronary systems including the 50-micron systems (Advanced Interventional Systems, Inc.) and the 100–150-micron systems (Spectranetics; USCI). This technique is particularly beneficial on contact cutting delivery systems. The guidewire is manipulated to the target lesion using standard techniques developed by clinicians for balloon angioplasty. The laser delivery system can then be advanced over the wire and to the lesion. The guidewire serves as a track for the delivery system to follow, directs it, and keeps the distal tip of the delivery system pointed in a coaxial direction. The catheter can advance through the lesion, tracking the guidewire during laser ablation (Fig. 3.9). The wire is collinear with the vessel, and the distal tip of the catheter is collinear to the guidewire. Thus the guidewire keeps the active fiber area from directly contacting the vessel wall.

Summary and Future Directions

This chapter has reviewed the physical principles and properties of fiber-optic transmission of laser energy, including high-peak-power, pulsed energy. The characteristics of fiber-optic construction as well as the construction of clinically applied laser catheters were reviewed. The catheter design currently in clinical trial that has shown success is

Catheters for Laser Angioplasty—Design Considerations 67

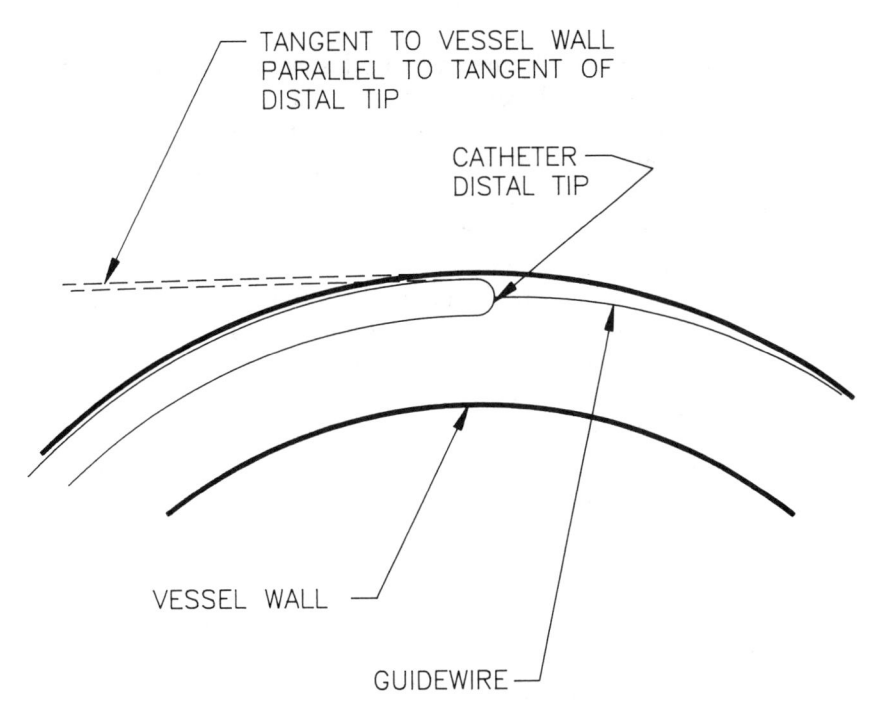

Figure 3.9. Depiction of the guidewire's role in steering an over-the-wire delivery system. Note that this technique is particularly effective with systems that use strongly absorbed laser energy. The guidewire keeps the distal tip of the delivery system from facing the vessel wall, in order for ablation to maintain a forward direction only.

the "over-the-wire" system constructed of multiple fiber-optics concentrically arranged about a guidewire lumen. The use of multiple fiber optics solves the apparent diametrically opposed design criteria of significant flexibility and ability to perform ablation on large areas. Highly flexible, multiple-fiber catheters can track standard coronary guidewires through most coronary segments while the catheter tip remains relatively coaxial with the artery. Currently available systems range from 1.3 mm to 2.4 mm in diameter. Drawbacks of this design include the need to first cross lesions with a guidewire (limiting efficacy in chronic total occlusions) and the need for progressively larger coronary guide catheters as catheter diameter is increased, thereby allowing the creation of large-diameter lumens. Furthermore, catheters with concentric lumen for the coronary guidewire are not ideally suited for highly eccentric lesions. Future catheter designs for "over-the-wire" systems would include catheters with eccentric guidewire lumens for dealing with eccentric stenoses, catheters with tip deflection to allow for more direct aiming of the laser energy, and some method of tip expansion so that a catheter of 5 or 6 French can create a substantially larger diameter channel following ablation.

At present, no good system has yet been developed to treat chronic total occlusions. The balloon-coaxiallizing, single-fiber method has been associated with coronary perforation and dissection. Significant further improvement is necessary in these systems to allow safe recanalization with or without these adjunctive balloons in chronic total coronary occlusions. The use of steerable balloon-tipped catheters as well as intracoronary ultrasound or angioscope imaging is being evaluated but as yet has not been applied clinically.

References

1. Miller S, Chynoweth A. Optical fiber communications. Orlando, FL: Academic Press, 1979.
2. Schonborn K, Bader H. Advantages of using thin fiber. Optical fibers in medicine III. *Proc SPIE* 1988;906:238–243.
3. Lawson KR, Cutler OR. UV cured coatings for optical fibers. *J Radiat Curing* 1982;9:4–10.
4. Lawson KR, Ansel RE, Stanton JJ. Optical fiber buffer coatings cured with ultra-violet light. Fiberoptic Communications 80 (newsletter), San Francisco, September 1980.
5. McGinniss VD. Photo initiation of acrylate systems for UV curing, Association of Finishing Processes of the Society of Manufacturing Engineers Technical Paper FC, 760486. 1976;476–486.
6. Ansel RE, Stanton JJ. Conference on physics of fiber optics. American Ceramic Society, April 1980.
7. Nevis EA. Alteration of the transmission characteristics of fused silica optical fibers by pulsed ultra-violet radiation. *Proc SPIE* 1985;540:181–185.
8. Taylor RS, Leopold KE, Mihailov S, et al. Damage and transmission measurements of fused silica fibers using long optical pulse XeCl lasers. *Optics Commun* 1987;63:26–31.
9. Beck WB, Hodge MH, Skutnik BJ, et al. Hard-clad silica (HCS) fibers for

data and power transmission. Proceedings of the European Fiberoptic Communications and Local Area Networks Exposition (EFOC/LAN) 85, 1985;146–151.
10. Skutnick BJ, Hodge MH, Nath DK. High strength, reliable, hard-clad silica (HCS) fibers Proceedings of the European Fiberoptic Communications and Local Area Networks Exposition (EFOC/LAN) 85, 1985;232–236.
11. Skutnick BJ, Hille RE. Environmental effects on hard clad silica optical fibers. Fiber optics in adverse environments II. *Proc SPIE* 1984; 506:184–188.
12. Tran D, Levin K. Zirconium fluoride fiber requirements for mid-infrared laser surgery applications. Optical fibers in medicine. *Proc SPIE* 1986;713:36–37.
13. McCann B. Fiber holds the key to medical success. *Photonics Spectra* May, 1990: 127–136.
14. Gal D, Katzir A. Silver halide optical fibers for medical applications. Optical fibers in medicine. *IEEE J Quantum Elec* 1987 (CIO-23):1827–1835.
15. Singleton DL, Paraskevopoulos G, Taylor RS, et al. Excimer laser angioplasty: tissue ablation, arterial response, and fiber optic delivery. *IEEE J Quant Elec* 1987;233(10):1772–1782.
16. Chutorian DM, Setzer PM, Kosek J, et al. The interaction between excimer laser energy and vascular tissue. *Am Heart J* 1986;112:739–745.
17. Grundfest W, Litvack F, Forrester J, et al. Laser ablation of human atherosclerotic plaque without adjacent tissue injury. *J Am Coll Cardiol* 1985;5:929–933.
18. Goldenberg T, Litvack F, Grundfest W, et al. Design criteria for in vivo laser angioplasty. Optical fibers in medicine. *Proc SPIE* 1987;713:53–55.
19. Isner J, Dov G, Steg G, et al. Percutaneous in vivo excimer laser angioplasty: Results in two experimental animal models. *Lasers Surg Med* 1988;8:223–232.
20. Srinivasan R. Ablation of polymers and biological tissue by ultraviolet lasers. *Science* 1986;234:559–565.
21. Allison SE, Gillies GT, Magnuson DW, et al. Pulsed laser damage to optical fibers. *Appl Optics* 1985;24(19):3140–3144.
22. Ready J. Effects of high-power laser radiation. Orlando, FL: Academic Press, 1971.
23. Lowdermilk WH, Milam D. Review of ultra-violet damage threshold measurements at Lawrence Livermore National Laboratory: excimer lasers, their applications and new frontiers in lasers. *Proc SPIE* 1984;476:143–162.

24. Lowdermilk H, Milam D. Laser-induced surface and coating damage. *IEEE J Quantum Elec* 1981;17(9):1888–1903.
25. Rainer F, Lowdermilk H, Milam D. Bulk and surface damage thresholds of crystals and glasses at 248 nm. *Optical Eng* 1983;22(4):431–434.
26. Bonner R, Smith P, Leon M. Quantification of tissue effects due to a pulsed Er:YAG laser at 2.9 (micron) with beam delivery in a wet field via zirconium fluoride fibers. Optical fibers in medicine II. *Proc SPIE* 1986;713:2–5.
27. Linsker R, Srinivasan R, Wynne J, et al. Far ultra-violet laser ablation of atherosclerotic lesions. *Lasers Surg Med* 1984;4:201–206.
28. Grundfest W, Litvack F, Goldenberg T, et al. Pulsed ultraviolet lasers and the potential for safe laser angioplasty. *Am J Surg* 1985;150:220–226.
29. Geschwind H, Monhkolsmai D, Stern J, et al. Laser angioplasty with contact sapphire probe. Optical fibers in medicine. *Proc SPIE* 1986;713:49–52.
30. Borst C. Percutaneous recanalization of arteries: status and prospects of laser angioplasty with modified fiber tips. *Lasers Med Sci* 1987;2:137.
31. Griscom D. Defect structure of glasses: some outstanding questions in regard to vitrious silica. *J Noncrystalline Solids* 1985;73:51–77.
32. Smith L, Bechtel J, Bloembergen N. Picosecond laser-induced breakdown at 5321 and 3547 A. Observation of frequency dependent behavior. *Phys Rev B* 1987;15:4039–4055.
33. Skutnik BJ. High strength large core pure silica fiber for laser power transmission. Optical fibers in medicine III. *Proc SPIE* 1988;906:204–250.
34. Abela GS, Seeger JM, Barbieri E, et al. Laser angioplasty with angioscopic guidance in humans. *J Am Coll Cardiol* 1986;8:184–192.
35. Ginsburg R, Wexler L, et al. Percutaneous transluminal laser angioplasty for treatment of peripheral vascular disease. *Radiology* 1985;156:619–624.
36. Moore G. Direct laser angioplasty. *Medical Electronics* October, 1988;92–95.
37. Nordstrom LA. Direct argon laser-assisted angioplasty: one year follow-up results in peripheral arteries and initial coronary experience. In: G. Biamino, ed. Advances in laser medicine. Second German Symposium on Laser Angioplasty, Berlin, 1989.
38. Stiles S. Laser angioplasty's ingenious hardware. *Cardiol* August, 1988;45–52.

39. Prince M, Deutsch T, et al. Selective laser ablation of atheromas. *Circulation* 1985;72 (suppl 3):401.
40. Leon MB, Smith PD, Bonner RF. Laser angioplasty delivery system: design considerations. In: White RA, Grundfest WS, eds. Lasers in cardiovascular disease. Chicago, Year Book Medical Publishers, 1987;52.

CHAPTER 4

Technique and Patient Selection for Excimer Laser Coronary Angioplasty

NEAL EIGLER

Introduction

OVER the past decade, improvements in equipment and technique have increased the number of patients who can be treated with balloon angioplasty (1). Despite these advances, several key limitations remain (see Table 4.1) that, if solved, would probably reduce the number of coronary bypass surgeries performed (2–10). These limitations have, in part, stimulated the development of new percutaneous devices such as the excimer laser that are capable of removing plaque from coronary arteries.

The purpose of this chapter is to extract from our early clinical experience a practical series of recommendations that will enable others to rapidly learn the technique of excimer angioplasty. In doing so, we wish to translate our beliefs concerning the indications and appropriate applications for excimer lasers. Our hope is that more widespread application of this device will advance the technology to achieve its ultimate role in coronary intervention.

Table 4.1. Limitations of Balloon Angioplasty

PATIENTS WITH:	small vessels
	diffuse disease
	long-segment stenoses
	calcified stenoses
	eccentric stenoses
	ostial stenoses
	bifurcation lesions
	bend points
	vein grafts
	complicated plaques with thrombus
	total occlusions
	multivessel disease
MORE FREQUENTLY HAVE:	suboptimal dilatation
	acute occlusion
	restenosis

Clinical Protocol

The following paragraphs summarize our initial clinical procedures and subsequent modifications to these procedures. Standard angioplasty guide catheters are used: 8 French catheters for angioplasty with 1.3- and 1.6-mm laser catheters and 9 French for 2.0-mm catheters (Schneider, Inc., Minneapolis, Minn.). Selective intracoronary nitroglycerin (200 mcg) is given prior to control angiography and following lasing, for three reasons: to reduce resting vascular tone for laser catheter sizing, for consistent quantitative angiography, and because coronary vasospasm was observed in early cases.

Stenoses are crossed with 0.016- or 0.018-inch coronary guidewires under fluoroscopic guidance (USCI, Inc., Billerica, Mass.; ACS, Inc., Temecula, Calif.). It has not been necessary to protect major side branches of the treatment artery with a second guidewire. Laser energy emitted from the catheter tip is precalibrated prior to insertion. The laser catheter is advanced over the guidewire until its tip is 3–5 mm proximal to the lesion. Under fluoroscopic control, the laser catheter is advanced slowly across the lesion ($\leq$ 1 mm/second) as laser pulses are delivered at 20 Hz. After each passage through the lesion, the catheter is withdrawn and angiographic contrast is injected. Early in our experience, multiple (one to five) passes were made through the lesion at the operator's discretion. The laser catheter is then totally withdrawn from the guiding catheter and cineangiography performed. If the posttreatment stenosis is visually estimated to be satisfactory, the guidewire is removed and completion angiograms performed. If the residual stenosis is judged not to be sufficiently improved, a larger-diameter laser fiber is attempted or adjunctive balloon angioplasty is performed prior to completion angiography.

Following laser angioplasty, patients are transferred to a monitored unit for 24 hours. Postprocedure care, including heparinization and aspirin, is identical to that for balloon angioplasty.

Training Issues

The risk of coronary artery perforation and its potential sequelae means that laser angioplasty is less "forgiving" than conventional balloon angioplasty. Excimer laser angioplasty should not be practiced by novice or occasional angioplasters. Presently, we recommend that operators possess a high level of experience and skill before performing this procedure. The practitioner should have performed a minimum of 1000 diagnostic coronary arteriograms and more than 500 percutaneous transluminal coronary angioplasties (PTCAs). This should include extensive experience with complex angioplasty cases. The operator should be familiar with the technical details and clinical use of all catheterization laboratory angiographic, angioplasty, and support equipment.

Specific training in excimer angioplasty includes completion of a basic course where different types of lasers are described and laser-tissue interactions, laser hardware, indications, patient selection, procedural technique, and management of laser-specific complications are discussed. "Hands-on" experience under the supervision of experienced operators is crucial because there are substantive differences from PTCA that may affect outcome. It is each operator's responsibility to keep thorough records of indications, anatomy, results, and complications so that quality-assurance parameters can be assessed and comparisons made with the experience of other laser angioplasters.

To maintain proficiency, the operator should perform at least 100 PTCAs and 30–40 laser procedures per year. These guidelines should be viewed as preliminary because they reflect the nature of the procedure at an early stage of its evolution.

Configuring a Catheterization Laboratory for Excimer Coronary Angioplasty

We have found that several modifications to the catheterization laboratory enhance the procedure. The first consideration is the physical size and operating specifications of the laser itself. The current AIS system measures 73 inches long by 32 inches wide by 4 inches tall and weighs 1500 lbs. Spectranetics, Inc. (Boulder, Colorado), manufactures a slightly different but smaller device. Two people are required to move the AIS device between laboratories. The laser is most conveniently located either across the table from the angiographer or behind the angiographer's back. The foot of the table should be reserved for systemic support devices such as an intra-aortic balloon pump. The laser is powered from a 20-amp 200–240-volt AC single-phase source. No special external cooling is needed such as the high-flow water and drain systems required for some continuous lasers.

The laboratory must be fully equipped to handle complex interventional cases in critically ill patients. There should be adequate floor space to accommodate sophisticated support and resuscitation equipment such as a volume-cycled respirator, anesthesia machine, intraaortic balloon pump, percutaneous cardiopulmonary bypass machine, etc. Additional space is required for the laser-gas exchange cabinet and for storage of special disposable equipment needed specifically for excimer angioplasty. This requires that the procedure room be a minimum of 550 square feet, and ideally it should be larger. The ideal dimensions for the procedure room are 30 ft long by 24 ft wide.

The specific requirements of excimer angioplasty should be considered when purchasing new radiographic equipment. We recommend that the procedure table be 10 ft long versus the usual 7-ft cardiac table. This facilitates the handling of 300-cm-long exchange guidewires or extended wires, which are more frequently used than in balloon angioplasty.

Biplane fluoroscopic equipment is very helpful but not essential. Not only does this reduce the dose of contrast material, but orthogonal imaging more precisely localizes the tip of the laser catheter with respect to the stenosis prior to and during lasing. This is important because the tip is relatively blunt and can cause more mechanical trauma than conventional PTCA balloons.

The quality of fluoroscopic imaging should be emphasized. Digital imaging with real-time, spatial filtration for edge enhancement is helpful to determine catheter size and to rapidly detect complications such as dissection and thrombosis. Motionless still-frame road maps and cine-loop playback capabilities are useful adjuncts. Facilities to perform quantitative coronary angiography are helpful to document the results of procedures.

Ideally, the catheterization suite should be located adjacent to a cardiac operating room. The practice of performing complex interventional procedures when the operating room is remote should be discouraged. Establishing a smooth working liaison with the cardiac surgery department to rapidly deal with emergency complications is a prerequisite for undertaking coronary laser angioplasty.

The staffing needs of a catheterization laboratory are also affected. Two physicians are required to perform laser angioplasty. Catheter exchanges are more complex than with PTCA. More importantly, the experience and the responsibility for intraprocedural decisions should be shared with another individual to provide a greater amount of case experience. Additional input from a skilled operator can be very helpful in different cases and in an emergency.

A minimum support staff of three nurse-technicians is needed to assist. Two circulating assistants are required in the procedure room, one to attend to the needs of the patient and the other to attend to the laser and its physician operators. The laser technician can be a nurse, cardiovascular technician, or radiology technician. This person sets up and calibrates the laser and the catheter-delivery system. Laser-gas exchanges, quality control, and simple troubleshooting can also be performed by trained cath lab personnel.

Disposable Equipment for Excimer Laser Coronary Angioplasty

As with PTCA, a full selection of guiding catheter types and sizes is needed. The 1.3- and 1.6-mm-diameter laser catheters can fit through large-lumen 8 French guides, the 2-mm and 2.2-mm laser fiber uses a 9 French guide, and the prototype 2.4-mm system will require a 10 French guide catheter. All cases to date have employed the femoral approach.

Our preference is to use the Schneider Super High Flow guides. The 8 French catheter has a lumen diameter of 0.081 inches and the 9 French is 0.092 inches in diameter. These diameters offer sufficient lumen size for adequate hand injection assessment of vessel patency and run-off.

We prefer the short-tip Judkins shape because it can more easily be deep-seated or "Amplatzed" in the left main stem. Deep-seating is more often necessary with the laser than with PTCA because the laser catheters are as yet not as "pushable" or as "trackable" as the latest generation of PTCA balloons. Also, efficient tissue ablation requires good contact with the lesion. If we encounter difficulty with the Judkins shape, we quickly change to an Amplatz shape of the appropriate size.

One important drawback of these thin-walled, large-lumen catheters is that overmanipulation can result in twisting of the catheter shaft, or, worse, kinking and knotting. These problems are best avoided by translating applied torque through moving the catheter to and fro and by using long introducer sheaths when there is iliofemoral tortuosity. Kinking of the catheter can be recognized by damping of the catheter tip pressure when the tip is not engaged in a coronary ostia. These problems can be largely avoided by using the smaller-diameter 0.79-inch-lumen 8 French guides. The trade-off however, is much poorer visualization with contrast injections.

Care should be taken to withdraw the laser catheter several centimeters into the guide catheter before making test injections. This helps protect against a high-velocity jet of contrast material injuring the arterial wall. The 2.0-mm and larger laser catheters do not fit through all commercially available Y-adapters. It is best to confirm that all ancillary equipment is compatible prior to the procedure.

Guidewires

We learned from early animal experiments that 0.014-inch guidewires had insufficient shaft column strength to maintain the laser coaxial within the artery and were a cause of perforation. This problem has for the most part been corrected by using heavier-gage 0.016- or 0.018-inch guidewires.

The USCI 0.016 Hyperflex wire handles well and maintains good laser catheter coaxiality. The major drawback of this wire is its high radiopacity. This can cause difficulty in assessing lumen size prior to removing the guidewire, especially after using the smaller 1.6- and 1.3-mm laser catheters.

The ACS 0.018 high-torque floppy wire is generally unacceptable for excimer laser coronary angioplasty (ELCA). This wire has a relatively long taper in the shaft. When lasing is performed over the tapered portion, the potential for loss of coaxiality exists.

We most frequently use a special-order ACS 0.018-inch "Laser" guidewire, which has the shaft taper of the High Torque Standard model combined with a floppy tip design. For more tortuous stenoses and total occlusions, the ACS 0.018-inch High Torque Intermediate and High Torque Standard wires are acceptable. Lasing should be performed over the solid mandrel portions of the wire to maintain catheter coaxiality. Lasing should never be continued over the platinum spring coil tip of the guidewire because this may result in perforation.

PTCA Balloons

Standard PTCA balloons can be used to perform adjunctive balloon angioplasty following laser ELCA. It is advisable to have an adequate supply of balloons in various sizes that can be exchanged over a 0.018-inch guidewire so that repetitive wire placement is avoided.

Patient Selection

All patients should be evaluated for surgical candidacy. At the time of this writing we perceive no clear advantage of excimer laser in ACC/AHA type A lesions without complicating features. (See Chapter 5 for results of excimer laser coronary angioplasty with the AIS system.) Certain type B and C morphologies may, however, benefit from laser angioplasty, particularly aorto-ostial lesions, highly calcified narrowing long tubular lesions, or segments containing diffuse disease. The current generation of laser catheters is not ideally suited for lasing distal segments to tortuous vessels or for approaching highly eccentric lesions.

Patients with acute evolving myocardial infarction are probably best treated with either an intravenous thrombolytic agent or primary balloon angioplasty. Excimer laser angioplasty is not recommended at this time because 1) there is no experience with these patients, and 2) the additional time required to prepare the laser may delay opening of the artery by 15 minutes. Patients with severe rest angina not relieved by medical therapy and angiographically demonstrated thrombus are another high-risk group in whom the acute efficacy and safety of laser angioplasty is not known.

A recent unhealed PTCA balloon dissection is an absolute contraindication for excimer laser angioplasty. Worsening of the dissection has been observed and the potential for perforating through a dissection plane is enhanced.

Two types of coronary anatomy have been associated with perforation. First, a highly eccentric plaque originating on the lesser curvature of a tight bend may force the laser fiber into the normal wall of the greater curvature, resulting in perforation (Fig. 4.1). A multivariate analysis has shown that a highly eccentric lesion is the only morphologic predictor of acute complications, which include acute closure, myocardial infarction, emergency bypass surgery, and death.

A second situation deserving extreme caution is when the stenosis involves the origin of a bifurcation vessel where a laser catheter is unable to first selectively engage a branch. Perforation has occurred by ablating the "carina" between the two branches (Fig. 4.2). In such cases, undersizing the laser catheter may avoid problems.

Technique of Lasing

Patients are treated with a minimum of 324 mg of aspirin and a calcium-channel antagonist starting no later than the day prior to the procedure. Intravenous heparin boluses are administered (10,000–15,000 units) to raise the activated clotting time to greater than 350 seconds and maintain it at this level for the duration of the procedure. Failure to apply heparin has been associated with in-situ thrombosis.

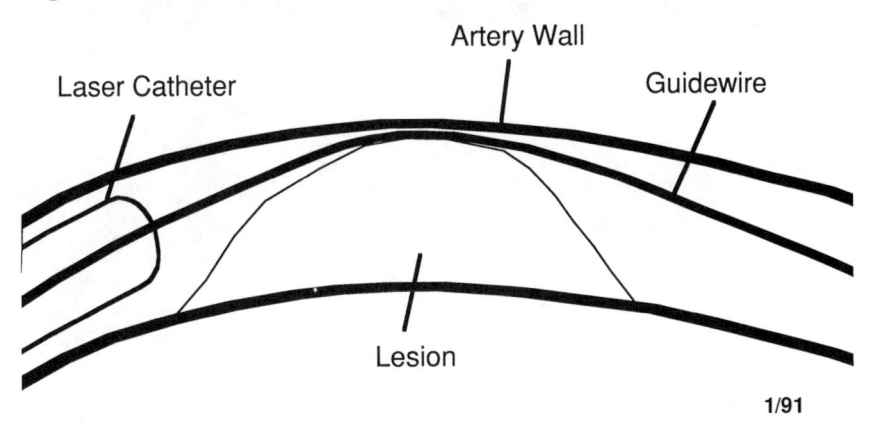

Figure 4.1. Highly eccentric stenoses on the inner curvature of a bend have been associated with perforations with current concentric catheter designs.

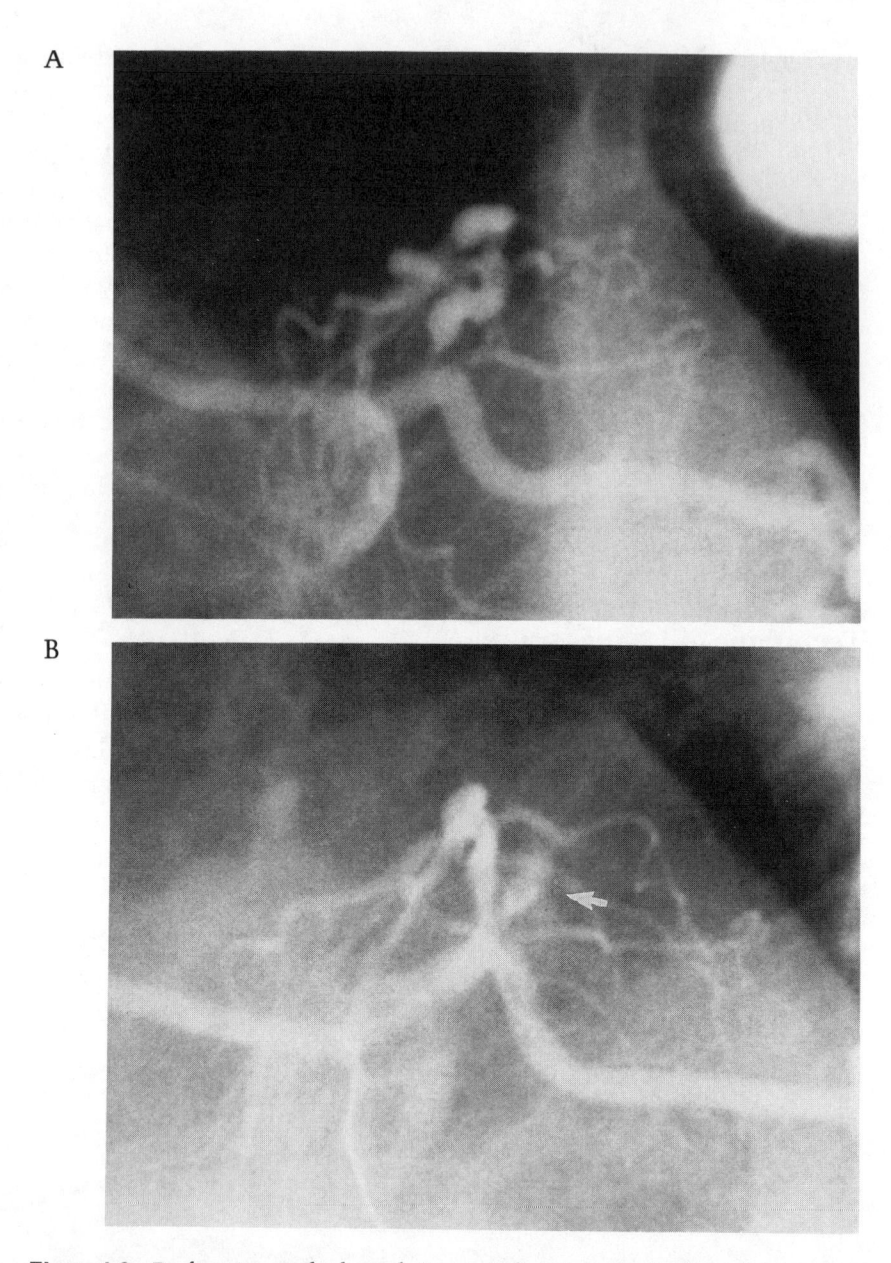

Figure 4.2. Perforation at the branch "carina" between the LAD and the ramus intermedius. *(A)* Prelasing LAO caudal view. The entrance to the LAD is at an abrupt angle from the left main and is involved with severe stenosis. *(B)* After lasing there is a localized perforation *(arrow)*.

Catheter Sizing

Catheters should be selected based on sizing the "normal" portion of the vessel with reference to the diameter of the guiding catheter (Table 4.2). This should be done after administering nitroglycerin 150–300 mg directly into the coronary. The size of the laser catheter is selected to leave at least a 30 percent residual stenosis (see Table 4.2). Oversizing the laser catheter has resulted in ablation of normal vessel wall dissection and perforation. For long or heavily calcified lesions, it is often easier to start with the 1.3-mm system at higher calibrated energy and then switch to a larger catheter size as needed.

Energy Selection

Preliminary results suggest that restenosis rates may be lower at higher catheter tip energies. This may be because there is more mechanical trauma at lower energies. We currently start at 45–50 mJ/mm^2 for the 1.6 and 2.0 multifiber catheters and 50–60 mJ/mm^2 for the 1.3-mm system. If the system fails to cross the stenosis and there is adequate guide-catheter support, the energy should be recalibrated and if accurate, the energy may be increased by 5 mJ/mm^2. We currently recommend that all de novo lesions exhibiting calcium or with a minimum lumen diameter of < 1.0 mm be "prelased" with the 1.3-mm catheter.

The laser catheter should be advanced to approximately 3 to 5 mm proximal to the stenosis. The radiopaque marker on the laser catheter is located 1.5 mm proximal to the tip. Tip position should be documented in two views. Lasing should be initiated from this location.

The laser should be advanced across the stenosis at a rate of < 1 mm/sec, because faster rates may cause insufficient ablation with additional mechanical trauma and resultant intimal dissection. The laser should be applied in bursts of pulses lasting 2–3 seconds with a 5-second

Table 4.2. Laser Catheter Sizing

LASER FIBER DIAMETER	MINIMUM VESSEL SIZE
1.3 mm	1.6–2.0 mm
1.6 mm	2.1–2.5 mm
2.0 mm	2.6–3.1 mm
2.2 mm	3.2–3.7 mm
2.4 mm	≥ 3.8 mm

interval between bursts. This allows the gaseous ablation products time to dissipate into the blood without building up in the subintimal tissue plains. Lasing is continued until the catheter tip emerges several millimeters past the end of the stenosis. If the laser does not progress across the stenosis with gentle forward pressure, more force may be necessary. Additional maneuvers include deep-seating of the guiding catheter and retraction of the guidewire during lasing. Further angiographic improvement sometimes occurs with a second slow pass of each catheter, but the complication rate for dissection and perforation may increase with multiple passes. Thus, we now limit the number of passes to one or two.

Control over catheter advancement proceeds as follows. The primary operator stands closest to the patient's groin and manipulates the laser catheter, the guiding catheter, and the laser on-off foot pedal. The assistant operator controls the guidewires and the x-ray foot pedals. The primary operator holds the laser fiber 2–3 mm from the Y-adaptor, limiting its advancement to this distance in each burst of pulses. This technique may limit mechanical trauma and minimize inadvertent forward lunging of the catheter as it exits the stenosis. Following lasing, a decision regarding adjunctive balloon PTCA is made. We currently recommend ballooning if the post laser stenosis is >30 percent. Should abrupt occlusion or severe dissection occur (never cross a dissection with a laser catheter), we switch immediately to balloon angioplasty, which most often results in successful completion of the case.

Hemodynamically significant perforations should be managed by placing a balloon or an autoperfusion balloon across the area of the perforation to tamponade the bleeding. If the patient is clinically stable, a pulmonary artery balloon catheter is inserted, and a two-dimensional echocardiogram is obtained. If there are signs of pericardial tamponade, needle aspiration is performed and the patient is taken to the operating room to repair the perforation and perform bypass surgery as needed. About one-third of the observed perforations have required immediate surgery. The most common occurs with perforation of a native vessel in the presence of an intact pericardium (i.e., no prior surgery). Laser balloon angioplasty (hot balloon) has been observed to worsen small perforations.

Following successful ELCA, postprocedure care is identical to that for patients with conventional balloon angioplasty. In uncomplicated cases on type-A lesions, heparin can be discontinued and the arterial-venous introducer sheaths removed after 4–6 hours. For patients with type B or

C lesions who presented with an unstable ischemic syndrome, or if there were intraprocedural problems such as transient closure or dissection, we currently maintain the patients on a heparin infusion for 24–48 hours before pulling the sheaths.

In summary, the techniques described in this chapter represent our collective experience from the first 2 years. The key to success for newer users is appropriate patient selection, operator experience, and exercise of good clinical judgment and common sense. The input of newer users will be instrumental in the further evolution of ELCA.

References

1. Detre K, Holubkov R, Kelsey S, and the Co-Investigators of the NHLBI PTCA Registry. Percutaneous transluminal coronary angioplasty in 1985–1986 and 1977–1981. *N Engl J Med* 1988;318:265–270.
2. Safian RD, McCabe CH, Sipperly ME, McKay RG, Baim DS. Initial success and long-term follow-up of percutaneous transluminal coronary angioplasty in chronic total occlusions versus conventional stenoses. *Am J Cardiol* 1988;61:23G–28G.
3. Kereiakes DJ, Selmon MR, McAuley BJ, McAuley DB, Sheehan DJ, Simpson JB. Angioplasty in total coronary artery occlusion: experience in 76 consecutive patients. *J Am Coll Cardiol* 1985;6:526–533.
4. Ellis SG, Shaw RE, Gershony G, et al. Risk factors, time course and treatment effect for restenosis after successful percutaneous transluminal coronary angioplasty of chronic total occlusion. *Am J Cardiol* 1989;63:897–901.
5. Bredlau CE, Roubin GS, Leimgruber PP, Douglas JS, King SB, Gruentzig AR. In-hospital morbidity and mortality in patients undergoing elective coronary angioplasty. *Circulation* 1985;72:1044–1052.
6. Ellis SG, Roubin GS, King SB, et al. Angiographic and clinical predictors of acute closure after native vessel coronary angioplasty. *Circulation* 1988;77:372–379.
7. Topol EJ, Ellis SG, Fishman J, et al. Multicenter study of percutaneous transluminal coronary angioplasty for right coronary artery ostial stenosis. *J Am Coll Cardiol* 1987;9:1214–1218.
8. Vandormael MG, Deligunl U, Kern MJ, et al. Multilesion coronary angioplasty: clinical and angiographic follow-up. *J Am Coll Cardiol* 1987;10:246–252.
9. Hollman J, Gruentzig AR, Douglas JS, King SB, Ischinger T, Meier B.

Acute occlusion after percutaneous transluminal coronary angioplasty—a new approach. *Circulation* 1983;68:725–732.
10. Sinclair IN, McCabe CH, Sipperly ME, Baim DS. Predictors, therapeutic options and long-term outcome of abrupt reclosure. *Am J Cardiol* 1988;61:61G–66G.

CHAPTER **5**

Results of Excimer Laser Coronary Angioplasty

Neal Eigler

WE performed the first excimer laser coronary angioplasty in August 1988 (1). Subsequent reports demonstrated the acute efficacy and relative safety of this procedure in small numbers of patients (2–5). This chapter describes the experience at Cedars-Sinai Medical Center in our first 100 patients. Shortly after our initial experience, a nonrandomized multicenter trial was initiated.

The goals of our research program are to determine the safety and efficacy of excimer laser coronary angioplasty as an alternative or adjunct to balloon angioplasty, to develop and refine the technique of excimer laser angioplasty as catheter technology improves, and to define appropriate indications for excimer laser angioplasty by assessing results for specific lesion types and locations.

Clinical Protocol

Between July 1988 and March 1990, excimer laser coronary angioplasty was attempted in 100 patients at Cedars-Sinai Medical Center and in 1284 patients in the multicenter trial (Table 5.1). There were two en-

Table 5.1. Multicenter Trial; Participating Centers and Investigators

Cedars-Sinai Medical Center, Los Angeles	F. Litvack	N. Eigler
South Miami Hospital, South Miami	J. Margolis	D. Krauthamer
St. Vincent's Hospital, Indianapolis	D. Rothbaum	T. Linnemeier
Emory University Hospital, Atlanta	S. King	J. Douglas
Mayo Clinic, Rochester	D. Bresnahan	J. Bresnahan
Georgetown University Hospital, Georgetown	K. Kent	L. Satler
Methodist Hospital, Houston	W. Spencer	A. Raizner
Hoag Hospital, Newport Beach	R. Haskell	P. McNalley
Philadelphia Heart Institute, Philadelphia	W. Untereker	
St. Luke's Hospital, Phoenix	M. Vawter	
St. Luke's Hospital, Milwaukee	F. Cummins	G. Dorros
Mercy Hospital, Pittsburgh	V. Krishnaswami	

trance criteria: first, patients were considered if they had symptomatic coronary artery disease, objective evidence of myocardial ischemia, or both, sufficient to warrant either balloon angioplasty or bypass surgery. Second, we required angiographically documented stenoses or occlusions of native coronary arteries or bypass grafts thought to be traversible by angioplasty guidewires. Patients with evolving myocardial infarction or with resting ischemia unrelieved with medical therapy were excluded.

We used a magnetically switched Thyratron-driven 308-nm xenon-chloride pulsed excimer laser manufactured by Advanced Interventional Systems, Irvine, California. This device has a pulse width of 180–220 ns with an output of more than 200 mJ at 20 Hz (6).

Laser energy was delivered through multifiber catheters 1.3 (4.0 Fr.), 1.6 (4.7 Fr.) or 2.0 mm (6.0 Fr.) in diameter (Advanced Interventional Systems, Irvine, Calif.). The 2.0-mm catheters became available in August 1989 and the 1.3-mm catheters in October 1989. The silica fibers are concentrically arranged around a central lumen that accepts a 0.018-inch guidewire. Early-generation 1.6-mm catheters were constructed of twelve 100-micron fibers with 200-micron fused silica tips (7). Currently available catheters have over 200 individual 50-micron fibers in a concentric array.

Patients were treated with a minimum of 324 mg of aspirin and a calcium-channel antagonist starting no later than the day prior to the procedure. Intravenous heparin boluses (10,000–15,000 units) were administered to raise the activated clotting time to greater than 350 seconds and maintain it at this level for the duration of the procedure. Standard angioplasty guide catheters were used: 8 French catheters for angioplasty with 1.3- and 1.6-mm laser catheters and 9 French for 2.0-mm catheters (Schneider, Minneapolis, Minn.). Selective intracoronary nitroglycerin (200 mcg) was given prior to control angiography and following lasing. This was adopted to reduce resting vascular tone for laser catheter sizing; for consistent quantitative angiography; and because coronary vasospasm was observed in early cases.

The lesion was crossed with a 0.016- or 0.018-inch coronary guidewire under fluoroscopic guidance (USCI, Billerica, Mass.; ACS, Temecula, Calif.). Major side branches of the treatment artery were not protected with a second guidewire. Laser energy emitted from the catheter tip was calibrated at 35 to 60 millijoules/mm^2. The laser catheter was then advanced over the guidewire until its tip was immediately proximal to the lesion. Under fluoroscopic control, the laser catheter was advanced slowly across the lesion ($\leq$ 1 mm/second) as laser pulses were delivered at 20 Hz. After each passage through the lesion, the catheter was withdrawn and angiographic contrast injected. Multiple (one to five) passes were made through the lesion at the operator's discretion. The laser catheter was then withdrawn and orthogonal-view cineangiography performed. If the posttreatment stenosis was visually estimated to be less than 50 percent, the guidewire was removed and completion angiograms were performed. If the residual stenosis was equal to or greater than 50 percent, a larger-diameter laser fiber was attempted or adjunctive balloon angioplasty was performed prior to completion angiography.

Following laser angioplasty, patients were transferred to a coronary care unit where they were monitored by telemetry for 24 hours. Heparin (800–1000 units/hour) was infused until the next morning when heparin was discontinued and the sheaths removed.

Acute laser success was defined as a greater than 20 percent improvement in the minimal stenotic diameter and a resultant vessel diameter of greater than 0.8 mm with the 1.3-mm catheter, 1.0 mm with the 1.6-mm catheter, and 1.5- mm with a 2.0-mm catheter following excimer laser angioplasty alone. Acute procedural success was defined as final diameter stenosis of less than or equal to 50 percent, determined by caliper measurements.

Lesion morphology was recorded using the BARI morphology classification as one of the following: single discrete, multiple discrete, diffuse, tubular, discrete aneurysmal, diffuse aneurysmal, or complete occlusion (8).

Lesions were also classified using guidelines established by the joint American College of Cardiology/American Heart Association Task Force on Assessment of Diagnostic and Therapeutic Cardiovascular Procedures as type A, B, or C (9, 10; see Table 5.2). Total occlusions were assigned to type C except when the occlusion was known from a prior angiogram to be more than 3 months old or had other type-C attributes.

Early Results

The demographic and clinical characteristics of our first 100 consecutive patients and from the multicenter trial are shown in Table 5.3. There was a male predominance with a mean age of 62 years. The ma-

Table 5.2. ACC/AHA Classification of Type A, B, and C Lesions

LESION-SPECIFIC CHARACTERISTICS	
TYPE-A LESIONS	
○ Discrete (<10 mm length)	○ Little or no calcification
○ Concentric	○ Less than totally occlusive
○ Readily accessible	○ Not ostial in location
○ Nonangulated segment, <45°	○ No major branch involvement
○ Smooth contour	○ Absence of thrombus
TYPE-B LESIONS	
○ Tubular (10 to 20 mm length)	○ Moderate to heavy calcification
○ Eccentric	○ Total occlusions <3 months old
○ Moderate tortuosity of proximal segment	○ Ostial in location
○ Moderately angulated segment >45°, <90°	○ Bifurcation lesions requiring double guidewires
○ Irregular contour	○ Some thrombus present
TYPE-C LESIONS	
○ Diffuse (>2 cm length)	○ Total occlusion >3 months old
○ Excessive tortuosity of proximal segment	○ Inability to protect major side branches
○ Extremely angulated segments >90°	○ Degenerated vein grafts with friable lesions

Table 5.3. Demographic and Clinical Characteristics of Patients Treated

	CSMC	MULTICENTER TRIAL
Patients	100	1284
Male (%)	79	77
Age (mean)	62 ± 13	62 ± 10 (range 29–87)
Number of lesions	119	1519
CCSFC (%)		
0	0	6
I	9	8
II	17	20
III	33	33
IV	41	33
Previous balloon angioplasty (%)	42	36
1	20	
2	16	
3	4	
≥4	2	
Location (%)		
LM	0	2
LAD	42	41
LCX	15	16
RCA	30	28
Vein graft	13	13
Lesion type (%)		
Stenosis	82	91
Total occlusion	18	9

CSMC = Cedars-Sinai Medical Center
CCSFC = Canadian Cardiovascular Society functional class

jority of the patients were Canadian Cardiovascular Society functional class III or IV for anginal symptoms. At Cedars-Sinai, 42 percent of patients had undergone one or more prior balloon angioplasties of the lesion that received the laser angioplasty. One patient had six previous percutaneous transluminal coronary angioplasty (PTCA) procedures, stent placement, and two directional atherectomy procedures to a saphenous vein graft to an obtuse marginal. The distribution of vessels treated included the proximal and mid segments of all portions of the coronary anatomy. The demographic and clinical characteristics of our patients appear to be similar to those of a typical balloon angioplasty population.

Table 5.4. Success of Excimer Laser Angioplasty by Lesion Location

	CSMC		MULTICENTER TRIAL	
	Laser success	Procedure success	Laser success	Procedure success
Location				
LM	—	—		85%
LAD	86%	95%		92%
LCX	87%	90%		91%
RCA	77%	93%		92%
Vein graft	100%	100%		95%
All vessels	85%	94%	81%	92%
Adjunctive balloon angioplasty		47%	56%	

The laser and procedural success rates by lesion location are shown in Table 5.4. At Cedars-Sinai, acute success was obtained with laser angioplasty in 85 percent. Procedural success was obtained in 94 percent. Reasons for laser failure were inability to cross the lesion with the guidewire (three patients), inability to advance the laser catheter through tortuosity proximal to the lesion (two patients), inability to completely cross the lesion with the laser catheter (four patients), acute closure of lesion (five patients), and severe dissection of the artery (one patient). Similar results were documented in the multicenter trial. The observed success rates are comparable to reports in the balloon angioplasty literature (10).

Adjunctive balloon angioplasty was performed in 47 percent of our patients. This proportion decreased to 41 percent in the 88 patients treated after the 2-mm laser catheters became available. The data show that laser and procedural success is high regardless of lesion location. Our lower frequency of laser success in the right coronary artery (RCA) was related to the higher proportion of total occlusions attempted in this vessel (30 percent vs. 13 percent) in other locations. Laser success

Figure 5.1. *(A)* Frequency distribution of percentage diameter stenosis at baseline after angioplasty and at the end of the procedure. *(B)* Frequency distribution of minimal stenotic diameter. Reprinted with permission from Percutaneous excimer laser coronary angioplasty of lesions not ideal for balloon angioplasty. *Circulation* 1991; 84(2):640.

Results of Excimer Laser Coronary Angioplasty 91

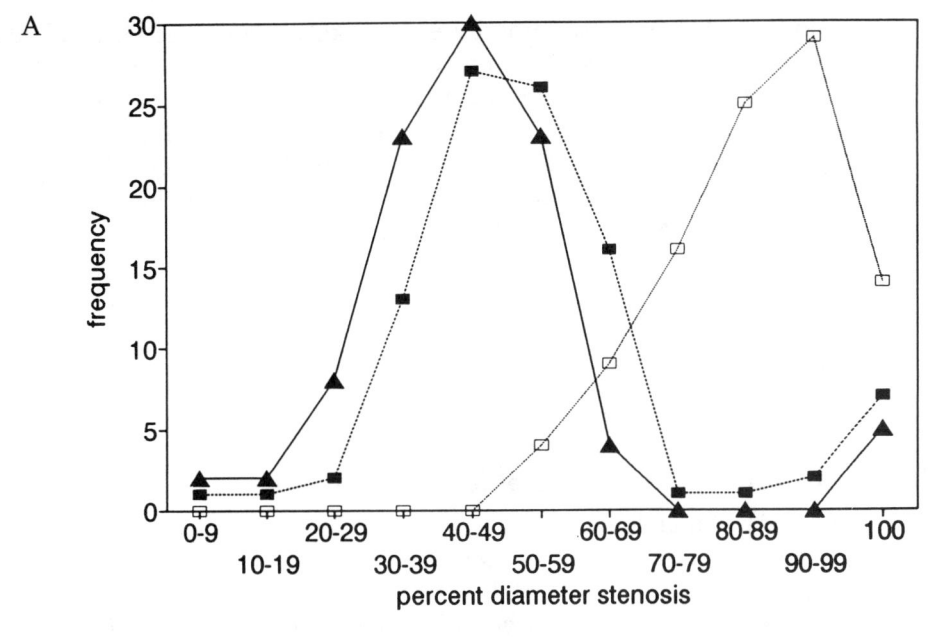

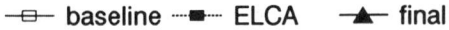

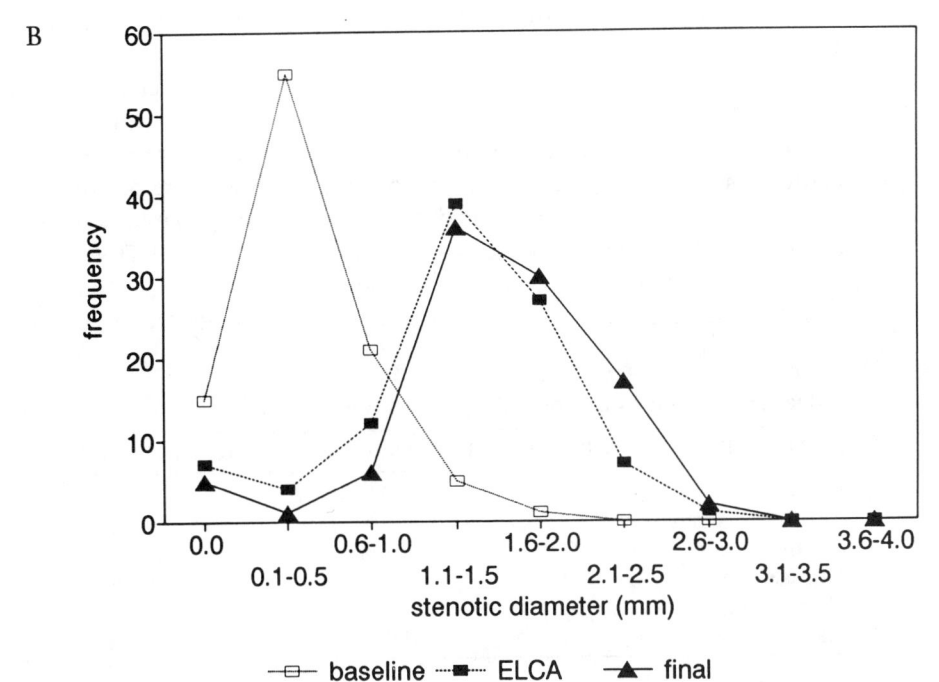

and "stand-alone" laser procedures are likely to increase with refinements in equipment and technique.

Figures 5.1A and 5.1B show the frequency distribution of percentage diameter stenosis and minimal stenotic diameter at baseline after laser angioplasty, and at the end of the procedure with or without PTCA in 98 of the first 100 patients. On average, laser angioplasty produced a significant fall in percentage diameter stenosis and a significant (greater than threefold) increase in minimal stenotic diameter. Adjunctive PTCA produced further improvement. Absolute stenotic diameter data indicate that, on average, the laser fiber creates a channel equal to its diameter.

Laser Angioplasty of Unfavorable PTCA Lesions

At Cedars-Sinai, 65 percent of lesions treated were identified as unfavorable for PTCA due to morphology (tubular, diffuse, or total occlusions) or ostial location (Table 5.5). Laser success was obtained in all eight ostial lesions (100%); adjunctive balloon PTCA was not performed in any cases. The overall laser success rate in this group was 86 percent and 91 percent in nonoccluded arteries. Procedural success rate was 94 percent. Laser and procedural success rates did not differ significantly between favorable (discrete) and unfavorable lesions. Laser was successful in 90 percent of the long (tubular and diffuse) lesions, with procedural success obtained in 97 percent. In this unfavorable subgroup, there were three acute closures (4.6%), no emergency bypass surgeries, one perforation without clinical sequelae, and no deaths. Six patients had excimer laser angioplasty following an unsuccessful attempted balloon PTCA. Excimer angioplasty was successful in four cases (67%).

In the multicenter trial, excimer laser coronary angioplasty (ELCA)

Table 5.5. Success by Stenosis Morphology (Cedars-Sinai)

STENOSIS TYPE	NUMBER	LASER SUCCESS	PROCEDURE SUCCESS
Discrete	38	87%	97%
Multiple discrete	5	80%	80%
Tubular lesion	10	100%	100%
Diffuse disease	29	86%	97%
Total occlusion	18	72%	83%
Ostial	8	100%	100%

was performed on 15 aorto-ostial stenoses with a successful outcome in 14 (93%). This group included eight patients with RCA, two patients with protected left main, and five patients with vein graft ostial lesions. Stand-alone ELCA was performed in nine (60%). Failure occurred in one patient due to inability to cross the stenosis with the laser. There was one complication, the small perforation mentioned above. Published data for PTCA of aorto-ostial stenosis have reported a low success rate (79%) and a high requirement for emergency bypass surgery (9%) (11). Although preliminary, our data suggest that ELCA of aorto-ostial stenosis appears to be a safe procedure with a high initial angiographic and clinical success rate.

Other angiographic variables previously shown to adversely affect acute success and complication rates of PTCA are calcification, eccentricity, presence of a bend greater than 45 percent, and side branches originating within a lesion (12–18). Of 11 moderately or heavily calcified stenoses, 10 (91%) were treated successfully with laser angioplasty. The eleventh could not be crossed over its entire length with the laser catheter at 42 mJ/mm^2. Its terminal portion was successfully dilated with the balloon. Eight eccentric lesions were successfully treated with laser angioplasty. Two further lesions containing bend points had successful stand-alone laser procedures without evidence of dissection or perforation. No side branch occlusions occurred in the 15 cases in which one or more side branches originated within the lesions.

Of the lesions treated, 26 percent were ACC/AHA type A, 47 percent type B, and 27 percent type C. Acute laser success for each type was type A—85 percent, type B—85 percent, and type C—85 percent. Procedural success for each type was type A—96 percent, type B—96 percent, and type C—89 percent (Fig. 5.2). Two acute closures occurred in type-A lesions, three in type-B lesions, and none in type-C lesions. Compared to a typical angioplasty population, the multicenter trial had a large proportion of patients (52%) with stenosis 10 mm in length or longer (Table 5.6). In contradistinction to PTCA, the success rate was not influenced by lesion length.

Follow-Up

Of the 279 patients eligible for 6-month follow-up, data are available in 99.4 percent, and 159 (61%) have undergone repeat angiography. Angiographic restenosis was detected in 51 percent; in the remainder, a

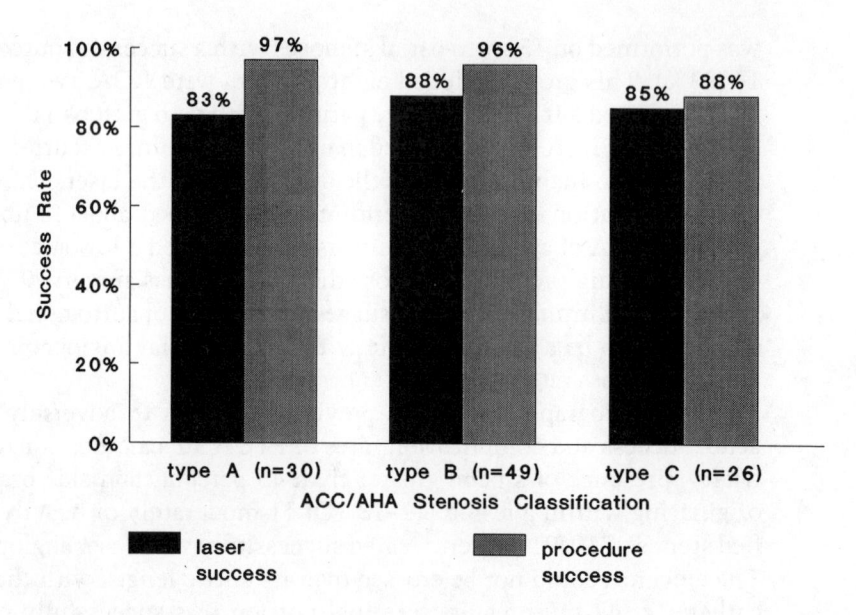

Figure 5.2. Procedural success for ACC/AHA lesion type A, B, and C.

positive follow-up stress test was noted in 14 percent and death or acute myocardial infarction (MI) was documented in another 3.1 percent. Thus, the overall restenosis rate was 41.8 percent. For the total follow-up population, 8.5 percent went on to coronary bypass surgery and 10 percent had a repeat catheter intervention.

Complications

Table 5.7 summarizes the incidence of complications in the multicenter study. Although not a randomized comparison, it is apparent that

Table 5.6. Lesion Length (excluding total occlusions)

	% OF LESIONS	% PROCEDURAL SUCCESS
<10 mm	47%	93%
10–20 mm	31%	96%
>20 mm	21%	92%

Table 5.7. Complications (n = 1284)

Death (in hospital)	0.4%
Emergency CABG	3.1%
Myocardial infarction (CK > 200u) (excludes CABG patients)	2.1%
Perforation	1.6%
Spasm	1.6%
Acute occlusion	6.5%
Dissection	12.1%
Embolism	0.8%
Aneurysm	0.5%

the rates of major complications, death, myocardial infarction, and emergency bypass surgery, compare favorably with those published in the NHLBI PTCA registry 1985–1986, where death was 1 percent, emergency surgery coronary artery bypass grafting (CABG) was 5.6 percent, and nonfatal MI was 4.3 percent.

Summary

Our initial experience suggests that excimer laser coronary angioplasty is acutely effective and safe therapy for lesions favorable and not favorable for balloon angioplasty. Excimer laser may be used either as standalone therapy or as an adjunct to balloon angioplasty. Presently, we do not perceive an advantage over balloon angioplasty for treatment of discrete stenoses without complicating features. Even at this very early juncture, however, we feel that excimer laser angioplasty is effective and safe and particularly well suited for long tubular lesions, diffuse disease, calcified plaque, ostial stenosis, chronic occlusions crossable by a guidewire, lesions that involve major side branches, and stenoses that cannot be crossed or dilated with a balloon. Restenosis appears to be comparable to PTCA. Much remains to be learned with respect to specific clinical subsets.

References

1. Litvack F, Grundfest W, Eigler N, et al. Percutaneous excimer laser coronary angioplasty (letter). *Lancet* 1989(II);102–103.

2. Litvack F, Grundfest WS, Segalowitz J, et al. Interventional cardiovascular therapy by laser and thermal angioplasty. *Circulation* 1990;81(suppl IV):IV-109–IV-116.
3. Litvack F, Grundfest WS, Goldenberg T, Laudenslager J, Forrester JS. Percutaneous excimer laser angioplasty of aortocoronary saphenous vein grafts. *J Am Coll Cardiol* 1989;14:803–808.
4. Karsch KR, Haase KK, Voelker W, Baumbach A, Mauser M, Sepel L. Percutaneous coronary excimer laser angioplasty in patients with stable and unstable angina pectoris. *Circulation* 1990;81:1849–1859.
5. Litvack F, Eigler NL, Margolis JR, et al. Percutaneous excimer laser coronary angioplasty. *Am J Cardiol* 1990;66:1027–1032.
6. Pacala TJ, McDermid JS, Laudenslager JB. Ultranarrow line-width, magnetically switched long pulse xenon chloride laser. *Appl Phys Lett* 1984;44:658–660.
7. Litvack F, Grundfest WS, Goldenberg T, Laudenslager J, Forrester JS. Excimer laser angioplasty. In: Topol EJ, ed. Textbook of interventional cardiology. Philadelphia: WB Saunders, 1990; 682–699.
8. BARI Manual of Operations, unpublished material.
9. Ryan TJ, Faxon DP, Gunnar RM, and the ACC/AHA Task Force on Assessment of Diagnostic and Therapeutic Procedures (Subcommittee on Percutaneous Transluminal Coronary Angioplasty). Guidelines for percutaneous transluminal coronary angioplasty. *Circulation* 1988;78:486–502.
10. Ellis, SG. Elective coronary angioplasty In: Topol EJ, ed. Textbook of interventional cardiology. Philadelphia: W.B. Saunders, 1990;199–222.
11. Topol EJ, Ellis SG, Fishman J, et al. Multicenter study of percutaneous transluminal coronary angioplasty for right coronary artery ostial stenosis. *J Am Coll Cardiol* 1987;9:1214–1218.
12. Bredlau CE, Roubin GS, Leimgruber PP, Douglas JS, King SB, Gruentzig AR. In-hospital morbidity and mortality in patients undergoing elective coronary angioplasty. *Circulation* 1985;72:1044–1052.
13. Ellis SG, Roubin GS, King SB, et al. Angiographic and clinical predictors of acute closure after native vessel coronary angioplasty. *Circulation* 1988;77:372–379.
14. Meier B, Gruentzig AR, Hollman J, Ischinger T, Bradford JM. Does length or eccentricity of coronary stenoses influence the outcome of transluminal dilatation? *Circulation* 1983;67:497–499.
15. Cowley MJ, Dorros, Kelsey SF, Van Raden M, Detre KM. Acute coronary events associated with percutaneous transluminal coronary angioplasty. *Am J Cardiol* 1984;53:12C–16C.
16. Ischinger T, Gruentzig AR, Meier B, Galan K. Coronary dissection and

total coronary occlusion associated with percutaneous transluminal coronary angioplasty: significance of initial angiographic morphology of coronary stenoses. *Circulation* 1986;74:1371–1378.
17. Meier B, Gruentzig AR, King SB, et al. Risk of side branch occlusion during coronary angioplasty. *Am J Cardiol* 1984;53:10–14.
18. Potkin BN, Robert WC. Effects of percutaneous transluminal coronary angioplasty on atherosclerotic plaques and relation of plaque composition and arterial size to outcome. *Am J Cardiol* 1988;62:41–50.

CHAPTER **6**

. . . .
Percutaneous Transluminal Coronary Excimer Laser Atherectomy— The German Experience

Karl R. Karsch

IN the 13 years prior to 1990, we have seen tremendous development in the treatment of atherosclerotic heart disease and considerable evolution of mechanical interventions. In 1977, Andreas Grüntzig introduced percutaneous transluminal coronary angioplasty (PTCA) for treatment of atherosclerotic obstructions, and this method has subsequently shown impressive clinical results in the acute setting (1). Increased experience and rapid advances in technology have resulted in a primary success rate of 90–95 percent. Despite the tremendous growth and success of angioplasty, restenosis remains the predominant problem, with an overall incidence of 25 to 35 percent (2,3). There are four major mechanisms associated with balloon angioplasty: 1) plaque splitting, 2) plaque compression, 3) stretching and overdistention of the arterial wall, and 4) plaque desquamation. Each mechanism contributes to the final angioplasty result and may be the trigger for the occurrence of restenosis (4). The extent and severity of vessel wall injury ultimately determines the incidence of subsequent platelet aggregation and muscle cell proliferation (5). A variety of new mechanical devices are being developed to address these problems, but their efficacy at this time does not appear to be superior to that of angioplasty alone. These devices can be separated into two main categories based on their effects on coronary luminal shape: 1) remodeling, and 2) removal.

Laser therapy has been developed to alter the degree of luminal obstruction by removing atherosclerotic tissue. In the earliest work with this technology, laser angioplasty was used for recanalization, but it produced a high, clinically unacceptable incidence of mechanical perforation, primarily due to the use of inflexible bare fibers (6). Subsequently the problem was solved by a novel tip design with a metal tip cap applied to the distal end of the optical fiber (7). This design, however, proved to be nearly impossible to use in small-diameter vessels such as the coronary arteries since the heated cap induced vascular spasm and thrombosis.

The mid-1980s marked the advent of clinically useful pulsed lasers such as the excimer laser as an alternative power source. These lasers offered the possibility of tissue ablation without pathologic heating of boundary tissue (8,9). It was shown that excimer laser energy is indeed capable of cutting through tissue without creating thermal injury. The ablation is accomplished by a photochemical disruption of the molecular bonds in tissue induced by the high peak power (10). Initial studies and pathologic analysis from our laboratory and others showed that the excimer laser is superior to the conventionally used medical lasers since incision margins are sharp and adjacent tissue damage is minimal (11,12). Although initial attempts to use the excimer laser for ablation of atherosclerotic tissue in humans had been limited by the difficulties in transmitting the high peak powers via silica fibers, novel means of laser-fiber coupling permitted successful fiber-optic transmission at 308-nm wavelength via commercially available fused silica fibers (13).

Part I

Initial Clinical Experience

In a first pilot study our combined clinical experience with coronary excimer laser angioplasty in ten patients with coronary artery disease undergoing elective percutaneous transluminal angioplasty was evaluated. All ten patients had been selected for elective balloon angioplasty on the basis of symptoms and coronary angiographic findings. Nine patients had exertional angina pectoris despite medical therapy. One patient had unstable angina and reversible ST-T elevation in the precordial leads that did not respond to vigorous medical therapy with intravenous nitrates, calcium antagonists, beta-receptor-blocking agents, and intravenous heparin. In this patient, bypass grafting was not indicated because of diffuse coronary artery disease with two previous myocardial infarctions. The baseline clinical and angiographic characteristics are depicted in Table 6.1. Permission to perform excimer laser angioplasty was obtained from our Institutional Review Board and Ethical Committee at the University of Tübingen. Informed consent for excimer laser angioplasty and balloon dilatation was obtained from each patient before the procedure.

A commercial excimer xenon chloride laser (Technolas, MAX-10, Munich, FRG) that delivered pulses at a pulse width of 60 nsec and at a wavelength of 308 nm was used. The laser was operated at a frequency of 20 Hz. The beam was coupled into a specially designed 1.3-mm catheter device consisting of 20 concentric 100-μm quartz fibers around a central lumen for a 0.014-inch-diameter flexible guidewire. The fibers were fixed at the proximal and distal end only to ensure maximal catheter flexibility. Energy transmission per pulse was approximately 5 mJ/mm^2. Before and after each irradiation series the actual transmitted energy at the catheter tip of each system was measured. In prior in-vitro studies the ablative threshold of this device was found to be approximately 4 mJ/mm^2 (14).

The patients were prepared for laser angioplasty using standard angioplasty techniques by way of the percutaneous femoral approach. After a heparin bolus (10,000 U given intraarterially) and intracoronary nitroglycerin application (100 μg left coronary artery, 50 μg right coronary artery), biplane control angiography of the ischemia-related artery was performed and confirmed the severity of the lesion in all but one patient, who had shown a total occlusion of the right coronary artery at the site of a subtotal lesion 1 week before at diagnostic catheterization. After intervention, all patients were monitored for 24 hours in the coronary care unit; ECGs and blood samples for enzyme levels of CK and CKMB were taken every 3 hours. The introducer sheath was left in place for 24 hours until control angiography was performed. Intravenous heparin was administered for 24 hours after intervention at a rate of approximately 1000 IU/hour. During all interventions a surgical team for emergency bypass operation was available.

With a 9 Fr. lumen guiding catheter (ACS) in place, a 0.014-inch-diameter, 180-cm-long steerable guidewire (USCI) was advanced through the lesion or total occlusion into the distal vessel and the location was con-

Table 6.1. Clinical Baseline Characteristics of the Study Population

PAT. #	SEX	AGE (YEARS)	EXTENT OF CORONARY ARTERY DISEASE	PRIOR MYOCARDIAL INFARCTION (LOCATION)	GLOBAL EJECTION FRACTION (%)	ISCHEMIA-RELATED VESSEL	ANGIOGRAPHIC MORPHOLOGY OF THE STENOSIS	LENGTH OF STENOSIS (MM)
1	M	44	1-vd	Anterior	54	LAD	Concentric	160
2	F	44	1-vd	—	78	CIRC	Concentric	178
3[a]	M	72	3-vd	Anterior	40	LAD	Eccentric	120
4	M	58	1-vd	Inferior	72	LAD	Eccentric	81
5	M	65	2-vd	Inferior	62	RCA	Total occlusion	—
6	M	64	1-vd	—	67	RCA	Concentric	105
7	F	62	1-vd	—	59	RCA	Concentric	160
8	M	55	1-vd	Anterior	50	LAD	Total occlusion	—
9	M	50	1-vd	—	68	LAD	Concentric	101
10	M	65	1-vd	Anterior	62	LAD	Eccentric	12

[a]Unstable angina

CIRC = left circumflex artery, LAD = left anterior descending artery, RCA = Right coronary artery.

firmed by angiography. The tip of the laser catheter was then positioned close to the lesion. In all cases, further advancement of the laser catheter across the lesion was performed with gentle pressure and during 8–10 seconds excimer laser energy delivery. The advancement was slowly performed up to the end of the lesion. After the lesion was passed, additional irradiation of the lesion was performed during slow withdrawal of the catheter. This procedure was repeated at least twice for approximately 10–15 seconds per cycle. After each cycle the laser catheter was pulled back into the guiding catheter and control angiography was performed. Laser angioplasty was stopped if no visible change in comparison to the result of the previous laser energy delivery was observed.

Balloon Angioplasty Procedure: Following excimer laser angioplasty, conventional balloon angioplasty was performed to ensure an adequate lumen. In nine patients the laser catheter device including the guidewire was exchanged and conventional balloon angioplasty was performed.

Qualitative Coronary Analysis: The coronary angiograms were reviewed by three experienced angiographers unaware of the clinical data. The coronary lesions were classified by a consensus of the three angiographers on the basis of qualitative analysis of the lesion in at least two projections.

Excimer Laser Angioplasty Results in the First Pilot Study: In two patients the laser catheter could not be advanced across the distal end of the lesion due to vessel tortuosities. Laser recanalization of the complete lesion was accomplished in eight patients. In these patients a stepwise increase of the central lumen between the irradiation cycles could be documented angiographically and implied ablation of plaque tissue by the device rather than effects due to mechanical catheter manipulations (Dotter mechanism). After completion of laser irradiation, residual stenoses of 80 percent and 70 percent were found in two patients, 50 percent in two patients, and less than 50 percent in four other patients (Table 6.2). Slight intraluminal lucencies and lesion irregularities were seen in two patients. In one patient a moderate coronary dissection occurred. In the first two patients total irradiation time was kept below 40 seconds to avoid vessel perforation. Since no evidence of perforation or severe damage of the adjacent tissue was seen at control angiography,

Table 6.2. Effects, Duration, and Complications of Laser Irradiation and Balloon Angioplasty

PAT. #	LUMINAL DIAMETER PRE–LASER ABLATION (MM)	LUMINAL DIAMETER POST–LASER ABLATION (MM)	NUMBER OF LASER IRRADIATIONS	TOTAL DURATION OF IRRADIATION (SECONDS)	COMPLICATION AFTER LASER IRRADIATION	BALLOON SIZE (MM)	INFLATION PRESSURE (ATMOSPHERES)	LUMINAL DIAMETER POST–BALLOON DILATATION (MM)	LUMINAL DIAMETER AT THE 24-HOUR CONTROL ANGIOGRAPHY (MM)
1	0.38	1.88	2	40	—	2.5	7	2.5	2.35
2	1.10	Unable to pass	1	38	Occlusion	2.5	5	2.35	2.5
3	1.00	Unable to pass	1	160	Occlusion	2.0	9	2.0	—
4	0	1.60	3	185	—	3.0	1	2.5	2.3
5	0.39	2.4	4	220	—	3.5	6	2.6	2.5
6	0.54	2.0	2	40	Dissection	—	—	—	2.0
7	0.25	1.25	4	215	—	3.5	5	2.5	2.8
8	0	1.25	3	167	—	3.0	5	1.96	2.15
9	0.35	1.75	4	210	—	3.0	4	2.5	2.7
10	0.54	1.8	3	187	—	—	—	—	1.5

irradiation time was subsequently prolonged in the following eight patients as was felt necessary for an optimal result. Although maximum irradiation time in this pilot study was increased up to 220 seconds, no adverse effects such as vessel perforation or embolization occurred in any patient.

The result of excimer laser angioplasty, however, seemed to depend on coronary morphology. In patients with concentric long lesions and in vessels with minimal tortuosities, the central channel created by laser ablation showed no irregularities, whereas in eccentric lesions the laser-induced channel had irregular borders and contrast opacification was reduced. In two patients in whom the lesion could not be passed completely by the laser catheter, tortuosities of the vessel were present. Fluoroscopy revealed a total occlusion, probably as a result of coronary spasm, in both patients. Although laser irradiation resulted in a definite lumen increase in the proximal part of the stenosis, the procedure was stopped to avoid vessel injury.

To ensure an adequate lumen, conventional balloon angioplasty was subsequently performed in eight patients after excimer laser angioplasty. In one patient with a dissection and in a second patient with a residual stenosis of less than 30 percent after laser treatment, additional balloon angioplasty was avoided. The individual angiographic data, balloon diameters, and inflation pressures are provided in Table 6.2. In both patients with unsuccessful laser passage, however, the lesion could be passed with a balloon catheter, and conventional balloon dilatation was successful. Subsequent balloon angioplasty resulted in a residual stenosis of 50 percent in one, of 40 percent in one, of 30 percent in two, and of 10 percent in four patients. A minor coronary dissection occurred in two patients at the distal end of the lesion. In two patients contrast opacification of the plaque area was persistently reduced even after balloon angioplasty.

Control angiography 24 hours after intervention was performed in nine patients and demonstrated a patent vessel in all cases without evidence for thrombus formation or persistent intraluminal lucencies. The residual stenosis was comparable to control angiography performed immediately after the procedure in eight and increased in only one patient from a less-than-30-percent to a 50 percent stenosis of the left anterior descending artery. In this patient subsequent balloon angioplasty was not performed.

All nine patients with stable angina tolerated the entire procedure well and were discharged home within four days. No significant ECG changes or rise in CK and CKMB levels occurred within the control period.

One patient with unstable angina and severe triple-vessel disease developed anterior ST segment elevation, hypotension, and ventricular tachycardia 3 hours after intervention and could not be resuscitated. At necropsy, diffuse and severe atherosclerosis, a recent myocardial infarct in the anteroseptal region next to a prior anterior scar, and a previous transmural inferior infarct were noted. There was a residual stenosis of about 75 percent of the luminal cross-section area at the end of the proximal segment of the left anterior descending artery at the origin of the second diagonal branch (Plate III). In the proximal part of the lesion just before the origin of the diagonal branch, discrete intimal laceration (Plate IV) and fibrin formation with platelet aggregation on the intimal layer were found. This probably resulted from laser ablation (Plate V). Serial histological evaluation of the lesion revealed plaque disruption and intimal hemorrhage associated with intraluminal thrombus at the distal end of the plaque where subsequent balloon angioplasty was performed (Plate VI).

The Early Experience

The combined use of intracoronary excimer laser angioplasty and balloon dilatation in ten patients with coronary heart disease was encouraging. The novel 1.3-mm fiber-optic laser-delivery catheter proved effective in partially reducing high-degree lesions and occlusions. All patients tolerated the intervention well without symptoms such as chest pain or burning sensations.

We learned through this early series that with careful technique, the risk of perforation with this device in comparison to the bare fiber technique or thermal laser angioplasty is minimal. The possibility of undue thrombogenesis, however, cannot be ruled out in this limited series, although we saw that the incidence of occluding thrombi seems low, at least in the acute setting.

We were unable to cross the lesion in two patients due to tortuosities of the vasculature. Although only gentle pressure was used, coronary occlusion occurred at the distal end of the lesion, most probably as a result of mechanical manipulations.

In this series, eight lesions were crossed during application of excimer laser energy and a definite lumen was produced. Interestingly, the lumen diameter achieved by excimer laser irradiation was larger than the diameter of the laser catheter itself. In the majority of our patients, repeat coronary angiography demonstrated a still-relevant residual lesion after laser ablation. To ensure an optimal result, subsequent balloon angioplasty was performed in eight patients, which was complicated by late occlusion and cardiogenic shock due to plaque disruption and thrombus formation in one patient.

The histologic specimen from this patient suggests that occlusion resulted from balloon angioplasty. Additional injury by laser irradiation, however, cannot be ruled out, since in the proximal part of the stenosis where ablation was performed, fibrin formation and platelet deposition were noted.

From this initial series, we concluded only that coronary excimer laser angioplasty is feasible and can be performed to remove coronary atherosclerotic tissue. We felt, however, that the clinical utility of this new technology would be dependent on further device modifications to enhance steerability and to achieve a more complete result.

Increasing Operator Experience and the Second Clinical Study

The characteristic learning curve associated with coronary angioplasty has been well documented in reports from the NHLBI PTCA Registry (15). On the basis of this phenomenon it was concluded that, although the flexibility of the catheter device was limited, further clinical experience was necessary. In the following clinical study, coronary excimer laser atherectomy was performed in 50 additional patients. As part of this study all patients underwent control angiography at least 6 months following the intervention. The results of this study have been published (16). All 60 patients in the first two studies had been previously selected for angioplasty on the basis of symptoms and angiographic findings. Forty-nine patients were markedly limited by severe exertional angina pectoris, and 11 patients had unstable angina with reversible ST-T segment changes at rest despite a therapy with nitroglycerin, beta-blocking agents, and calcium antagonists. In 41 patients the left anterior descending artery, in 7 patients the left circumflex artery, and in 10 patients the right coronary artery was the target vessel. As in the first ten patients, the extended protocol of excimer laser angioplasty was approved by the Institutional Review Board Committee at the University of Tübingen. Informed consent was obtained from each patient before the intervention.

The study protocol was slightly changed in an attempt to reduce the necessity of additional conventional balloon dilatation. All patients were on long-term treatment with acetylsalicylic acid (250 mg/day). After a heparin bolus (10,000 U given intra-arterially), the site of the lesion was visualized and intracoronary nitroglycerin (100 μg) was administered. With a 9 Fr. large lumen guiding catheter (ACS) placed in the ostium of the target vessel, the 0.014-inch-diameter flexible guidewire was advanced across the lesion into the distal vessel. In nine patients with total occlusion of the target vessel, recanalization was achieved by guidewire alone. Six of these patients had had a previous myocardial infarction in the perfusion area of the target vessel. The laser catheter was advanced over the guidewire through the proximal vessel up to the lesion. Advancement of the laser catheter through the lesion was attempted during 10–30 seconds of laser energy delivery, depending on lesion length. The catheter was advanced by applying only moderate pressure. Additional irradiation of the lesion was performed during slow withdrawal. This procedure was repeated at least twice. The procedure was terminated if no visible change of lumen diameter in comparison to the previous cycle was observed. Angiography of the target vessel was repeated after a control period of at least 20 minutes to confirm lesion morphology after intervention. Decisions to perform additional balloon angioplasty were based on the qualitative judgment of the lesion severity after laser atherectomy. In patients with an unsatisfactory result after laser angioplasty, subsequent balloon angioplasty was performed. Balloon angioplasty was also performed when vessel occlusion during or after laser treatment occurred. Twenty-four to 36 hours after the intervention, early follow-up angiography was performed in the majority of these patients. Forty-seven of the 55 patients underwent follow-up angiography between 30 to 212 days postintervention only. Five patients refused the invasive follow-up study. Computer-based coronary quantitative angiographic analysis was employed to analyze the cineangiograms of all patients. Quantitative analysis of the lesion before and after each irradiation cycle, at the early follow-up and late follow-up angiograms, was performed using identical angiographic projections by means of a computer-based coronary angiographic analysis system. The minimal stenotic diameter and percentage stenosis were calculated. Success of laser angioplasty and balloon dilatation was defined as a reduction of lesion severity of more than 50 percent.

The early and late follow-up angiograms of the target vessel were performed using a standardized acquisition and analysis. The angular settings of the x-ray gantry and the various height levels were readjusted according to the values previously documented to correspond as much as possible to the projections used during the previous angiographies. To minimize possible blurring effects, only end-diastolic cineframs were analyzed.

Two definitions of restenosis were applied: 1) a loss of at least 50 percent gain in luminal diameter achieved at PTCA, and 2) a decrease in minimal luminal diameter of greater than or equal to 0.72 mm with respect to the postintervention situation (17).

Results of the Expanded First Trial: In 5 of 60 patients, excimer laser angioplasty could not be performed because of vessel tortuosities proximal to the lesion and at the site of the lesion. Thus, it was impossible to place the catheter in a coaxial position within the vessel and laser irradiation was not initiated to reduce the risk of perforation. In the residual 55 patients, percentage stenosis decreased from 81 ± 57 percent before to 37 ± 17 percent after laser atherectomy. Correspondingly, the minimal lumen diameter increased from 0.45 ± 0.36 mm to 1.66 ± 0.47 mm. In 23 of these 55 patients no additional balloon angioplasty was performed. Percentage stenosis decreased from 76 ± 14 percent before to 27 ± 17 percent after laser angioplasty and was 34 ± 15 percent at the 24-hour control angiogram. The minimal lumen diameter increased from 0.53 ± 0.34 mm to 1.78 ± 0.45 mm after laser angioplasty and was 1.77 ± 0.6 mm 24 hours later. In 32 patients percentage stenosis decreased from 85 ± 14 percent to 44 ± 14 percent after coronary excimer laser atherectomy and balloon angioplasty was performed resulting in a residual percent stenosis of 24 ± 15 percent. At the early follow-up angiography, however, percentage stenosis increased to 32 ± 24 percent in 27 patients.

Coronary occlusion after laser angioplasty occurred 2–20 minutes later in 11 patients (20%) and was treated with balloon dilatation. The initial result immediately after laser angioplasty was 42 ± 15 percent diameter stenosis and 1.45 ± 0.55 mm minimal lumen diameter in these 11 patients. In none of these patients was angiographic evidence of intracoronary thrombi or severe dissection found. Intracoronary nitroglycerin failed to relieve vessel closure in all cases. In nine patients, balloon angioplasty was successful with persistent patency of the target vessel. In two patients (4%) the vessel could not be reopened by balloon dilatation. Both patients developed Q-wave infarctions in the perfusion area of the target vessel with a typical rise in CK and CKMB.

In the subgroup of 11 patients with unstable angina, laser irradiation of the ischemia-related lesion was impossible in one patient, could be performed in ten, and was successful in two patients only. In the remaining eight patients additional balloon angioplasty was necessary due to acute vessel closure in four patients and due to an insufficient result in the residual four patients. Serious complications occurred in all three patients with unstable angina.

The clinical course in 44 patients was uneventful. Early follow-up angiography demonstrated a patent vessel in all patients. The severity of the residual lesion was comparable to the angiographic result immediately after intervention. Stress tests performed before hospital discharge were unremarkable in all but two patients, who had triple-vessel disease and exertional angina at maximum exercise.

In the last patient of this series we encountered a technical problem of the catheter tip. The gold marker at the tip separated from the laser catheter during slow withdrawal after initially successful lesion ablation, and the vessel wall was perforated. Subsequent spasm and vessel occlusion were managed by immediate balloon dilatation and patency of the vessel was achieved and still present at the early follow-up angiography. Neither pericardial effusion nor recurrent ischemia occurred during follow-up.

Reliability of the Transmission Device: Initial energy transmission of the laser catheter was found to be 30 ± 5 mJ/mm^2. Energy transmission was above the ablative threshold in all catheters preintervention. Mean irradiation time was 123 ± 65 sec. Energy fluence after treatment was found to be significantly decreased to 16 ± 19 mJ/mm^2.

Additionally, the angiographic success and incidence of complications were not dependent on the energy threshold of the catheter pre- and postintervention.

Late Follow-Up: During the 6-month follow-up period no patient died. Myocardial infarction did not occur within this period in any patient. In 22 patients quantitative analysis of the target lesion revealed a restenosis according to the applied criteria. In six of these patients a total occlusion at follow-up was found. Reintervention by either balloon angioplasty or aortocoronary bypass grafting was performed in 15 patients. Five patients refused the late follow-up angiography. All five patients had had no episodes of recurrent chest pain and no signs of ischemia during treadmill exercise at maximum workload.

Of the 23 patients treated with laser ablation only, 19 underwent late follow-up arteriography, which revealed angiographic restenosis in six patients. PTCA was performed in four patients and bypass surgery in one patient.

Twenty-eight of the 32 patients with laser ablation and balloon angioplasty underwent late follow-up angiography. Sixteen of these patients fulfilled the criteria of restenosis. In ten patients reintervention was performed.

Discussion and Perspectives

The strategy of directional atherectomy using excimer laser energy in patients with coronary artery disease was facilitated by the advent of clinically useful catheters. The difficulties in transmission of high peak powers via 100-μm diameter fibers and the problems of energy coupling were formidable. Novel means of laser-fiber coupling, however, permitted transmission of even 60-nsec pulse-duration excimer light via these small-diameter fibers and facilitated energy transmission even in fiber bundles. An additional problem was fixation of fibers within a catheter suitable for coronary treatment. We decided that the first approach should be an over-the-wire system with a central lumen for a 0.014-inch guidewire. The fibers were concentrically arranged around this central lumen to avoid vessel perforation. Fixation of the fibers at the distal catheter tip, however, resulted in a stiff and inflexible end for at least 5–8 mm. These features of the prototypical catheter resulted in a high number of patients with left anterior descending artery target lesions in our treatment group. Catheter flexibility and trackability was improved and in the latest series of our patients in the current protocol, standard wires instead of high-torque wires are used to ensure better guiding facilities for the laser catheter. In the majority of our patients, however, the LAD is still the target vessel. Current catheter design in Germany is still in a stage of development comparable to the initially used prototype balloon catheters of the late 1970s and early 1980s. Treatment is limited to patients with disease of the proximal two-thirds of the coronaries presenting with only minor tortuosities.

A key question is the residual luminal diameter narrowing after treatment with stand-alone laser using this small-diameter catheter atherectomy (18). As a result of the small increase of diameter with the initial device, additional balloon angioplasty was necessary in the majority of our patients.

The results of the current trial employing catheters with a diameter of 1.8–2.0 mm suggest that the primary success rate can be improved to 60–70 percent with stand-alone coronary excimer laser procedures. Besides the laser catheter diameter, two additional limitations of this prototypical multifiber catheter became obvious: 1) The ablative area of the fibers effective for tissue removal was only 15 percent compared to the total catheter tip area, and 2) fiber-face damage occurred during treatment resulting in a significant decrement in energy output during the intravascular treatment period (19).

The first limitation, relation of the cross-sectional fiber face to the total cross-sectional area of the catheter tip, is still in the early stage of innovation and investigation and will probably be solved with the use of a higher number of smaller-diameter fibers or augmented spot size with lens-tipped fibers. Whatever the ultimate solution of this problem might be, the purely mechanical "Dottering" effect will be reduced in favor of effective tissue ablation, thereby reducing phenomena such as spasm and dissection that might result from mechanical vessel injury. The impact of improved ablative area at the catheter tip is even more important with the larger catheters currently under investigation since the Dotter effect of catheters with 1.8–2.3 mm diameter will be more pronounced.

Concerning the second limitation, in the majority of our cases, postprocedural testing of our fiber-optic catheters revealed a significant decrease in energy output compared to the preprocedure energy output. This reduced energy transmission probably represents fiber damage due to light back-scattered from the lesion during the ablative processes. It can be speculated that this effect might occur more often in heavily calcified than in fibromuscular plaque. Additionally, direct mechanical trauma from tortuosities or bends of the vasculature in diffusely diseased arteries cannot be excluded.

Although the overall "technical" success rate in all three ongoing clinical multicenter trials is above 90 percent, the need for adjunctive balloon angioplasty is obvious. This holds true not only for vessels with occlusion during the first 20 minutes after the procedure but also for an unsatisfying angiographic result. The initial idea of reduced trauma to the arterial wall by ablation rather than disruption and overdistention of the vessel implies that the only successful procedures are those that do not necessitate additional mechanical interventions.

The contribution of adjunctive balloon angioplasty to the incidence of restenosis may be considerable. Thus, the strategy is to avoid a second injury even if the initial angiographic result shows a luminal diameter narrowing between 35–50 percent, since it has been shown that the incidence of restenosis is an independent function of the residual luminal diameter narrowing (20). Whether the latter finding will also hold true for the incidence of restenosis following excimer laser atherectomy remains open to question, but investigations of this topic have been incorporated into all clinical trials (21,22). Analysis of a small subgroup among our patients suggests that the restenosis rate after stand-alone excimer laser atherectomy is comparable to that of balloon angioplasty, since in 6 of 19 patients angiographic restenosis was found by quantitative and clinical criteria (16). Even though the subgroup of patients was small, it has to be stated that restenosis will occur even after excimer laser atherectomy. However, any assessment of restenosis must be regarded as premature until the technical problems of the currently used catheter devices are solved and a stage of development similar to that of balloon angioplasty catheters is reached.

The results of our early experience and of the other two clinical multicenter trials convincingly confirm that excimer laser coronary atherectomy is a realistic form of treatment for atherosclerotic heart disease. Whether this form of therapy will be superior to other mechanical alternative techniques will have to be determined in further investigations.

In terms of control, it must be stated that conventional angiography is limited. Further techniques such as spectroscopy or even intravascular ultrasound may be necessary to ensure on-line control of ablation for an optimal result. The safety and efficacy of pulsed laser atherectomy by improved catheter devices combined with on-line diagnostic techniques will definitely open new horizons for percutaneous transluminal coronary atherectomy in the treatment of atherosclerotic heart disease.

Part II

In this section the clinical, angiographic, and technical data of four patients are reported. All patients underwent excimer laser coronary atherectomy for treatment of symptomatic atherosclerotic heart disease.

Case 1

A 65-year-old white woman presented with single-vessel disease. She had had an inferior myocardial infarction 3 months previously and a history of angina for 5 years. She was in stable condition with recurrent angina and signs of ischemia on the treadmill. She remained symptomatic on therapy with beta-blockers, Ca-antagonist, sublingual nitrates, and 100 mg aspirin. At angiography, a subtotal lesion of the proximal right coronary artery was visualized. Only mild hypokinesia of the posterobasal area was found at biplane cineventriculography. Thallium-201 scintigraphy revealed a small area of subendocardial infarction and considerable redistribution of the inferior wall. Although it was felt that the lesion in the proximal bend was not ideal for excimer laser atherectomy, the concentric appearance of the lesion (Fig. 6.1A) was attractive. After ostial intubation of a 9 Fr. Metronic Giant guiding catheter, a 0.014 inch high-torque floppy wire was placed in the periphery of the vessel and laser ablation was initiated after a 1.2-mm Technolas, Inc., laser catheter was placed directly in front of the lesion. Preprocedural energy output was 9 mJ/mm^2 at the catheter tip. Energy was applied for 33 seconds during slow advancement with only moderate pressure on the device and during slow withdrawal. Control angiography revealed an increase of lumen at the lesion site; however, the residual lumen diameter was still reduced (Fig. 6.1B). Thus, an extension was docked to the 0.014 inch wire and the 1.2-mm-diameter laser was exchanged for an 1.8-mm-Ceramoptec, Inc., (Bonn, FRG) laser catheter with a preprocedural energy output of 11 mJ/mm^2 at the catheter tip. Additional ablation of the lesion was performed for 39 seconds. Control angiography revealed a less-than-50-percent lesion after treatment (Fig. 6.1C). Twenty-four-hour control angiography was identical to the immediate postprocedural morphology. The patient was asymptomatic at treadmill exercise 3 days later and free of pain for the following 6 months. She underwent control angiography as part of the treatment protocol 6 months later. The vessel was patent, and a 40 percent residual stenosis was found at the identical projection (Fig. 6.1D). To date, 12 months after treatment, the patient is still asymptomatic.

Case 2

A 52-year-old white man presented with recent-onset angina that had been increasing in frequency and intensity during the prior three months. His history was unremarkable; he had not had previous myocardial infarctions. As a pilot, every year he underwent regular stress tests, which did not present evidence of ischemia during recent years. At initial coronary angiography, single-vessel disease and normal left

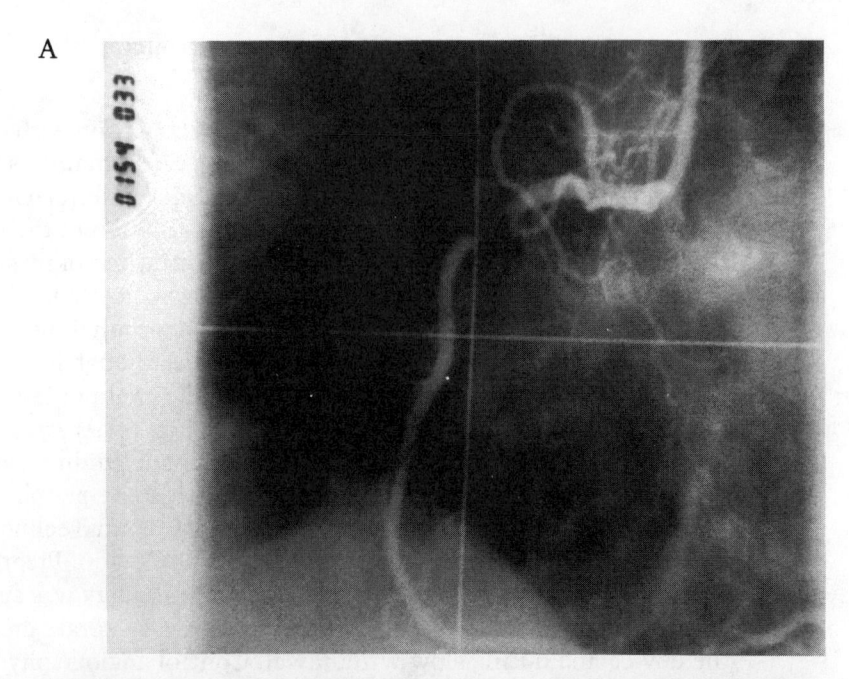

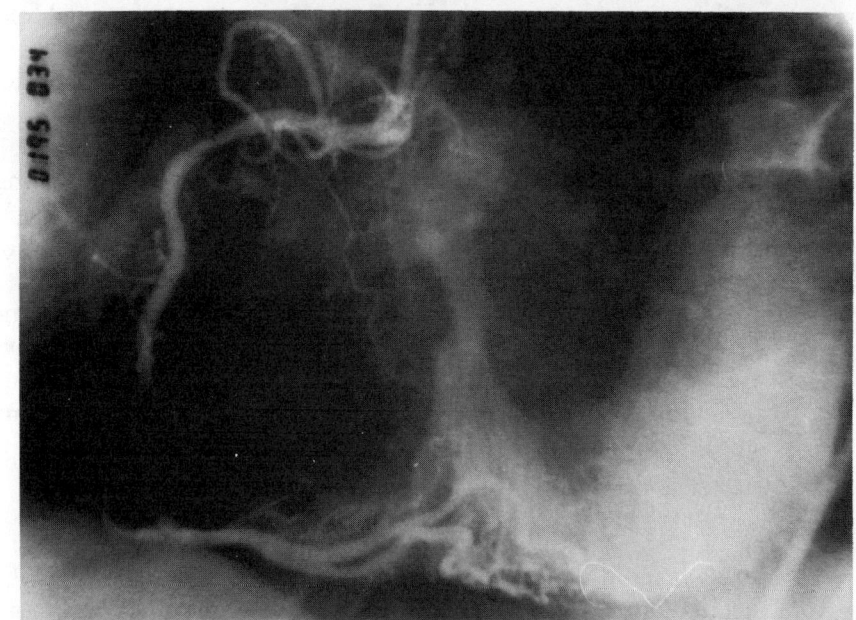

Figure 6.1. (*A*) Right coronary artery of a 65-year-old woman demonstrating a tight, concentric lesion of moderate length in the proximal right coronary artery. (*B*) Following excimer laser angioplasty with a 1.2-mm catheter, moderate improvement in luminal caliber is seen.

C

D

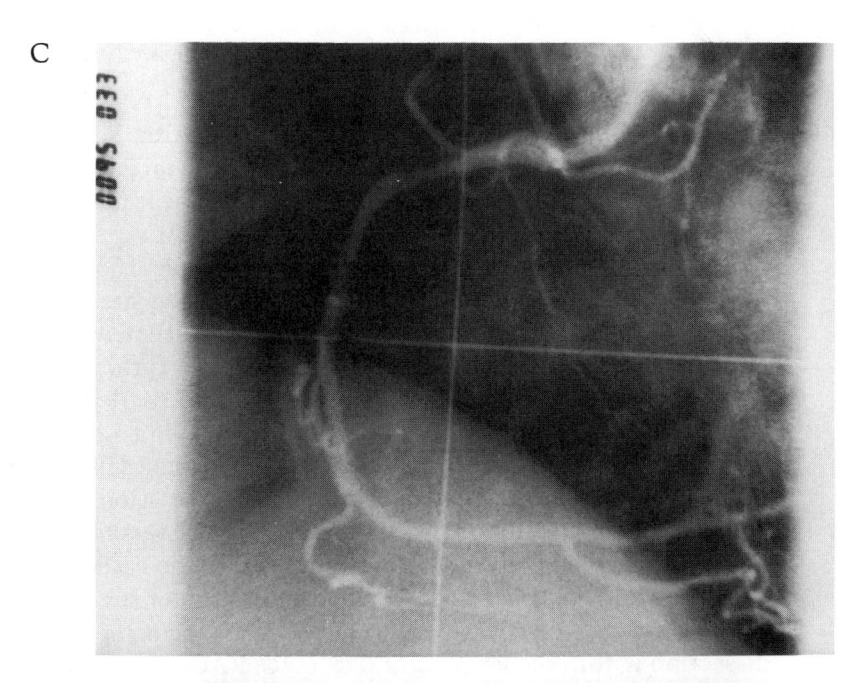

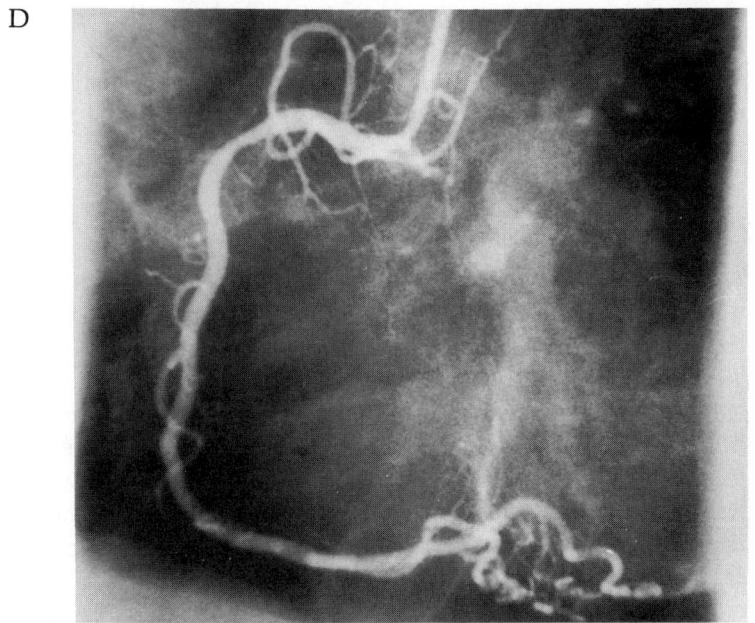

Figure 6.1 (cont.) (C) Following excimer angioplasty with a 1.8 mm diameter catheter, a stenosis of less than 50% results. (D) At 6 months, there has been no diminution of luminal caliber.

ventricular function were found. He was transferred for intervention and scheduled for excimer laser atherectomy. The target vessel was the left anterior descending artery with a very eccentric lesion after the origin of the first diagonal (Fig. 6.2A, 15° RAO projection, 15° craniocaudal view; Fig. 6.2B, 45° RAO projection, 15° craniocaudal view). Although the angle of the vessel at the lesion site was felt to be crucial for laser atherectomy, the vessel diameter seemed to be ideal for treatment with a 2.0-mm Technolas, Inc., laser catheter. A 9 Fr. 4 Metronic Giant guiding catheter was placed into the left main stem, and after intracoronary administration of 0.1 ms of nitroglycerin, a 0.018-inch high-torque flexible guidewire was advanced into the periphery of the left anterior descending artery and its location confirmed by angiography. Subsequently the 2-mm laser catheter was advanced to the lesion. Initial energy output was 10 mJ/mm^2 at the catheter tip. Slow advancement through the lesion with application of energy for 57 seconds over two cycles was performed. Control angiography revealed a dissection within the lesion area (Fig. 6.2C, RAO, and Fig. 6.2D, LAO, identical views). Flow was not compromised and the residual luminal diameter was less than 50 percent. The procedure was terminated. The results of an exercise test 3 days later were unremarkable and the patient remained asymptomatic. He is to undergo final follow-up angiography.

Case 3

A 63-year-old white man with a long history of recurrent angina presented with single-vessel disease of a very proximal high-grade eccentric lesion of the left anterior descending artery. He had had previous balloon angioplasty at the lesion site and recurrent symptoms indicative of restenosis for 5 months. Control angiography was performed, and it was decided to perform excimer laser atherectomy based on the location (no tortuosities) and length of the lesion. Additional disease with a second lesion in the mid LAD was found, but the proximal stenosis was identified as the target lesion (Fig. 6.3A). Following the same protocol as in cases 1 and 2, we used a 1.5-mm Ceramoptec catheter. The initial preprocedural energy output was 15 mJ/mm^2 at the catheter tip. Initial ablation was performed over 57 seconds with two passes at the lesion site. The initial result was a moderate increase of lumen diameter (Fig. 6.3B). Five minutes later, however, apparent spasm occurred and antegrade flow reduced, although intracoronary nitroglycerin had been adminis-

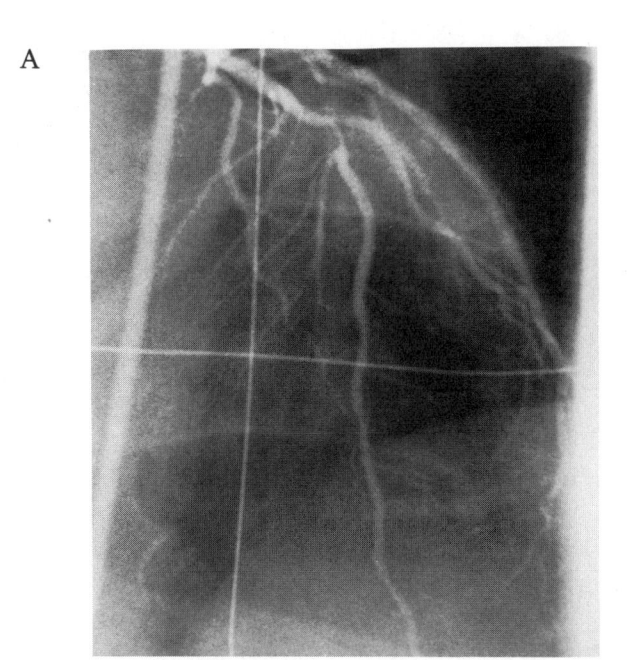

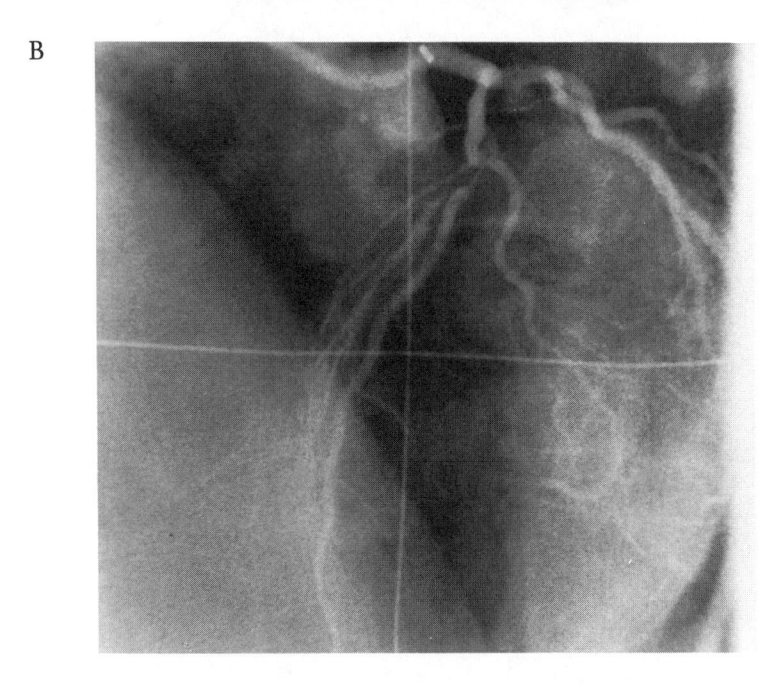

Figure 6.2. (A) Baseline coronary angiogram of a 52-year-old pilot who presented with increasing angina. (B) The culprit lesion is a somewhat eccentric stenosis of the proximal left anterior descending involving the take-off of the first diagonal.

C

D

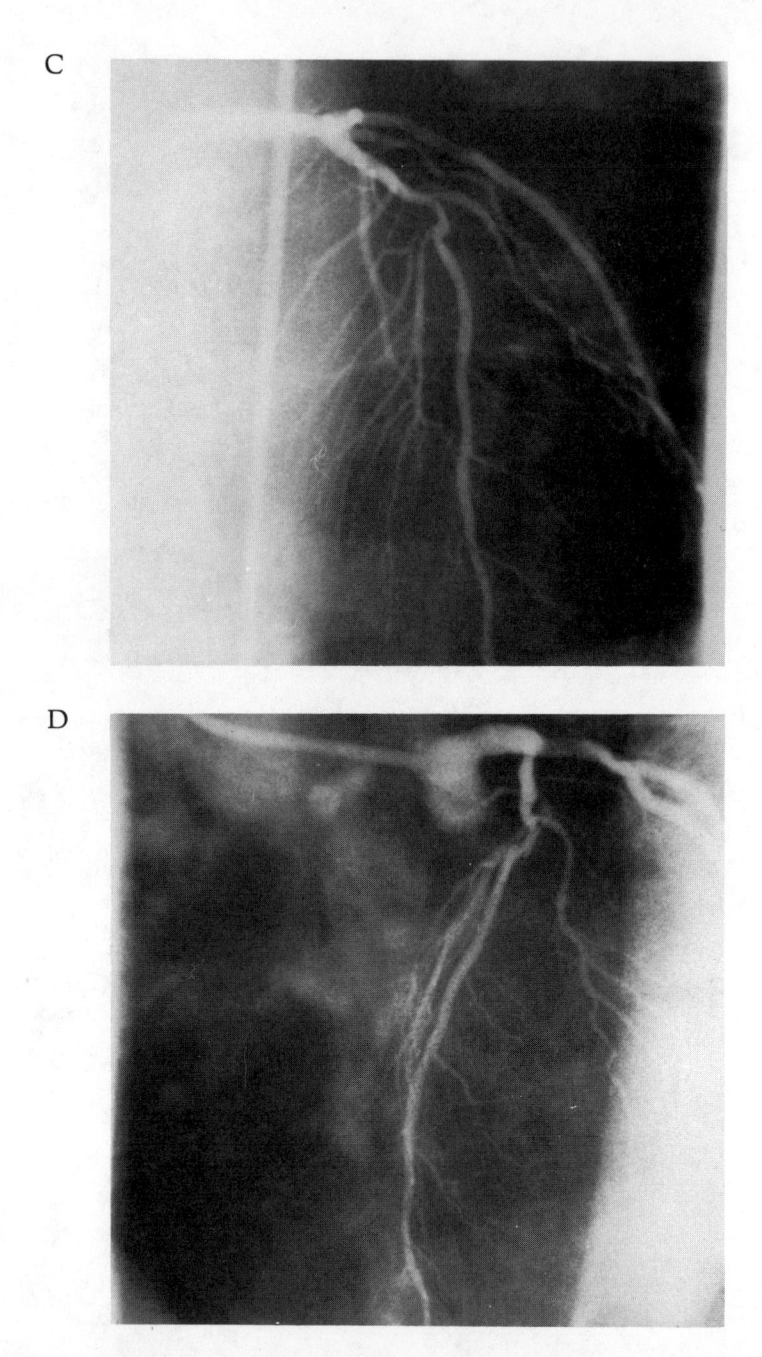

Figure 6.2 (*cont.*) (C) Following 2 passes with a 2.0-mm catheter at 10 mJ from the tip, angiography reveals a dissection within the lesion. (D) Flow was not compromised and no adjunctive balloon angioplasty was performed. A follow-up stress test was negative within the first week.

Percutaneous Transluminal Coronary Excimer Laser Atherectomy   119

A

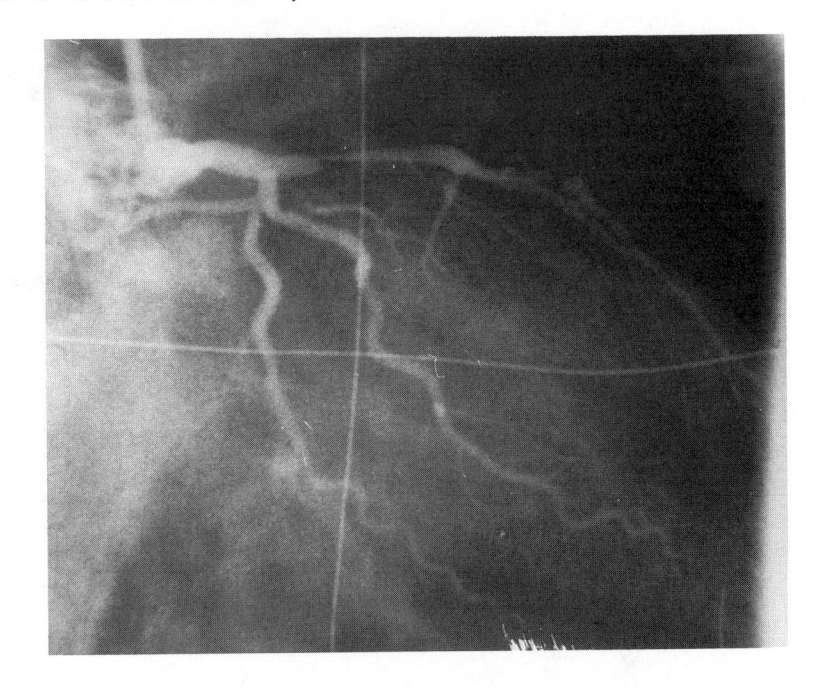

B

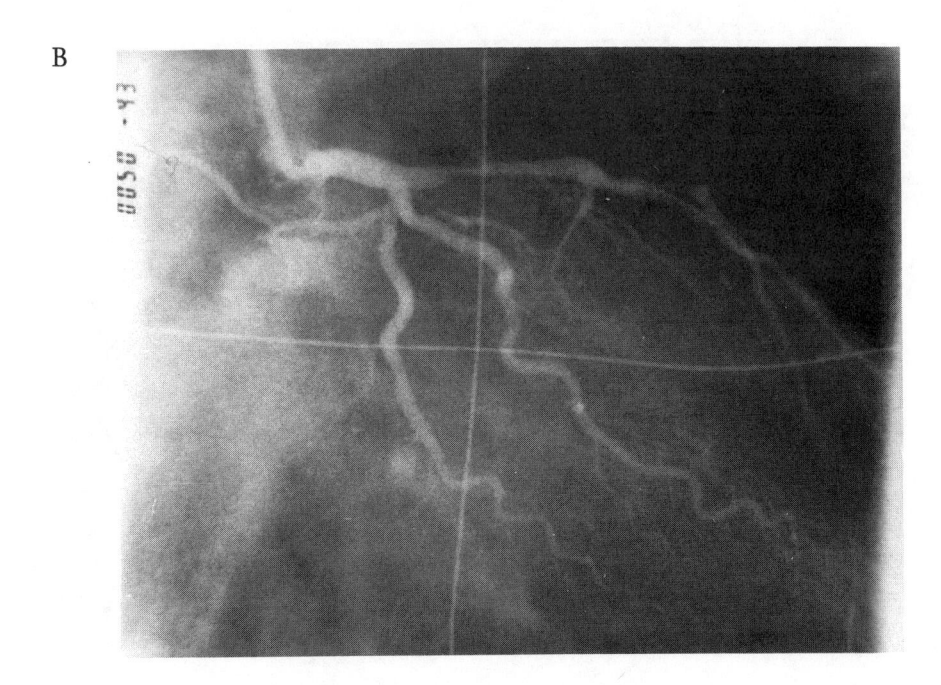

120 . . . . Coronary Laser Angioplasty

C

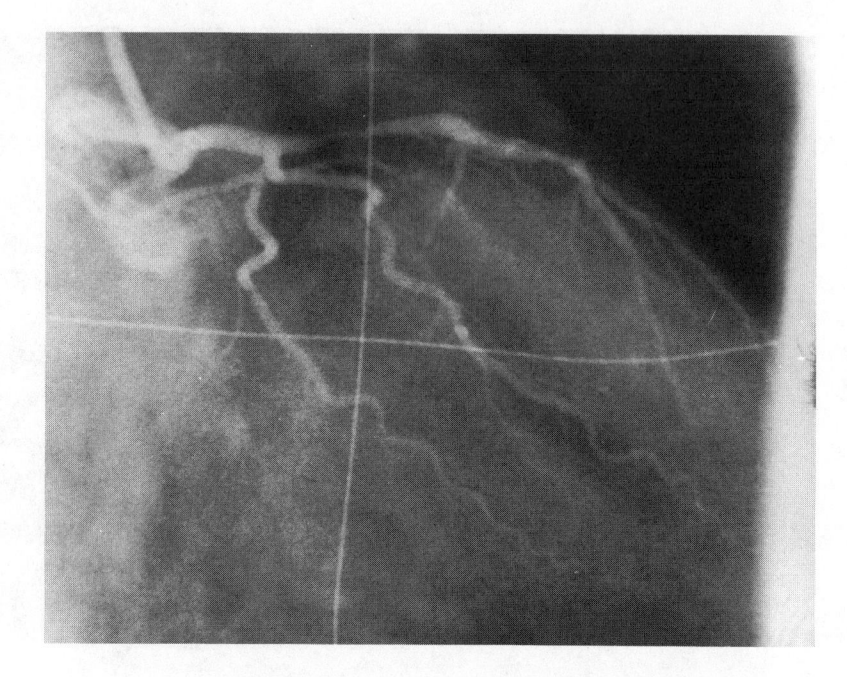

D

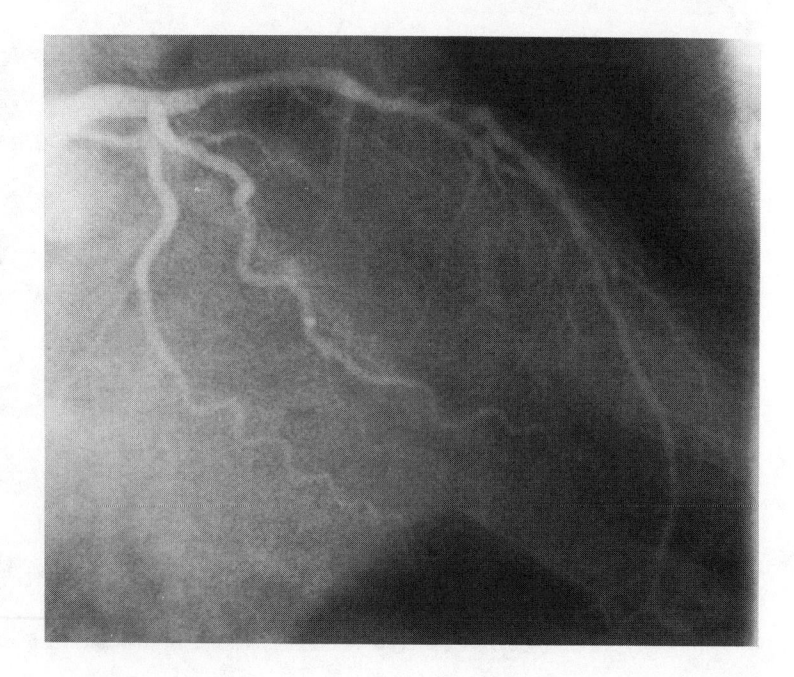

E

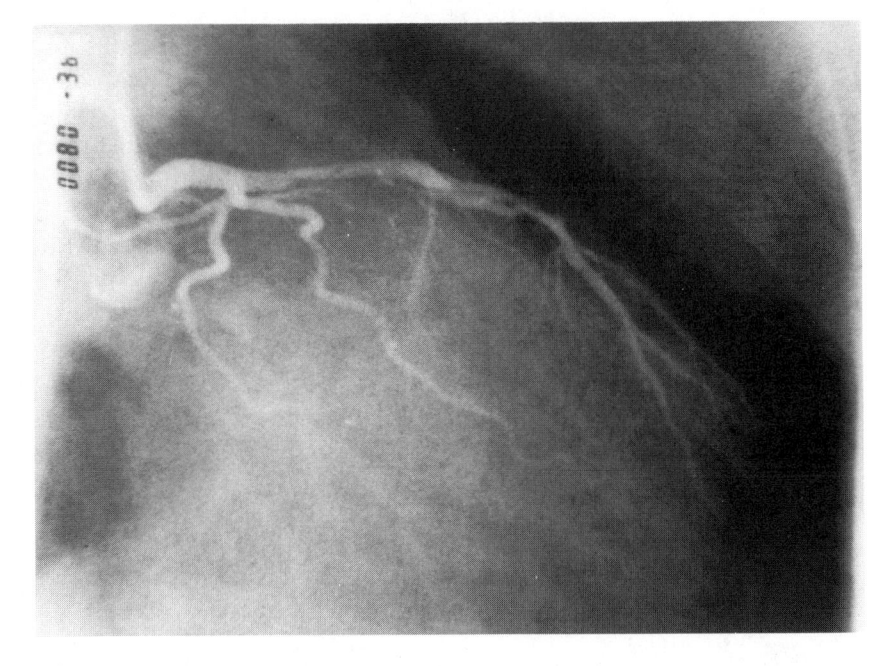

Figure 6.3. (A) Baseline angiogram of a 63 year old man with recurrent angina 3 months following balloon angioplasty. A long, proximal left anterior descending stenosis is seen. (B) Following excimer angioplasty with a 1.5 mm catheter and 15 mJ out the tip delivered over 57 seconds, a moderate increase in luminal diameter is seen. (C) Within 5 minutes, the luminal caliber was diminished with decreased flow in the left anterior descending. This may have been secondary to coronary spasm. Subsequently, excimer angioplasty with a 2.0 mm catheter and 20 mJ out the tip was performed over 46 seconds in 2 passes. (D) The post laser angiogram revealed a residual stenosis of 35% with good distal flow. The patient had a negative stress test and was discharged on day 3. He presented with recurrent angina at 4 months. (E) Repeat angiography revealed no significant restenosis at the proximal left anterior descending site but progression of a lesion in the mid left anterior descending. This lesion was treated with conventional balloon angioplasty as it was felt that it was on too angulated a segment for excimer angioplasty. Six months following the second intervention, the patient is asymptomatic.

tered at the beginning of the procedure and additional sublingual nifedipine (10 μg) was given (Fig. 6.3C). It was decided to move on and perform additional ablation using a 2.0 Technolas laser catheter device. The initial energy output was 20 mJ/mm^2 at the catheter tip. Ablation was performed for 46 seconds with only two passes. Crossing of the lesion was uncomplicated and facilitated virtually without applying pressure on the laser catheter. The initial and 24-hour control angiograms revealed a 35 percent residual luminal diameter narrowing (Fig. 6.3D). A stress test was negative and the patient was discharged home after 3 days. He presented with recurrent angina 4 months later. Control angiography (Fig. 6.3E) disclosed a still satisfying result at the site of the lesion treated but a worsening lesion severity in the mid third, which was subsequently treated by conventional balloon angioplasty. The decision not to perform excimer laser atherectomy on the second lesion was based on the two angles proximal to the lesion. Six months after the second intervention the patient is still asymptomatic and monthly stress tests are negative.

Case 4

A 46-year-old white man presented with an 18-month history of stable exertional angina. At stress test, left-bundle branch block occurred during exercise. Despite therapy with beta blockers, Ca-antagonists, nitrates, and aspirin, he remained symptomatic. He had not had a previous myocardial infarction and had stopped smoking 3 years earlier. Coronary angiography revealed two-vessel disease with a 60 percent lesion of the right coronary artery and a very short eccentric lesion in the proximal mid left anterior descending artery at the origin of the first septal perforator (Fig. 6.4A RAO, Fig. 6.4B LAO 45°, 15° cranio-caudal view). Thallium-201 scintigraphy was positive with redistribution of the tracer in the LAD perfusion area anterolateral and apical without persistent defects. Left ventricular function was normal. Although an angle of approximately 30° was present, the decision to perform excimer laser ablation was based on the poststenotic vessel diameter, which seemed appropriate for a stand-alone procedure using a 1.8-mm laser catheter. The energy output was 21 mJ/mm^2 at the catheter tip pre- and postintervention. Due to the proximal angle, a standard 0.018 inch wire was used and passed over the lesion without problems. The 1.8-mm laser catheter (Technolas) was advanced to the lesion. Passage of the catheter through the lesion, however, was complicated and could be achieved only after 40 seconds of energy application and considerable pressure on the device. Two passes of the lesion with a total exposure time of 78 seconds were necessary. At the end of the treatment period the residual luminal diameter was improved to 30 percent with some lumen irregularities in the area of ablation (Figs. 6.4C, D). The patient

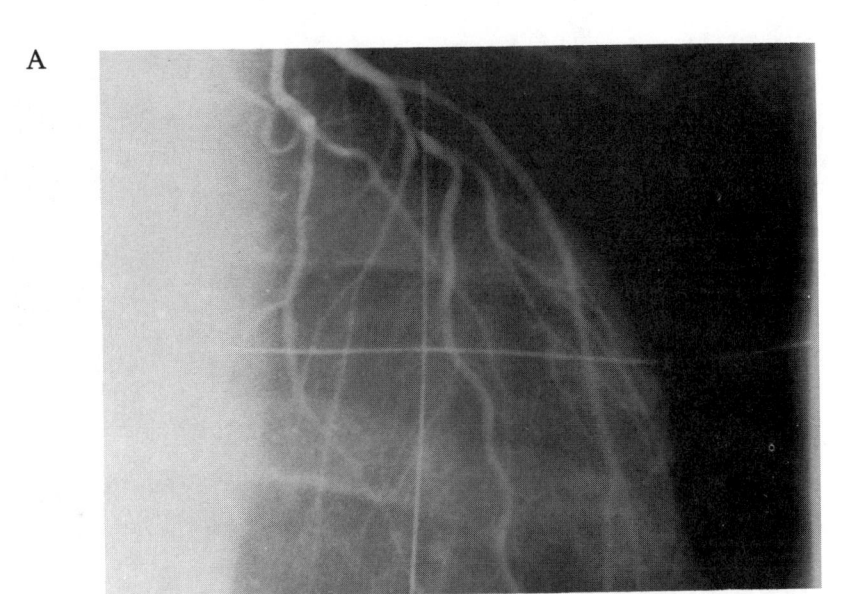

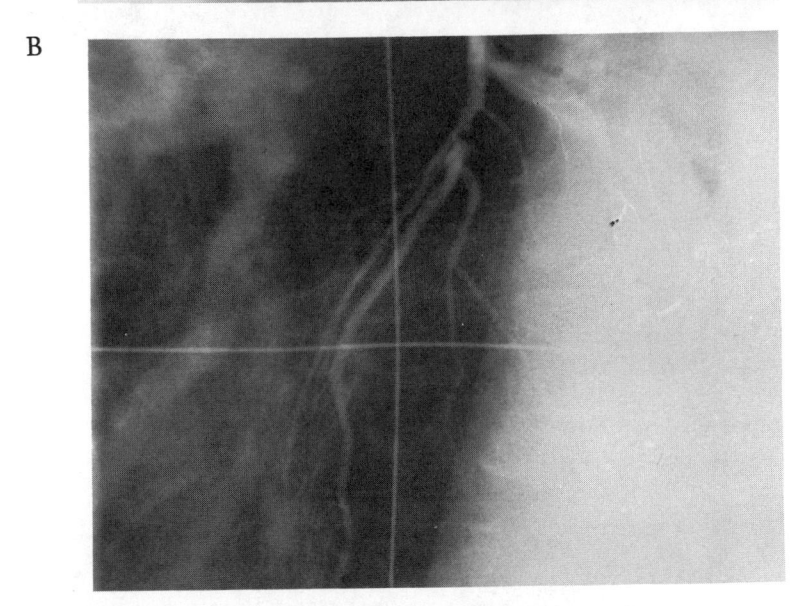

Figure 6.4. (A) Baseline angiograms from a 46 year old man who presented with an 18 month history of stable angina. Coronary angiography revealed a 60% lesion in the right coronary artery and a very short eccentric lesion in the proximal left anterior descending at the origin of the first septal perforator. (B) Excimer laser angioplasty was performed with a 1.8 mm catheter at 21 mJ. Passage of the catheter through the lesion was complicated and could be achieved only after 40 seconds of energy application and considerable pressure on the device. Two passes and a total of 78 seconds were used.

C

D

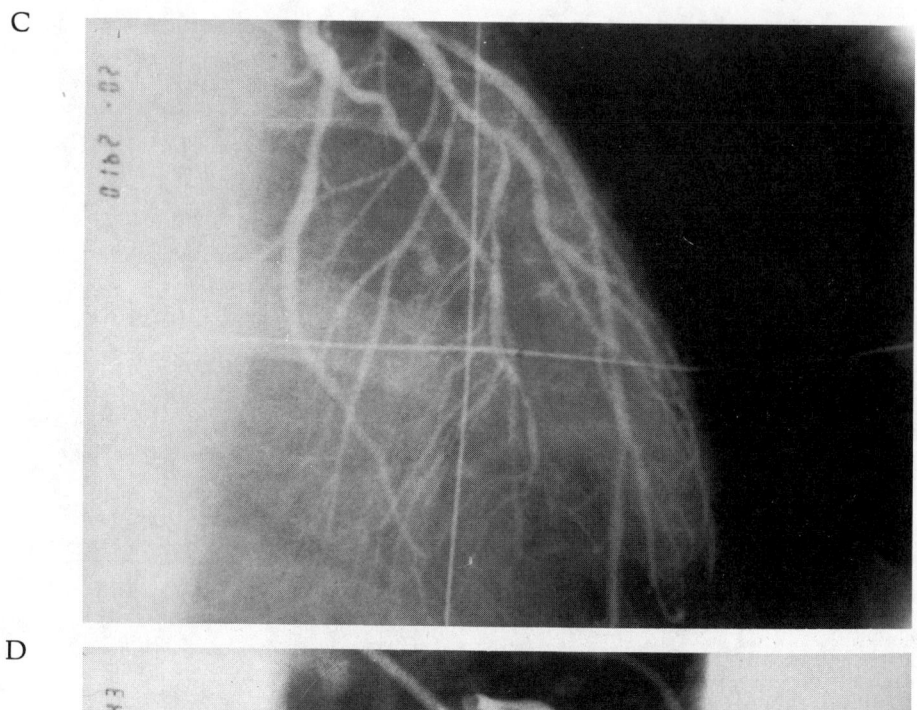

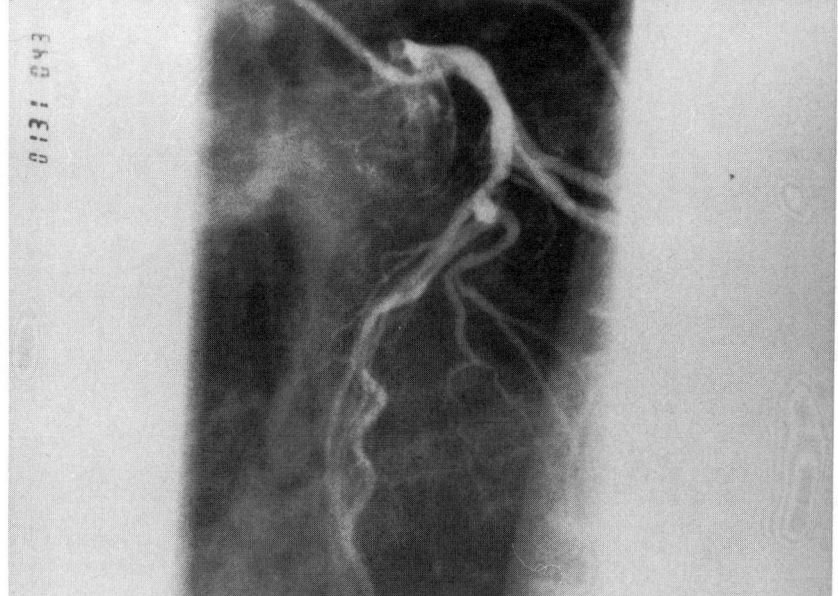

Figure 6.4 (*cont.*)(*C*) Following angioplasty, the residual luminal diameter was improved to approximately 30% stenosis with some irregularity. (*D*) No adjunctive balloon angioplasty was performed. The patient was discharged on the second operative day and was asymptomatic as of 4 month follow-up.

was free of pain and could be discharged home 2 days later. After 4 months he was still asymptomatic without specific therapy.

References

1. Grüntzig AR, Meier B. Percutaneous transluminal coronary angioplasty. The first five years and the future. *Int J Cardiol* 1983;2:319–323.
2. Kent KM, Bentivoglio LG, Block PC, et al. Long-term efficacy of percutaneous transluminal coronary angioplasty (PTCA): report from the National Heart, Lung, and Blood Institute PTCA Registry. *Am J Cardiol* 1984;53:27C-31C.
3. Holmes DR, Vlietstra RE, Smith HC, et al. Restenosis after percutaneous transluminal coronary angioplasty (PTCA): a report from the PTCA Registry of the National Heart, Lung, and Blood Institute. *Am J Cardiol* 1984;53:77C-81C.
4. Ming WL, Roubin GS, King SB III. Restenosis after angioplasty. Potential biologic determinants and role of intimal hyperplasia. *Circulation* 1989:79(6):1374–1387.
5. Hanke H, Strohschneider T, Oberhoff M, Betz E, Karsch KR. Time course of mitotic activity of smooth muscle cells in the intima and media of arteries following experimental angioplasty. *Circ Res* 1990; 67(3):651–659.
6. Sanborn TA. Laser angioplasty: what has been learned from experimental studies and clinical trials? *Circulation* 1988;78:769–774.
7. Hussein H. A novel fiberoptic laserprobe for treatment of occlusive vessel disease. *Proc SPIE* 1986;605:59–66.
8. Grundfest WS, Litvack F, Goldenberg T, et al. Pulsed ultraviolet lasers and the potential for safe laser angioplasty. *Am J Surg* 1985;150:220–226.
9. Murphy-Chutorian D, Selzer PM, Kosek J, Quay SC, Profitt D, Ginsburg R. The interaction between excimer laser energy and vascular tissue. *Am J Cardiol* 1986;112:739–745.
10. Linsker R, Srinivasan R, Wynne JJ, Alonso DR. Far-ultraviolet laser ablation of atherosclerotic lesions. *Lasers Surg Med* 1984;4:201–205.
11. Haase KK, Wehrmann M, Walz R, Duda S, Karsch KR. Intracoronary excimer laser angioplasty: study on postmortem hearts with angiographic control. *Z Kardiol* 1990:701–706.
12. Isner JM, Gal D, Steg G, et al. Percutaneous in vivo excimer laser angioplasty: results in two experimental animal models. *Lasers Surg Med* 1988;8:223–232.

13. Isner JM. Fibers. In: Isner JM, Clarke RH, eds. Cardiovascular laser therapy. New York: Raven Press, 1989:17–23.
14. Karsch KR, Haase KK, Mauser M, Ickrath O, Voelker W, Duda S. Percutaneous coronary excimer laser angioplasty: initial clinical results. *Lancet* 1989;647–650.
15. Bourassa MG, Aldermann EL, Bertrand M, et al. Report of the joint ISFC/WHO task force on coronary angioplasty. *Circulation* 1988;78:780–789.
16. Karsch KR, Haase KK, Voelker W, Baumbach A, Mauser M, Seipel L. Percutaneous coronary excimer laser angioplasty in patients with stable and unstable angina pectoris—acute results and incidence of restenosis during 6 months follow up. *Circulation* 1990;81:1849–1859.
17. Serruys PW, Luuten HE, Beatt KJ, et al. Incidence of restenosis after successful coronary angioplasty: a time-related phenomenon. A quantitative angiographic study in 342 consecutive patients at 1, 2, 3, and 4 months. *Circulation* 1988;77(2):361–371.
18. Karsch KR, Haase KK, Mauser M, Voelker W. Initial angiographic results in ablation of atherosclerotic plaque by percutaneous coronary excimer laser angioplasty without subsequent balloon dilatation. *Am J Cardiol* 1989;64:1253–1257.
19. Karsch KH, Haase KK, Mauser M, et al. Perkutane transluminale koronare Laserangioplastie. *Dtsch Med Wochenschr* 1989;114:1183–1187.
20. Liu MW, Roubin GS, King SB. Does an optimal luminal result after PTCA reduce restenosis? (abstract). *Circulation* 1989;80(suppl II):II-63.
21. Litvack F, Margolis J, Eigler N, et al. Percutaneous excimer laser coronary angioplasty: results of the first 110 procedures. *J Am Coll Cardiol* 1990;15(suppl A):25A.
22. Sanborn TA, Hershman RA, Siegel RM, et al. Percutaneous coronary excimer laser–assisted balloon angioplasty: initial multicenter experience. *J Am Coll Cardiol* 1990:15(suppl A):25A.

CHAPTER 7

Excimer Laser Coronary Angioplasty: Illustrative Cases and Applications

STEPHEN L. COOK
FRANK LITVACK

SINCE excimer laser coronary angioplasty (ELCA) is a new procedure, many of its technical aspects are still evolving. As operator experience increases and the laser catheters improve, ELCA is being performed on a wider range of coronary lesions, and the indications for the procedure are being defined. Initial experience suggests that excimer laser angioplasty may be useful in several types of lesions considered to be unfavorable for balloon angioplasty (PTCA) (1). These include long lesions, diffuse disease, and aorto-ostial stenoses.

The techniques of ELCA and PTCA are similar in many respects. For example, ELCA is performed using standard angioplasty guide catheters. Other aspects of the procedures differ, however. During ELCA, for example, the operator calibrates the energy emitted by the catheter tip based on the catheter being used and the lesion being treated.

The cases presented in this chapter have been chosen to emphasize the technical aspects of performing excimer laser angioplasty and the potential applications of this technology in the future. In addition, several complications are presented to show how they may be avoided, and if they occur, how they may be managed.

The cases were all performed using the laser and catheter systems manufactured by Advanced Interventional Systems, Inc. (Irvine, Calif.). The specifics of the cases presented may not necessarily be extrapolated to the equipment provided by other excimer laser angioplasty system manufacturers because the laser parameters and catheter designs vary significantly.

The clinical trial that commenced in late 1988 and continues to the time of this writing has included more than 1200 patients and 1500 lesions. As with any new procedure, equipment and dogma are still evolving. Prior to presenting specific case examples, we present some specific technical recommendations on the performance of ELCA. We expect these to continue to evolve but present them as general guidelines. For physicians planning to perform ELCA, the guidelines should not be considered a substitute for, but only a supplement to, a comprehensive training course.

I. ELCA—POTENTIAL CLINICAL INDICATIONS

1. Stenoses of native coronary arteries longer than 10–15 mm.
2. Stenoses or occlusions in saphenous vein grafts.
3. Rigid lesions not dilatable by conventional balloon angioplasty.
4. Aorto-ostial lesions, including those on vein grafts.
5. Left anterior descending ostial lesions.
6. Diffusely diseased coronary segments
7. Selected total occlusions that can be crossed by a coronary guidewire.

II. ELCA—CONTRAINDICATIONS

1. Unprotected left main coronary stenoses.
2. Patient not a candidate for bypass surgery (exception for patients with no other clinical options).
3. Laser catheter diameter >60–70 percent diameter of coronary segment being treated.
4. Lesion not crossable by a guidewire (for "over-the-wire" system).
5. Bifurcation lesions (to be differentiated from lesions involving a side branch).
6. Previously dissected lesions.

III. ELCA RELATIVE CONTRAINDICATIONS

1. Highly eccentric lesions, especially when on a bend. (Eccentricity index >30% [2] Roughly corresponds to lesions on the outer one-third of the artery lumen.)

Excimer Laser Coronary Angioplasty 129

2. Lesions on acute bend >45° (2).

IV. ELCA CATHETER SIZING

CATHETER DIAMETER	MINIMUM ARTERY DIAMETER
1.3 mm	1.8 mm
1.6 mm	2.2 mm
2.0 mm	3.0 mm
2.2 mm	3.3 mm
2.4 mm	3.6 mm

Case 1: Discrete Stenosis
M. W., 78-year-old female

HISTORY	October 1988	Coronary artery bypass grafting
	August 1989	Recurrence of angina; exercise ECG: exercised 4 minutes, 1.5 mm horizontal ST depression in a VF.
PAST HISTORY		Hypertension, claudication
MEDICATIONS		Verapamil, aspirin
CORONARY ANGIOGRAPHY	August 23, 1989	All

ELCA Procedure 8/23/89
Saphenous vein graft to right coronary artery

CASS SEGMENT	GUIDE CATHETER	GUIDEWIRE	LASER CATHETER	ENERGY DENSITY	PULSES	BALLOON CATHETER	NUMBER OF INFLATIONS
Graft to 3	8 Fr. Shiley Multipurpose	0.016" USCI Hyperflex	1.6 mm	42 mJ/mm^2	515	—	—

Discussion: This lesion, a discrete stenosis in a nondegenerated vein graft (Fig. 7.1A), could be treated with ELCA with high probability of acute success (3). Although saphenous vein grafts are often ≥ 4 mm in diameter, the relatively small caliber of this vessel permitted a stand-alone laser procedure with a 1.6-mm laser catheter (Fig. 7.1B). For larger-diameter grafts, the 2.0-mm, 2.2-mm, or 2.4-mm catheters may be used.

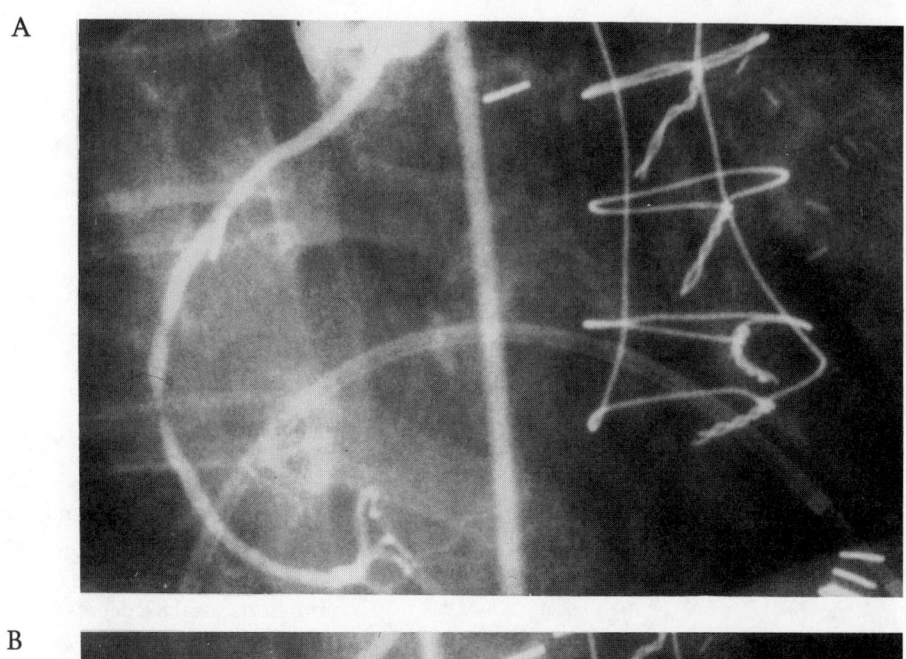

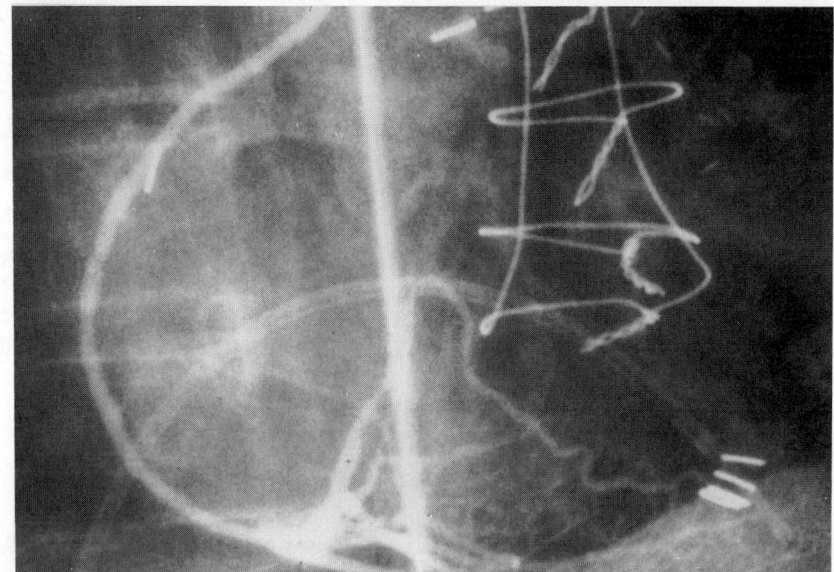

Figure 7.1. ELCA of a discrete stenosis in a saphenous vein graft. *(A)* Baseline angiogram. *(B)* Following ELCA.

Case 2: Ostial LAD Stenosis
C. D., 51-year-old male

HISTORY	July 1989	Asymptomatic. Routine screening exercise ECG: 4-mm downsloping ST depression. Exercise thallium: reversible anterior defect.
	September 8, 1989	Coronary angiography: 90% ostial LAD, 70% mid LAD. Refused bypass surgery.
PAST HISTORY		Total cholesterol 220.
MEDICATIONS		Diltiazem, aspirin.

ELCA Procedure 12/22/89
Left anterior descending artery

CASS SEGMENT	GUIDE CATHETER	GUIDE WIRE	LASER CATHETER	ENERGY DENSITY	PULSES	BALLOON CATHETER	NUMBER OF INFLATIONS
12	9 Fr. Shiley JL4	0.018" ACS laser wire	1.6 mm	35 mJ/mm^2	340 (proximal and mid)	—	—
12	9 Fr. Shiley JL4	0.018" ACS laser wire	2.0 mm	35 mJ/mm^2	160	—	—
13	9 Fr. Shiley JL4	0.018" ACS laser wire	1.6 mm	35 mJ/mm^2	340 (proximal and mid)	2.5-mm Medtronic Thruflex II	1

Discussion: PTCA of ostial lesions has a lower acute success rate and higher complication and restenosis rates (4). This patient has a severe ostial LAD lesion classified as ACC/AHA type B (Fig. 7.2A) as well as a mid-LAD stenosis (not shown) classified as type A. Following laser angioplasty with a 1.6-mm laser catheter, both lesions were improved, but there was a localized dissection of the mid-LAD stenosis. This dissection was "tacked up" with a single, long inflation. The ostial stenosis was then treated with a 2.0-mm laser catheter (Fig. 7.2B). Recent data has demonstrated high (>90%) acute success rates on ostial stenoses (5). Discrete lesions such as the one in CASS segment 13 of this patient

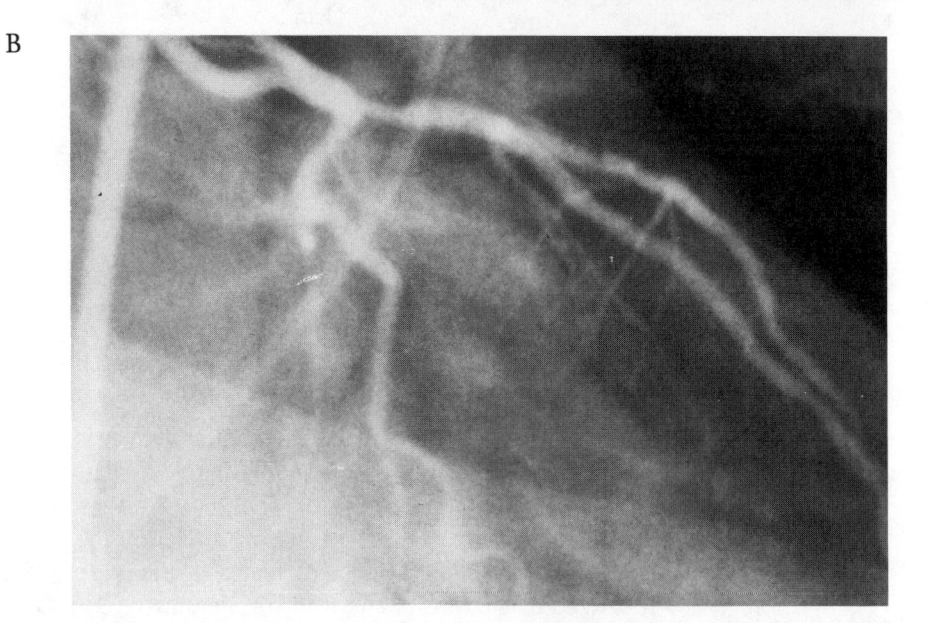

Figure 7.2. ELCA of an ostial LAD stenosis. *(A)* Baseline angiogram. *(B)* Following ELCA.

Excimer Laser Coronary Angioplasty 133

are probably best treated by conventional balloon angioplasty. In contrast to type B or C lesions, these type A lesions may have a higher acute occlusion rate and incidence of major ischemic complications when treated with ELCA as compared to PTCA (1,6). This data was not yet available at the time this patient was treated.

Case 3: Failed Balloon Angioplasty
Z. Y., 76-year-old male

HISTORY	February 1988	Acute inferior myocardial infarction
	August 1988	Admitted with unstable angina. Coronary angiography revealed a severe proximal stenosis of the right coronary artery. Refused balloon angioplasty.
	November 1988	Admitted with unstable angina. Refused interventional therapy.
	January 1989	Admitted with unstable angina.
PAST HISTORY		Hypertension, non–insulin dependent diabetes mellitus
MEDICATIONS		Verapamil, Metoprolol, aspirin
CORONARY ANGIOGRAPHY	January 24, 1989	Left ventriculography: inferior hypokinesis. LAD normal. 60% obtuse marginal. Severe proximal RCA stenosis.
ATTEMPTED BALLOON ANGIOPLASTY	January 24, 1989	Right coronary lesion crossed with guidewire, but could not be crossed with any balloon.

ELCA Procedure 1/26/89
Proximal right coronary artery

CASS SEGMENT	GUIDE CATHETER	GUIDEWIRE	LASER CATHETER	ENERGY DENSITY	PULSES	BALLOON CATHETER	NUMBER OF INFLATIONS
1	Interventional Medical AL .75	0.018" ACS High-torque Intermediate	1.6 mm	40mJ/mm^2	412	3.0-mm ACS Simpson-Robert	2

Discussion: Despite the continuing improvement of balloon- and guide-catheter technology, some coronary stenoses cannot be crossed with a balloon or adequately dilated (7). In this case, a long, calcified proximal RCA stenosis (Fig. 7.3A) could be crossed with a guidewire, but not with any balloon catheter, even fixed-wire systems. The lesion was crossed without difficulty with a 1.6-mm laser catheter at 40 mJ/mm^2 (Fig. 7.3B). If this catheter had not crossed the lesion, the next step would be to either 1) increase the energy density to 45 mJ/mm^2 (up to 55 mJ/mm^2, if necessary, with this catheter); or 2) perform laser angioplasty with a 1.3-mm catheter at 50–60 mJ/mm^2. At the time this procedure was performed, the 2.0-mm catheter was not yet available, so an adjunctive PTCA was performed to achieve a final stenosis of < 50% (Fig. 7.3C). This patient was treated relatively early in our experience. More recently, we would have approached this patient first with a 1.3-mm catheter at 55–60 mJ/mm^2 and then exchanged for a larger laser catheter.

A

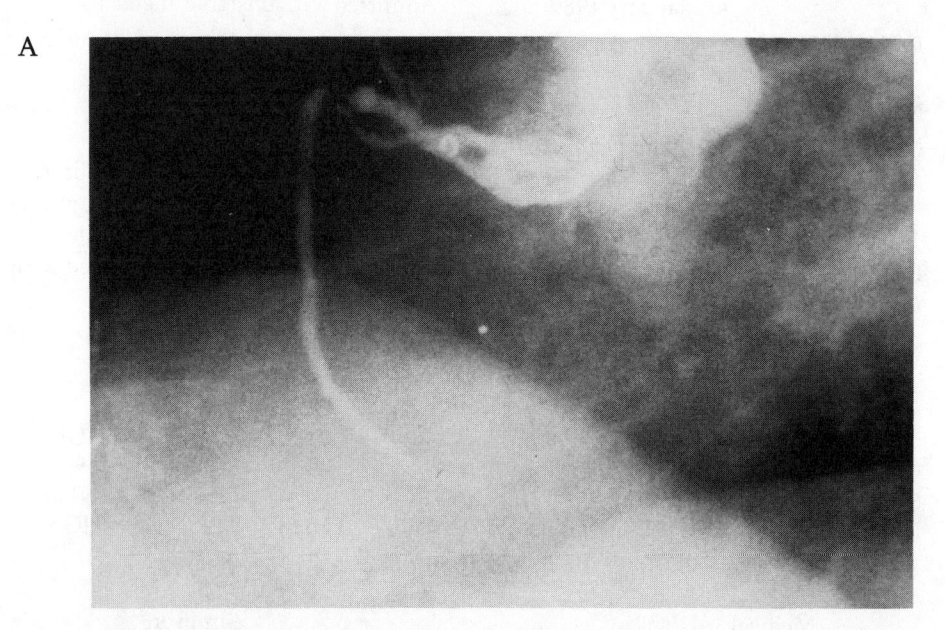

Figure 7.3. ELCA of a proximal right coronary artery stenosis following failed PTCA. *(A)* Baseline angiogram.

Excimer Laser Coronary Angioplasty 135

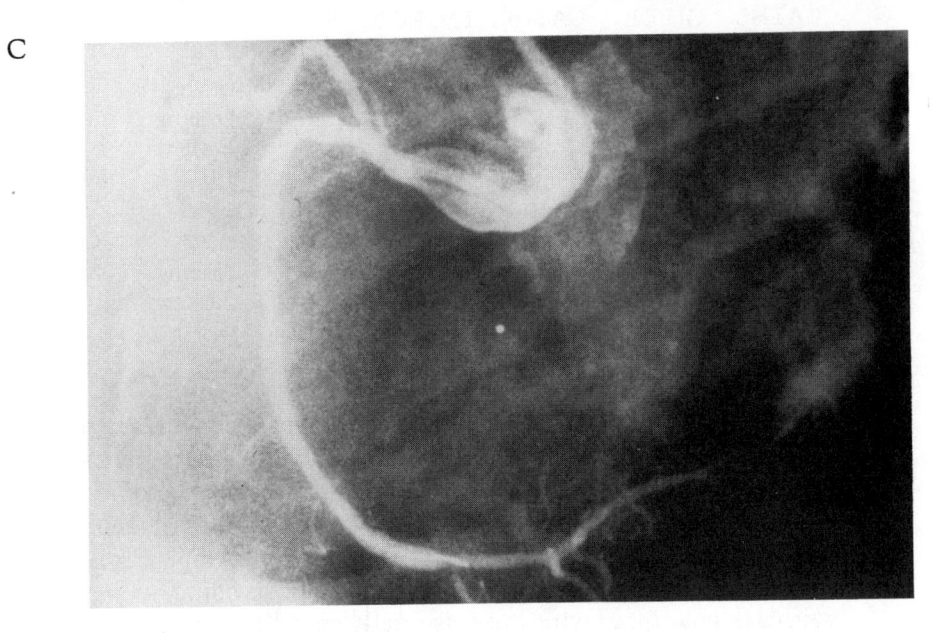

Figure 7.3. *(B)* Following ELCA. *(C)* Following adjunctive PTCA.

Case 4: Bend Point Lesion
D. Z., 66-year-old male

HISTORY	1982	Coronary artery bypass grafting
	May 7, 1989	Admitted with non–Q wave myocardial infarction (CPK 200 U, 17% MB)
PAST HISTORY		Hypertension
MEDICATIONS		Blocadren, Aldactizide, Persantine, aspirin
CORONARY AND GRAFT ANGIOGRAPHY	May 11, 1989	75% proximal LAD. 90% obtuse marginal. 100% proximal RCA. Grafts to LAD, diagonal, and RCA patent. Graft to obtuse marginal diffusely degenerated.

ELCA Procedure 5/18/89
Obtuse marginal

CASS SEGMENT	GUIDE CATHETER	GUIDEWIRE	LASER CATHETER	ENERGY DENSITY	PULSES	BALLOON CATHETER	NUMBER OF INFLATIONS
20	Interventional Medical AL-2	0.018" ACS High-torque Floppy	—	—	—	USCI Probing Catheter	—
20	Interventional Medical AL-2	0.018" ACS HT Intermediate	1.6	40	273	USCI Probing Catheter	—

Discussion: PTCA on major bend points is associated with a higher risk of dissection and vessel closure (8,9). In this case, a severe stenosis of an obtuse marginal immediately proximal to the distal anastomosis of an occluded bypass graft is between two sharp bends in the vessel (Fig. 7.4A). Because of the tortuosity of the vessel, a left Amplatz guide catheter was used for maximum support. The stenosis could not be crossed with a floppy-tipped wire, but was finally crossed with an intermediate wire with a USCI probing catheter used for additional support. Following laser angioplasty, there is a mild residual stenosis with no evidence of dissection or perforation (Fig. 7.4B).

Excimer Laser Coronary Angioplasty 137

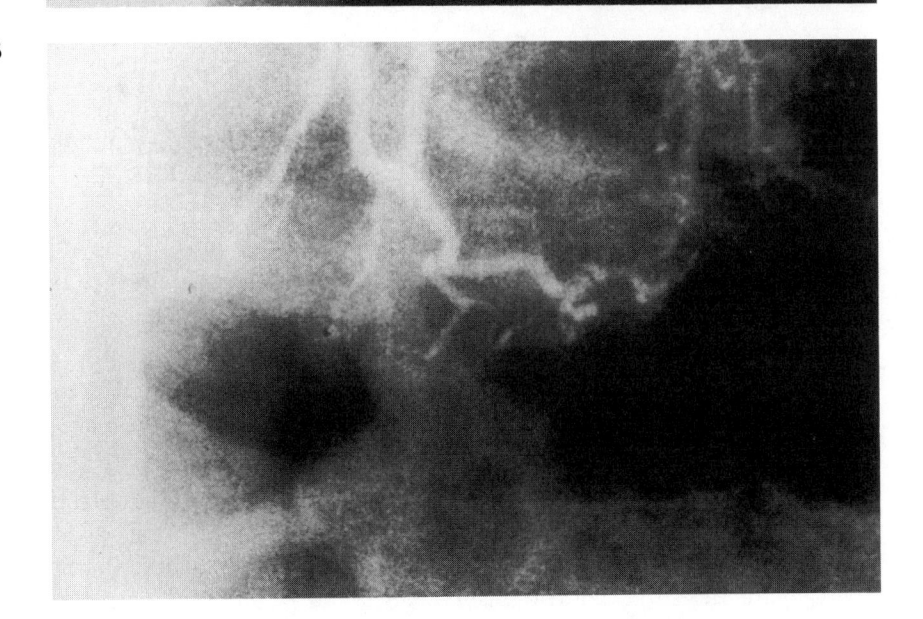

Figure 7.4. ELCA of a bend point lesion in an obtuse marginal. *(A)* Baseline angiogram. *(B)* Following ELCA.

Case 5: Long Stenosis
E. S., 29-year-old male

HISTORY	1987	Onset of exertional angina.
	September 1989	Complained of severe, daily angina.
	September 18, 1989	Exercise thallium: exercised 5:35, stopping due to severe chest pain at 61% maximum predicted heart rate. Thallium: reversible anterior defect.
PAST HISTORY		Hypercholesterolemia (288)
MEDICATIONS		Mevacor, niacin, Diltiazem, aspirin
CORONARY ANGIOGRAPHY	September 22, 1989	Normal left ventricular wall motion. Long, severe proximal LAD stenosis.

ELCA Procedure 9/22/89
Left anterior descending

CASS SEGMENT	GUIDE CATHETER	GUIDEWIRE	LASER CATHETER	ENERGY DENSITY	PULSES	BALLOON CATHETER	NUMBER OF INFLATIONS
12	8 Fr. Shiley SL4	0.018" ACS laser wire	1.6 mm	38 mJ/mm^2	780	—	—

Discussion: This lesion of the LAD is not ideal for PTCA due to its length and irregular borders (Fig. 7.5A) (8,9). Laser angioplasty alone with a 1.6-mm catheter achieved an adequate result (Fig. 7.5B) At the time this procedure was performed, the 2.0-mm catheter was not yet available, so no additional procedure was performed. At more than 6 months follow-up, this patient is asymptomatic with a normal stress test, but refuses angiographic follow-up. Currently, this procedure would probably be performed with the 2.0-mm- or 2.2-mm-diameter catheter following the 1.3-mm device.

Excimer Laser Coronary Angioplasty 139

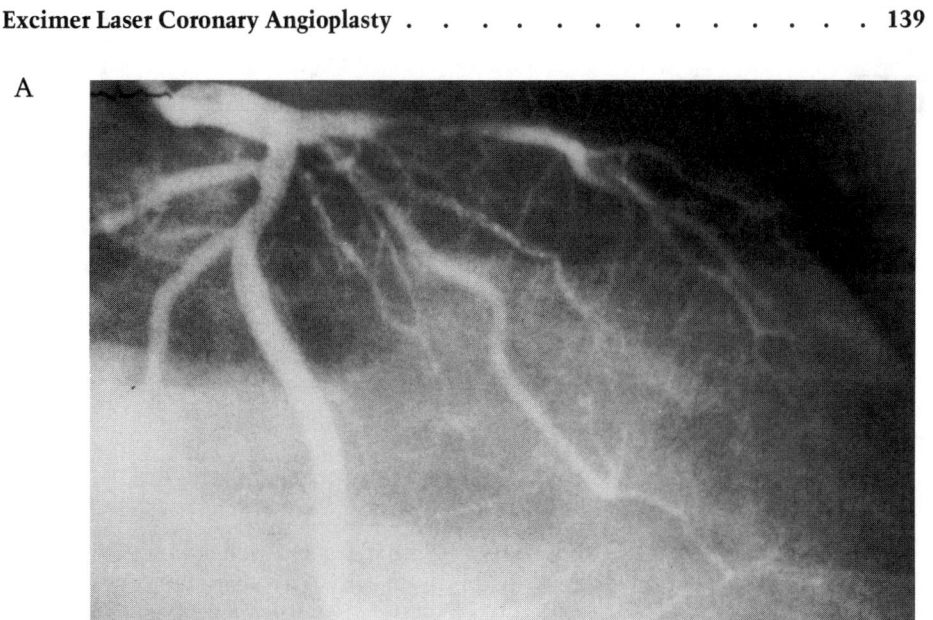

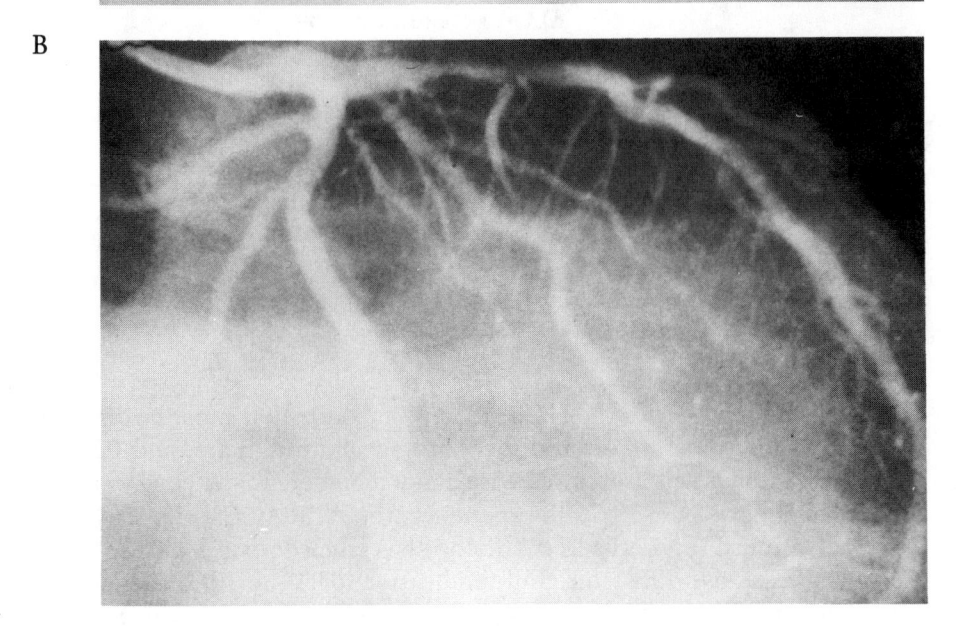

Figure 7.5. ELCA of a long, irregular stenosis of the proximal left anterior descending. *(A)* Baseline angiogram. *(B)* Following ELCA.

Case 6: Diffuse Disease
A. H., 53-year-old male

HISTORY	1989	New onset angina
	March 16, 1989	Exercise thallium: exercised 10:21. ECG: 2-mm down-sloping ST depression in V5. Planar and tomographic thallium imaging: severe, extensive reversible defect involving the inferior and posterolateral wall.
PAST HISTORY		Noncontributory
MEDICATIONS		Diltiazem, aspirin
CORONARY ANGIOGRAPHY	March 24, 1989	Normal left ventricular function. LAD normal. RCA nondominant. Severe, diffuse disease of circumflex.

ELCA Procedure 4/3/89
Obtuse marginal

CASS SEGMENT	GUIDE CATHETER	GUIDEWIRE	LASER CATHETER	ENERGY DENSITY	PULSES	BALLOON CATHETER	NUMBER OF INFLATIONS
18, 20	Interventional Medical AL-2	0.018" ACS High-Torque Floppy	1.6 mm	43 mJ/mm^2	2,239	—	—

Discussion: Due to the large amount of plaque that must be displaced, diffuse lesions are often difficult to adequately dilate, and PTCA of these stenoses is associated with a much higher incidence of vessel closure (4,9). Because of this experience, the ACP/ACC/AHA Task Force on Clinical Privileges in Cardiology has labeled severe, diffuse disease of a vessel as an absolute contraindication to PTCA (10). Diffuse lesions are often difficult to treat surgically as well, since the caliber of these vessels is frequently insufficient to permit implantation of a bypass graft. In this case, a diffusely diseased dominant circumflex (Fig. 7.6A) was successfully treated with laser alone (Fig. 7.6B) over its entire length. Due to the length of the lesion and some tortuosity of the vessel,

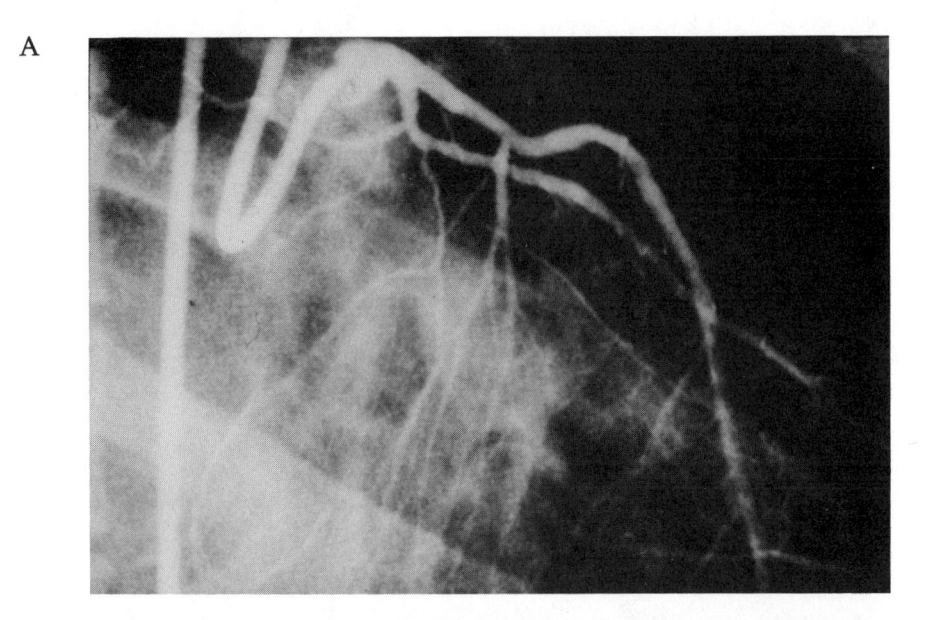

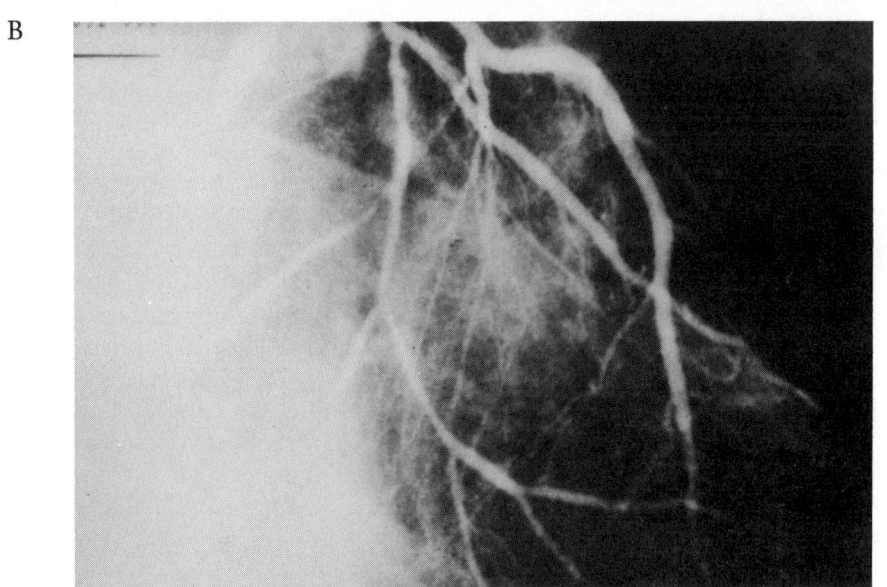

Figure 7.6. ELCA of a diffuse lesion of an obtuse marginal. *(A)* Baseline angiogram. *(B)* Following ELCA.

a left Amplatz guide catheter was used for maximal guide support. The large number of pulses used reflects the extensive length of the vessel treated. Currently, this procedure would be started with the 1.3-mm catheter at 50–70 mJ/mm^2 (not available in April 1989). This would probably be followed with a 1.6-mm catheter at 50 mJ/mm^2, conventional balloon angioplasty, or both.

Case 7: Aorto-ostial Lesion
A. W., 75-year-old male

HISTORY	1980	Inferior myocardial infarction. Coronary artery bypass surgery: saphenous vein grafts to LAD, OM1, OM2.
	October 1989	Developed rest and exertional angina.
PAST HISTORY		Hypertension. CVA 1985. Non–insulin dependent diabetes mellitus.
MEDICATIONS		Micronase, Isordil, Cardene, Lasix, aspirin.
CORONARY ANGIOGRAPHY	October 1989	RAO left ventriculogram: severe, diffuse hypokinesis. LAD, LCX, RCA all occluded proximally. Grafts to LAD and OM1: mild, diffuse disease. Graft to OM2: severe ostial stenosis.

ELCA Procedure 12/5/89
Saphenous vein graft to obtuse marginal

CASS SEGMENT	GUIDE CATHETER	GUIDEWIRE	LASER CATHETER	ENERGY DENSITY	PULSES	BALLOON CATHETER	NUMBER OF INFLATIONS
Vein graft to 21	9 Fr. Shiley JR4	0.018″ ACS laser wire	1.6 mm	35 mJ/mm^2	120	—	—
Vein graft to 21	9 Fr. Shiley JR4	0.018″ ACS laser wire	2.0 mm	35 mJ/mm^2	460	—	—

Excimer Laser Coronary Angioplasty 143

Discussion: Aorto-ostial stenoses are often difficult to treat with PTCA. Guide catheters often do not engage the vessel well enough to provide adequate support for crossing high-grade stenoses with a balloon (11,12). Because these lesions are frequently elastic, calcified, or both, high inflation pressures, oversized balloons, or both are often required, which increases the risk of dissection (12). This procedure on a discrete aorto-ostial stenosis of a saphenous vein graft to an obtuse marginal (Fig. 7.7A) was further complicated by extreme tortuosity in the patient's aortoiliac system, which made extensive guide catheter manipulation impossible. After the stenosis was crossed with a guidewire, however, guide catheter position was not important to the success of the procedure. Multiple passes were made with 1.6- and 2.0-mm catheters with the guide catheter disengaged from the ostium, giving a good stand-alone result (Fig. 7.7B). Excimer laser angioplasty of a calcified right coronary ostial stenosis is discussed in Case 9. More recently, a 2.2-mm or 2.4-mm catheter could have been used to complete the procedure.

A

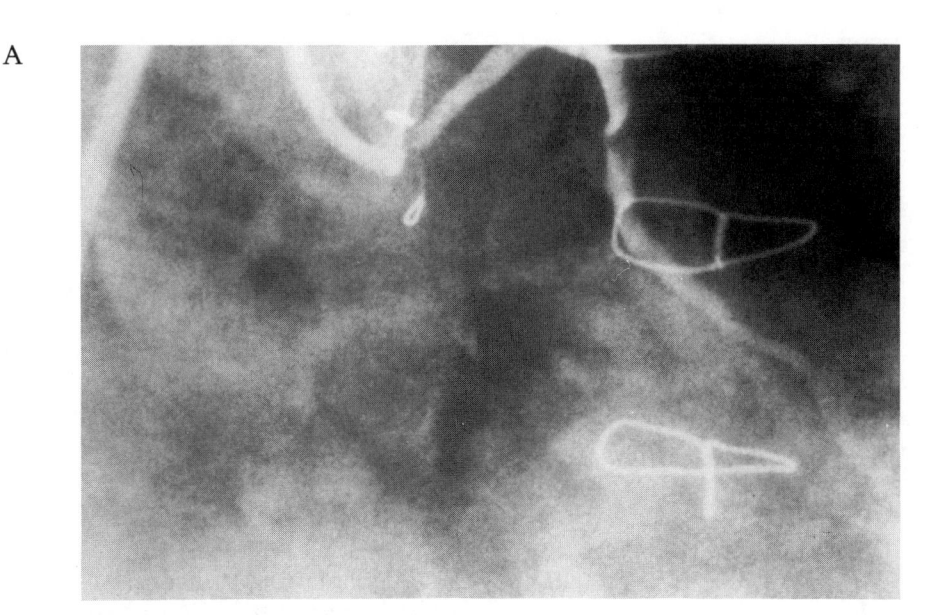

Figure 7.7. ELCA of an aortoostial stenosis of a saphenous vein graft to an obtuse marginal. *(A)* Baseline angiogram.

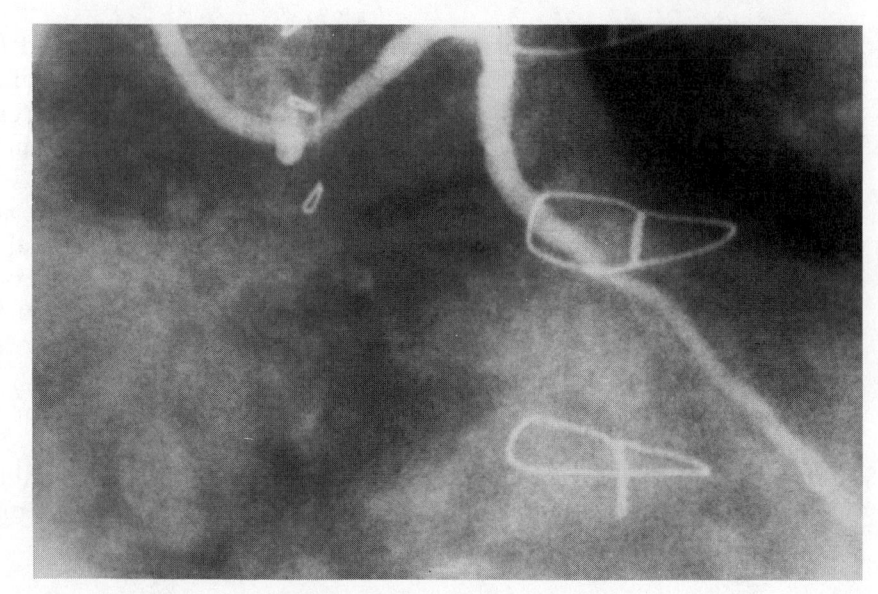

Figure 7.7. *(B)* Following ELCA.

Case 8: Long Total Occlusion
F. W., 39-year-old male

HISTORY	1989	New-onset angina.
	May 1989	Severe, prolonged episode of angina. Ruled out for myocardial infarction by ECG, enzymes. Subsequently had frequent, severe angina with minimal exertion.
	August 1989	Exercise thallium: exercised 3:00. ECG: ST depression in inferior leads. Planar thallium imaging: reversible inferior defect.
PAST HISTORY		Noncontributory.
MEDICATIONS		Diltiazem, aspirin.
CORONARY ANGIOGRAPHY	August 8, 1989	Normal left ventricular wall motion. LAD and circumflex normal. 100% occlusion of distal RCA with collaterals from circumflex.

ELCA Procedure 8/15/89
Distal right coronary artery and posterior descending artery

CASS SEG-MENT	GUIDE CATHE-TER	GUIDE-WIRE	LASER CATHE-TER	ENERGY DENSITY	PULSES	BALLOON CATHE-TER	NUMBER OF INFLA-TIONS
3	8 Fr. Interventional Medical AL .75	0.016" USCI Hyperflex	1.6	42	840 total pulses	3.0	2
4	8 Fr. Interventional Medical AL .75	0.016" USCI Hyperflex	1.6	42	840 total pulses	—	—

Discussion: Balloon angioplasty of chronic total occlusions has a lower acute success rate than PTCA of subtotal occlusions, mostly due to difficulty crossing the occlusion with a guidewire (13,14). As an over-the-wire system, the excimer laser system used in these cases shares the same limitation. In our experience, however, many total occlusions are long, occur in diffusely diseased arteries, or involve major side branches, situations in which laser angioplasty may be superior to PTCA. In this case, a chronic occlusion of the distal right coronary artery (Fig. 7.8A), the occlusion occurred in a diffusely diseased segment extending into the posterior descending artery. The PDA could not be entered with a guidewire, so another distal branch was wired. Following initial laser angioplasty, enough antegrade flow was established that the PDA could be visualized angiographically (Fig. 7.8B) and entered with a guidewire (Fig. 7.8C). Laser angioplasty was then repeated, extending into the diseased portion of the PDA. Following ELCA, adjunctive balloon PTCA was performed on the proximal portion of the lesion for the final result shown in Fig. 7.8D. In this case, ultimate success depended on not closing the PDA when performing laser angioplasty of the distal RCA with the guidewire in another branch. In our experience to date, we have not observed closure of any major ($\geq$ 1 mm in diameter) side branches originating from a lesion treated with excimer angioplasty. This difference between ELCA and PTCA is presumably due to plaque ablation (rather than plaque displacement) occurring during laser angioplasty.

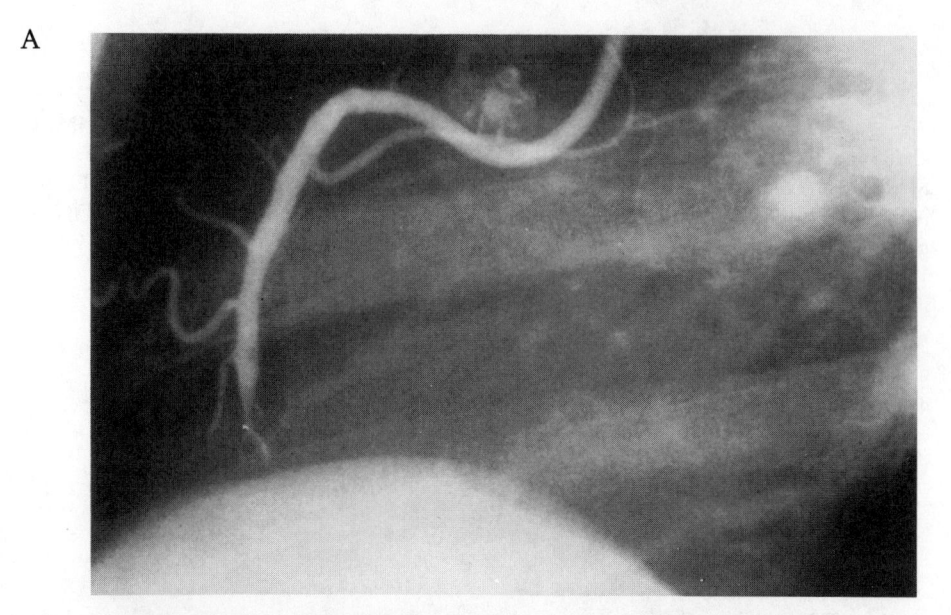

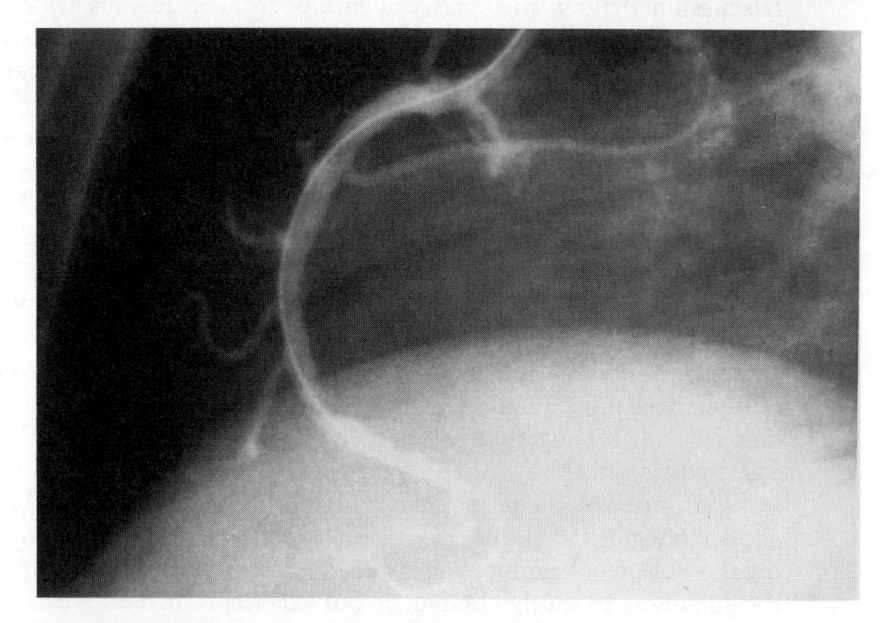

Figure 7.8. ELCA of a long total occlusion of a right coronary artery. *(A)* Baseline angiogram. *(B)* Following initial laser angioplasty.

Excimer Laser Coronary Angioplasty 147

C

D

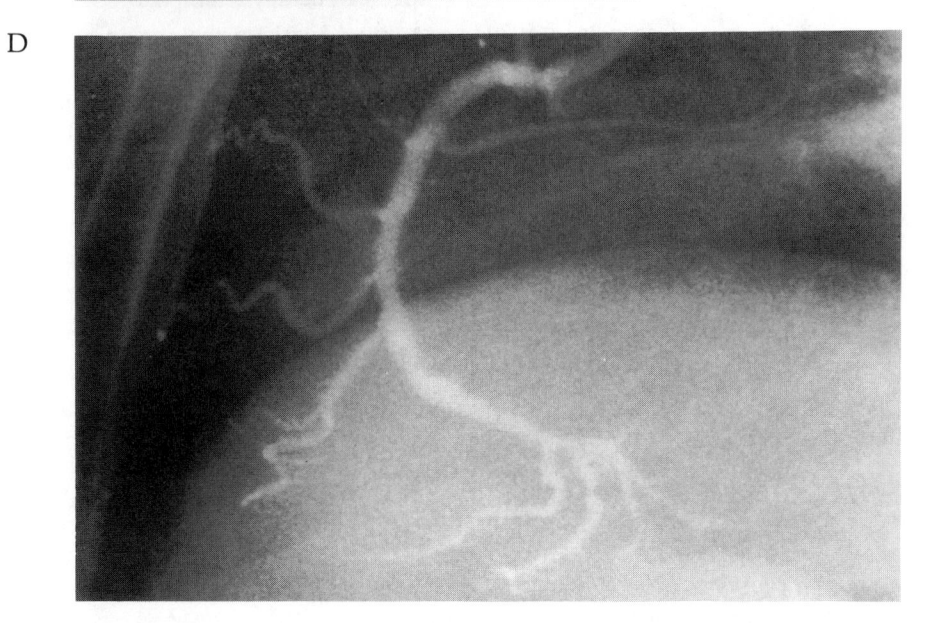

Figure 7.8. *(C)* Guidewire redirected into the posterior descending artery. *(D)* Following repeated ELCA and adjunctive PTCA of the proximal portion.

Case 9: Ostial Right Coronary
R. C., 41-year-old male

HISTORY	1987	Gradual onset of exertional angina and dyspnea.
	June 1989	Worsening symptoms. Exercise ECG: exercised 3:54, stopping due to angina. ECG: ST depression in inferior and lateral leads. Coronary angiography: severe calcification of aortic root, LV normal, left coronary system normal, severe ostial RCA stenosis.
	August 1989	Single-vessel bypass with right internal mammary artery bypass to RCA.
	October 1989	Recurrence of angina. Coronary angiography: right internal mammary graft closed, otherwise unchanged. Medical therapy attempted.
	December 8, 1989	Admitted with unstable angina. Transferred for ELCA.
PAST HISTORY		Metabolic disorder characterized by calcium deposition in arteries, gall bladder, joints, corneas. Metabolic work-up negative.
MEDICATIONS		Diltiazem, antenolol, nitroglycerin patch, aspirin

ELCA Procedure 12/15/89
Right coronary artery ostium

CASS SEGMENT	GUIDE CATHETER	GUIDEWIRE	LASER CATHETER	ENERGY DENSITY	PULSES	BALLOON CATHETER	NUMBER OF INFLATIONS
1	8 Fr. Shiley JR3.5	0.018" ACS High-Torque Intermediate	1.3 mm	50 mJ/mm^2	—	—	—

CASS SEG-MENT	GUIDE CATHE-TER	GUIDE-WIRE	LASER CATHE-TER	ENERGY DENSITY	PULSES	BALLOON CATHE-TER	NUMBER OF INFLA-TIONS
1	8 Fr. Shiley JR3.5	0.018" ACS High-Torque Intermediate	1.6 mm	40 mJ/mm^2	—	—	—
1	9 Fr. Shiley JR4	0.018" ACS laser wire	2.0 mm	—	—	—	—

Discussion: This patient had a heavily calcified aorto-ostial stenosis of the right coronary artery producing severe angina (Fig. 7.9A). Due to heavy calcification of the ascending aorta, routine coronary artery bypass surgery could not be performed. A right internal mammary bypass graft was placed to the RCA using femoral-femoral bypass, with initial resolution of symptoms. Within 2 months, however, his angina had recurred and angiography revealed closure of the graft.

At the beginning of the laser procedure, no guide catheter would intubate the right coronary ostium. A right Judkins catheter was manipulated to sit just outside the ostium, and the stenosis was crossed with a guidewire. Due to the heavy calcification of the lesion, it was decided to begin with a 1.3-mm catheter calibrated to have an energy density of 45 mJ/mm^2. After debulking the lesion with this catheter, ablation was repeated with a 1.6-mm catheter at 37 mJ/mm^2, leaving a moderate residual stenosis (Fig. 7.9B). Laser angioplasty with a 2.0-mm catheter produced further improvement. It was attempted to enlarge the lumen further by turning the guide catheter to change the angle at which the laser catheter entered the vessel on subsequent passes. During one pass, the catheter entered at an acute angle, producing a small perforation of the inferior surface of the vessel (Fig. 7.9C). No extravasation of contrast into the pericardium was observed. The patient's heparinization was immediately reversed with protamine. Serial echocardiograms revealed no pericardial effusion. Repeat coronary angiography the next day revealed no change in the appearance of the vessel. The patient has remained asymptomatic since ELCA. Follow-up angiography at 6 months revealed no restenosis (Fig. 7.9D).

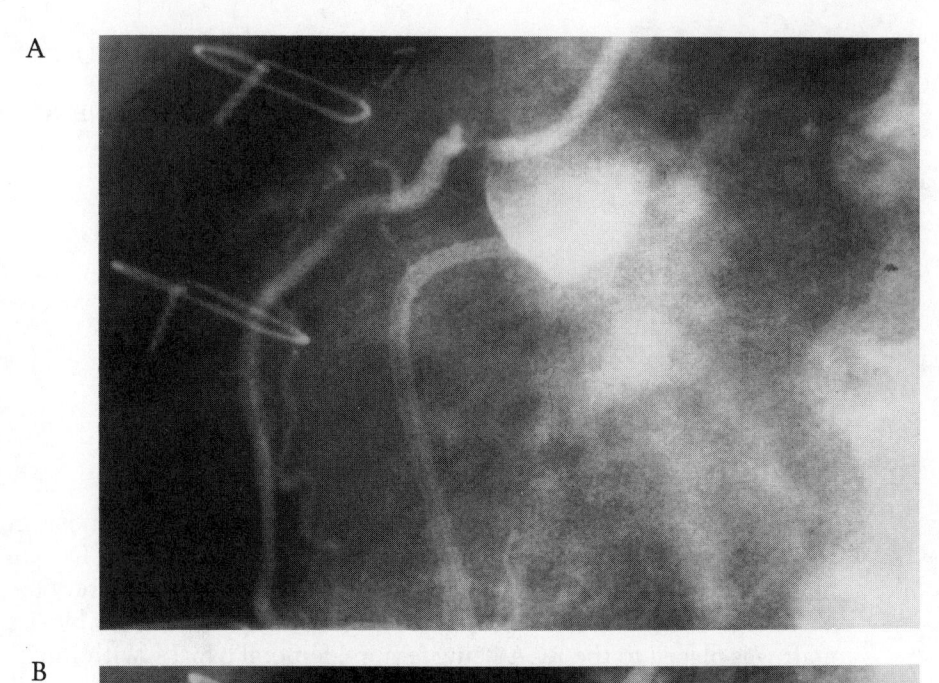

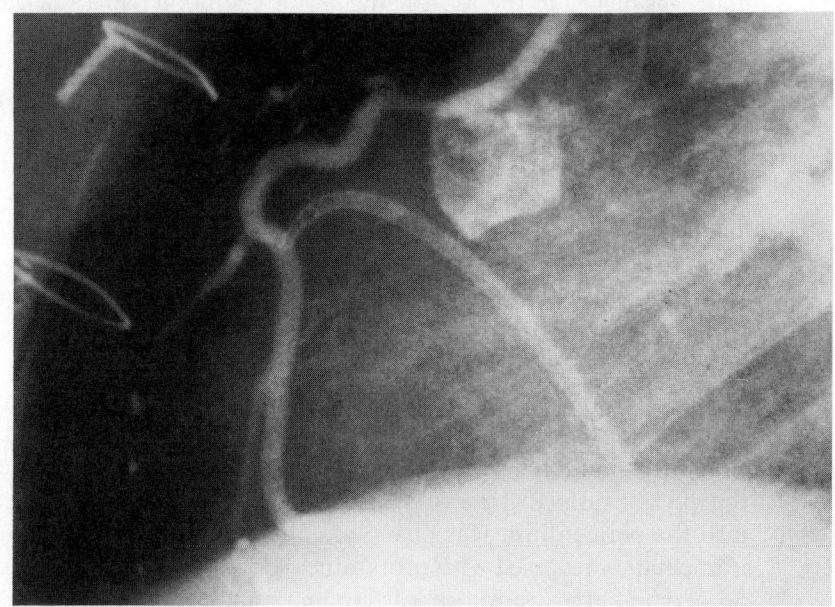

Figure 7.9. ELCA of a calcified right coronary ostial stenosis resulting in perforation. *(A)* Baseline angiogram. *(B)* Following ELCA with a 1.6-mm laser catheter.

Excimer Laser Coronary Angioplasty 151

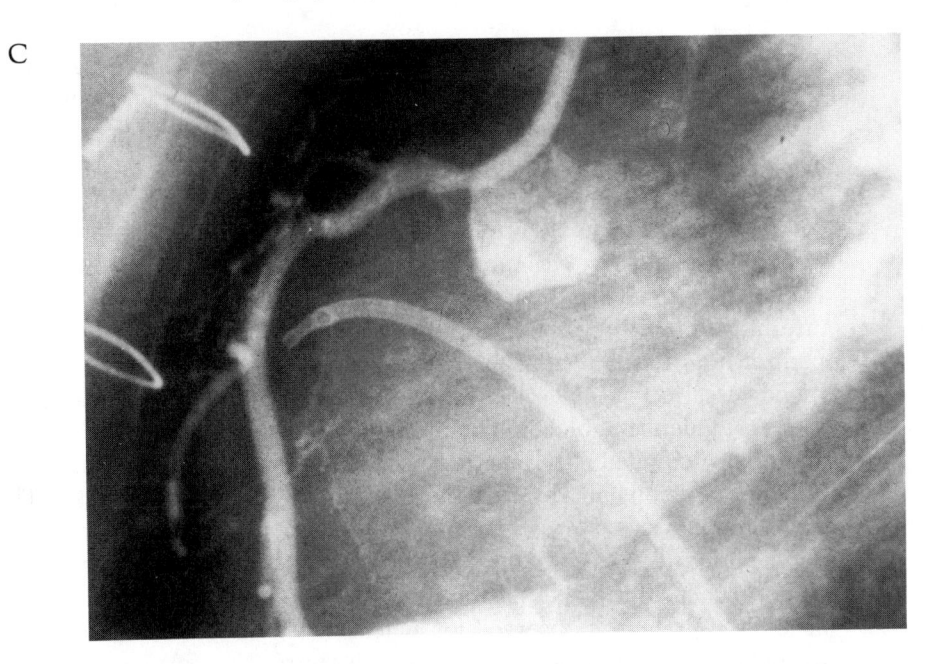

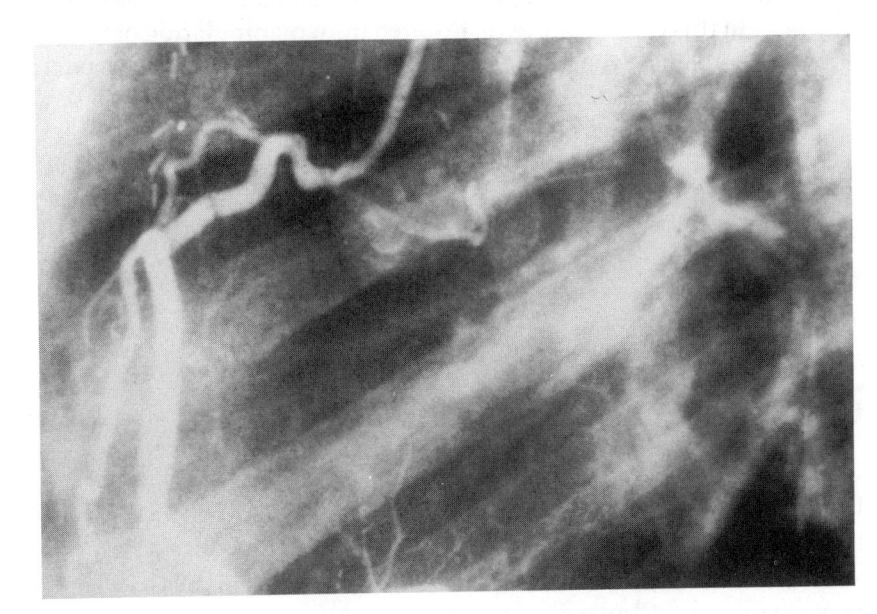

Figure 7.9. *(C)* Following ELCA with a 2.0-mm catheter. *(D)* Six-month follow-up.

The manifestations of coronary perforation complicating ELCA range from minor extravasation of contrast into the adventitia without clinical sequellae, such as in this case, to a massive leak into the pericardial space producing near-instantaneous cardiac tamponade. The incidence of this complication has been just over 1 percent. Most perforations can be avoided and have occurred in the following situations: multiple passes with the laser catheter; lasing of highly eccentric lesions, especially those on bends; using a laser catheter >70 percent of the normal arterial diameter; and lasing at bifurcation points. Successful therapy of perforations depends on immediate recognition. In all cases, we recommend cessation of the laser procedure and reversal of heparinization. If there is evidence of bleeding into the pericardial space, the perforation should be occluded with an inflated balloon. Preferably, this should be an autoperfusion balloon to maintain distal perfusion in the vessel. The patient should then have emergency bypass surgery with repair or ligation of the perforated vessel. If tamponade occurs, pericardiocentesis should be performed. If the leak is small and does not involve the pericardial space, the patient is observed for at least 24 hours in the ICU with a Swan-Ganz catheter and serial echocardiograms.

In this case, perforation resulted from manipulation of the guide catheter to make the laser catheter enter the vessel in a noncoaxial position and thus produce a lumen larger than the diameter of the laser catheter. This technique had been successful in several earlier cases of aorto-ostial lesions. Based on our experience with this case, however, we now recommend keeping the laser catheter coaxial with the vessel at all times.

Case 10: Laser Dissection
D.C., 65-year-old female

HISTORY		Class III angina
PAST HISTORY		Diabetes, hypertension
MEDICATIONS		ASA, Cardizem, NTG
CORONARY ANGIOGRAPHY	September 15, 1989	Normal left ventricular function. Normal LAD and circumflex. Severe stenosis of proximal RCA.

ELCA Procedure 12/15/89
Right Coronary Artery

CASS SEG-MENT	GUIDE CATHE-TER	GUIDE-WIRE	LASER CATHE-TER	ENERGY DENSITY	PULSES	BALLOON CATHE-TER	NUMBER OF INFLA-TIONS
1	9 Fr. Shiley JR4	0.018" ACS laser wire	1.6 mm	42 mJ/mm^2	480	—	—
1	9 Fr. Shiley JR4	0.018" ACS laser wire	2.0 mm	42 mJ/mm^2	500	—	—

Discussion: Dissection during ELCA is postulated to occur by three mechanisms: 1) mechanical disruption by the laser catheter, 2) disruption by gas bubbles produced during laser ablation of tissue, 3) disruption by photoacoustical shock waves produced by transmission of high-energy laser pulses through the catheter. Like dissections produced by balloon angioplasty, laser dissections can be minor or can lead to acute closure of a vessel.

In this case, a severe stenosis of the proximal right coronary artery (Fig. 7.10A) was treated with ELCA. Following laser angioplasty with the 2.0-mm catheter, there was a severe dissection extending back to the right coronary ostium (Fig. 7.10B). Because the lumen was adequate and flow into the distal vessel was unimpaired, it was decided not to perform adjunctive balloon angioplasty. The patient had an uncomplicated hospital course, and her symptoms and abnormal stress test were resolved. Angiographic follow-up 6 months following the procedure revealed that the dissection had healed with a good residual lumen.

Our approach to a dissection following laser angioplasty depends on the extent of the dissection and the effect on flow through the vessel. If, as in this case, the residual lumen is adequate (<30%) and flow is unimpaired, adjunctive balloon angioplasty is not performed. If, however, the dissection leaves significant stenosis or flow is sluggish, we attempt to tack down the dissection with a balloon. In our experience, attempting laser angioplasty on a disrupted artery (following balloon dissection) often results in a more severe or extensive dissection. We currently consider an acutely disrupted artery, due to either balloon or laser angioplasty, to be a relative contraindication to ELCA.

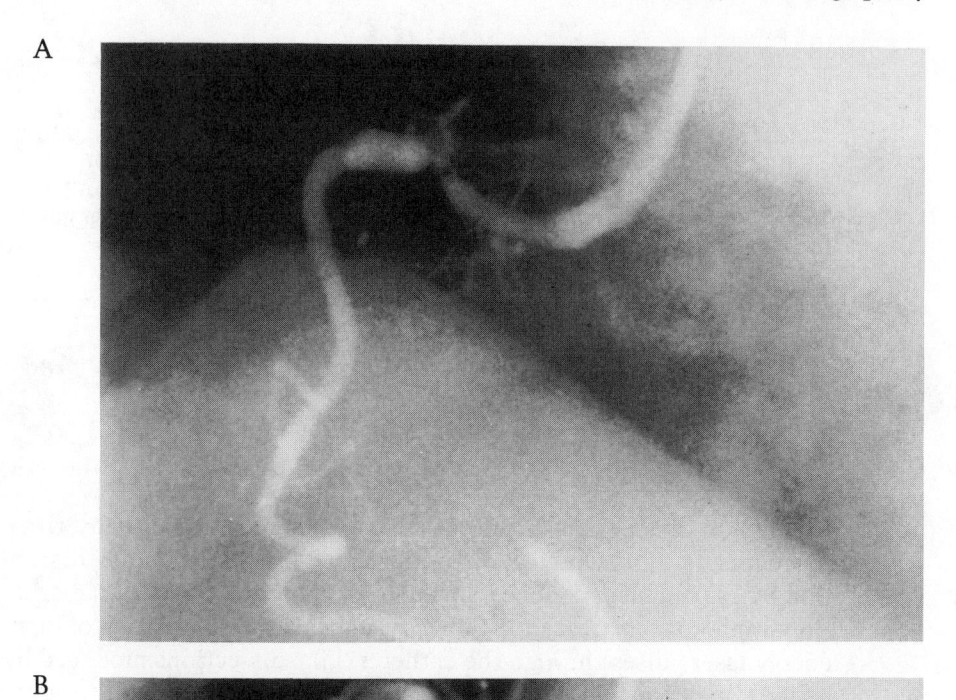

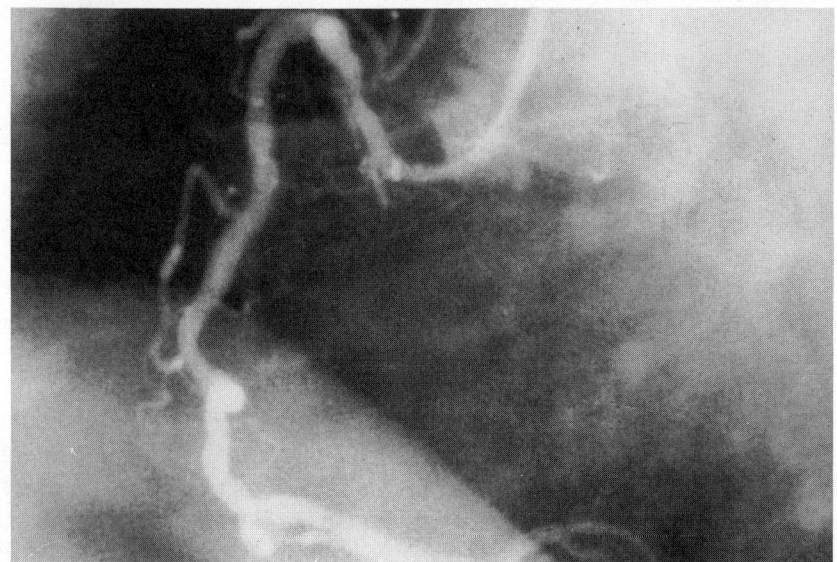

Figure 7.10. ELCA of a proximal right coronary artery stenosis, resulting in a dissection. *(A)* Baseline angiogram. *(B)* Following ELCA.

Case 11: Mechanical Dissection
E. P., 75-year-old male

HISTORY	April 1982	Saphenous vein bypass grafting to LAD and LCX.
	September 8, 1989	Recurrent angina pectoris functional class III. Coronary angiography—99% mid-RCA stenosis with 50% slightly more distal stenosis. Patent saphenous vein graft to LAD and LCX. Inferior wall hypokinesia on left ventriculography.
	September 11, 1989	RCA angioplasty complicated by large dissection extending over several centimeters. Subsequent total occlusion of angioplasty site with inferior subendocardial infarction (CPK 820) with no ECG changes.
	September–December 1989	Continued angina pectoris with positive thallium treadmill for inferolateral-wall ischemia.
PAST HISTORY		Peripheral vascular disease with claudication.
MEDICATIONS		Aspirin, Procardia, Persantine
CORONARY ANGIOGRAPHY	December 1989	Sequential 90% mid-RCA stenoses with good antegrade flow, patent SVG to LAD, LCX, marked inferior wall hypokinesia on left ventriculography.

ELCA Procedure 12/21/89
Right coronary artery

CASS SEGMENT	GUIDE CATHETER	GUIDEWIRE	LASER CATHETER	ENERGY DENSITY	PULSES	BALLOON CATHETER	NUMBER OF INFLATIONS
3	8 Fr. Shiley AL2	0.018" ACS HTS/F	1.6 mm	45 mJ/mm^2	0	2.5-mm ACS RX	Numerous inflations performed along the length of the vessel from the midportion to the posterior descending.

Quantitative Coronary Angiography

	BASELINE	POSTLASER	POSTBALLOON
MINIMAL ARTERIAL DIAMETER	.30 mm	N/A	1.29 mm
PERCENT STENOSIS	84%	N/A	18%

Discussion: Prior to laser catheter insertion, angiography with guiding catheter confirmed good guidewire positioning of the distal RCA with no evidence of dissection. Immediately after advancing the 1.6-mm–12-fiber AIS excimer laser catheter into the RCA proximal to the lesion, a test injection through the guiding catheter demonstrated extensive dissection of the RCA of the midportion just proximal to the lesion and extending distally into the posterior descending and posterolateral branches. No laser energy was applied. Despite multiple balloon inflations, it was not possible to seal the dissection (Fig. 7.11A–C). The patient had chest pain but no electrocardiographic or enzyme evidence of myocardial infarction.

It was felt that the dissection was produced by the mechanical effect

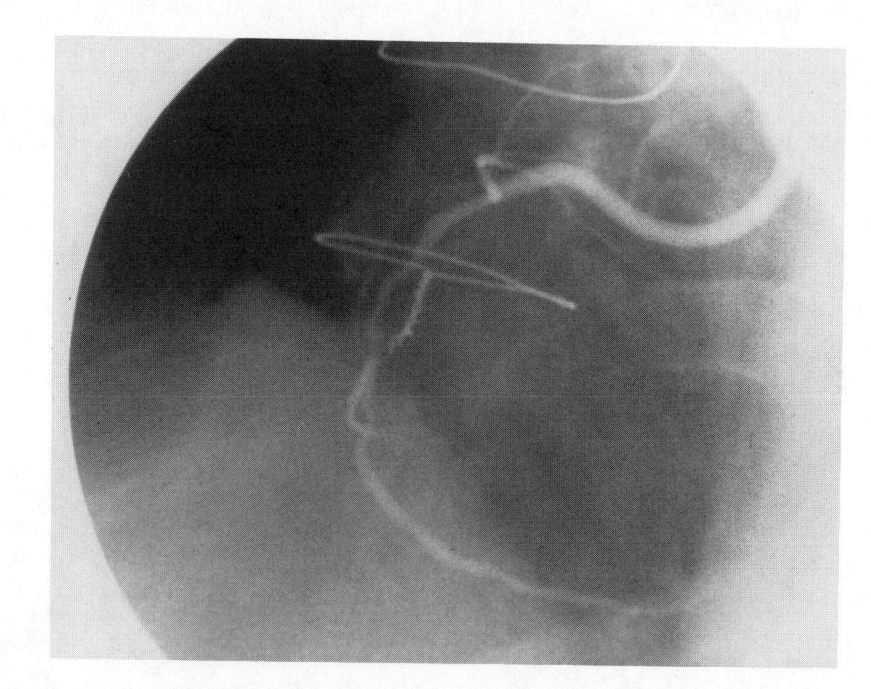

Figure 7.11. Demonstration of mechanical dissection. *(A)* Baseline angiogram.

Excimer Laser Coronary Angioplasty 157

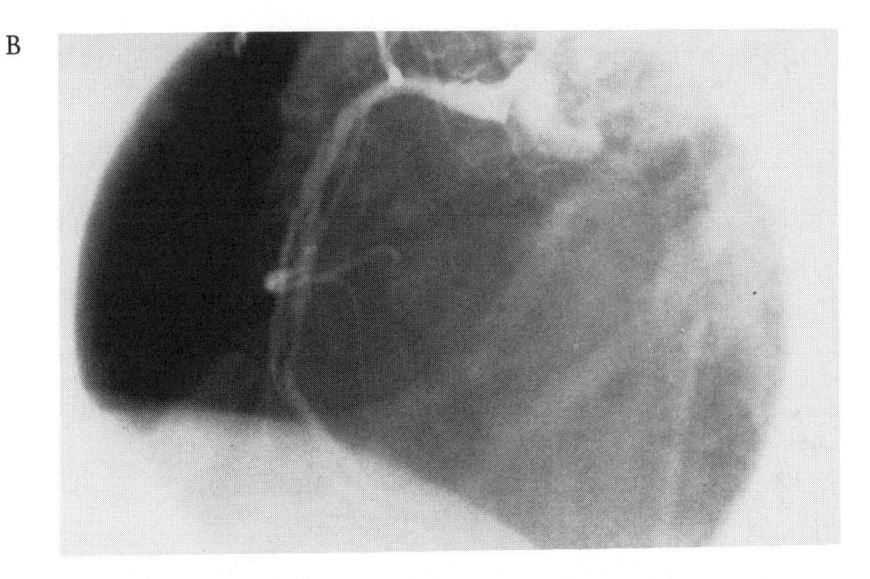

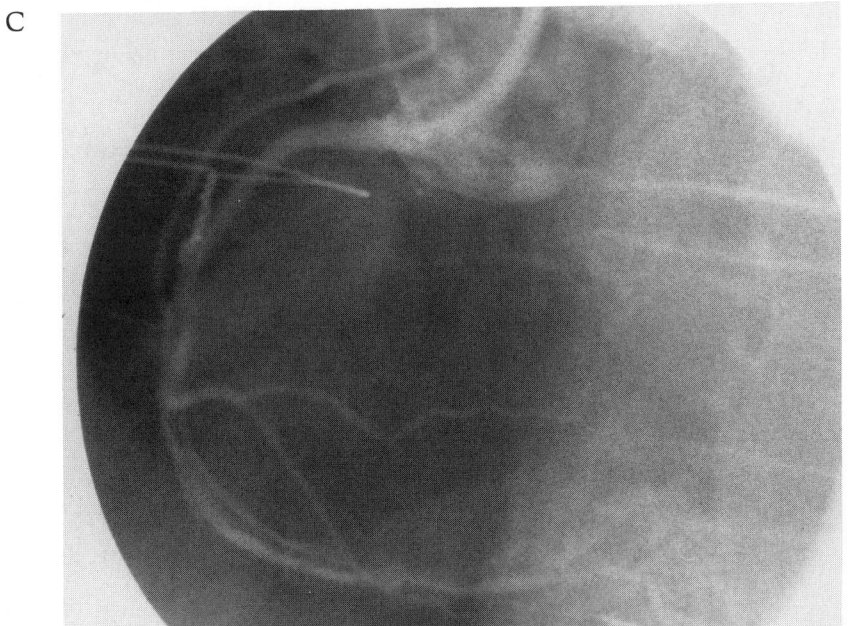

Figure 7.11. *(B)* Following dissection induced by dye jet. *(C)* Unsuccessful attempt to "tack-up" using PTCA.

of the guiding catheter being advanced into the RCA to a position just proximal to the lesion, or by contrast injected in a jet around the laser catheter. This may represent either a new dissection or reopening of the previous dissection plane from the balloon angioplasty procedure in September 1989, at which time significant dissection of the vessel had occurred. This case illustrates the point that contrast injection should not be performed when the laser catheter tip is just beyond the guide tip. This may create a jet, which could potentially induce or exacerbate coronary dissections.

Case 12: RPDA Graft

S. M., 80-year-old male

HISTORY	June 1970	Coronary artery bypass grafting; grafts to left anterior descending and right coronary artery.
	March 1980	Repeat coronary artery bypass grafting of LAD; graft to first diagonal, RPDA.
	September 1990	Developed unstable angina, acute pulmonary edema, and two subsequent episodes of CHF.
	October 1990	Acute myocardial infarction; cardiac catheterization shows patent LAD, first diagonal occluded, 90% RCA stenosis at midbody of graft.
PAST HISTORY		Insulin-dependent diabetes mellitus, hypertension, 40-pack-year smoking history.
MEDICATIONS		Mevacor, Cardizem, Isordil

ELCA Procedure 1/8/91
Saphenous vein graft to right posterior descending artery

CASS SEGMENT	GUIDE CATHETER	GUIDEWIRE	LASER CATHETER	ENERGY DENSITY	PULSES	BALLOON CATHETER	NUMBER OF INFLATIONS
Graft to 4	9 Fr. USCI	0.018" ACS	1.6 mm	45 mJ/mm^2	480	3.5-mm Medtronic	1
			2.2 mm	60 mJ/mm^2			

Excimer Laser Coronary Angioplasty 159

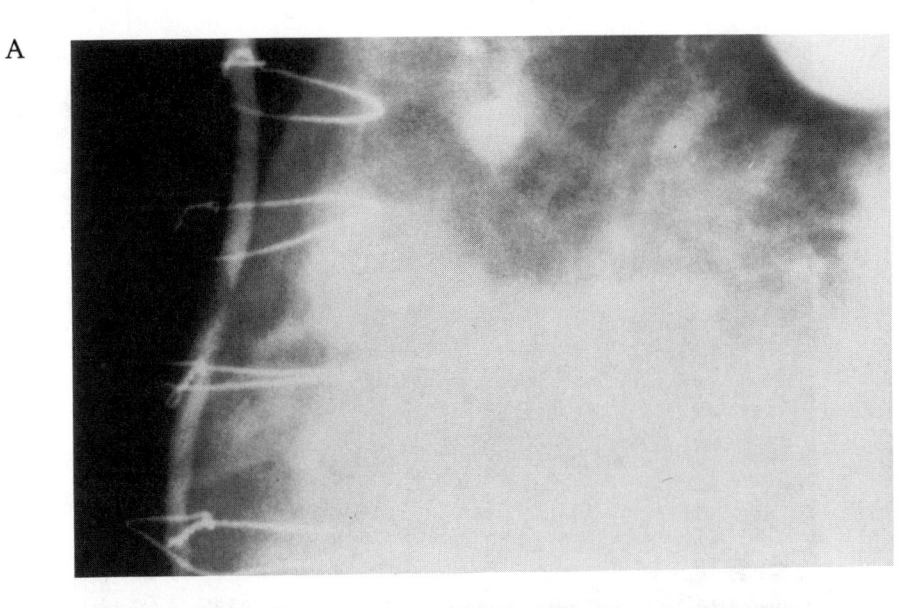

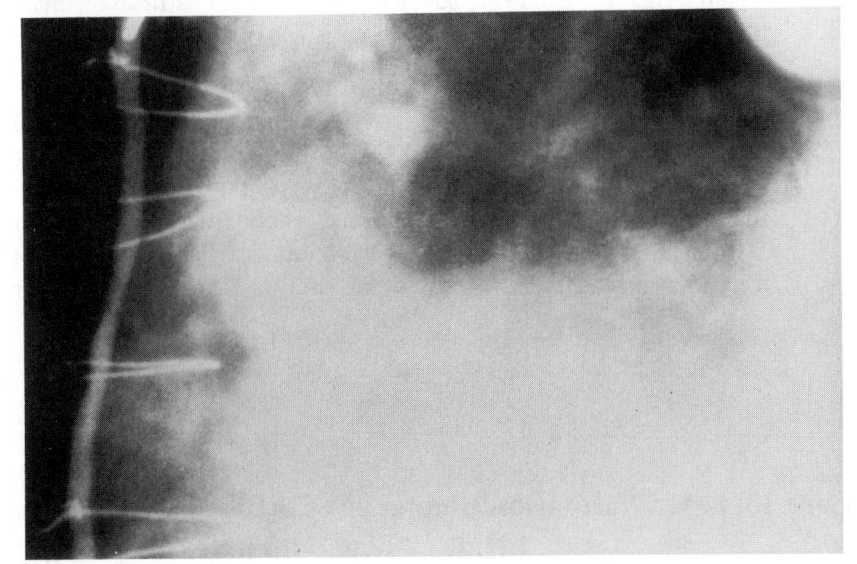

Figure 7.12. ELCA with the 2.2-mm catheter. *(A)* Baseline angiogram. *(B)* Following ELCA with a 2.2-mm catheter.

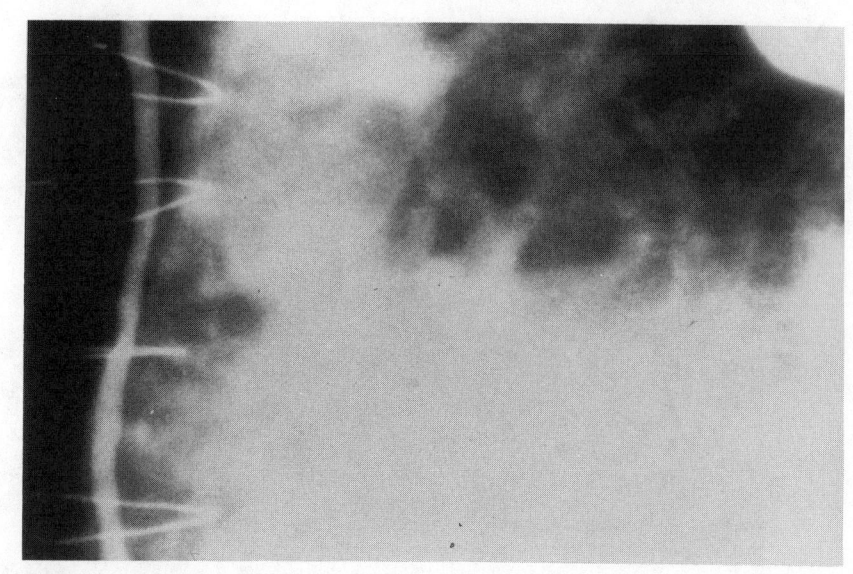

Figure 7.12. *(C)* Following adjunctive PTCA, there is little further improvement.

Discussion: This case shows a subtotal baseline stenosis on the midgraft (Fig. 7.12*A*). Following ELCA with a 1.6-mm and a 2.2-mm catheter, an excellent midgraphic result was obtained (Fig. 7.12*B*). Adjunctive balloon angioplasty was performed with little improvement (Fig. 7.12*C*). This case could probably been left as a "laser stand-alone" without adjunctive PTCA. This was the first use of the new 2.2-mm catheter.

Case 13: Laser Perforation/Emergency CABG
H. K., 73-year-old male

HISTORY	January 1989	Anterior myocardial infarction
	April 1990	Developed chest and arm discomfort. Routine thallium markedly positive with ST-T wave changes; reversible thallium defect of lateral wall.

Excimer Laser Coronary Angioplasty   161

May 1990	Coronary angiography reveals 100% occlusion of LAD; obtuse marginal has subtotal ostial obstruction at origin of circumflex.
PAST HISTORY	Noncontributory.
MEDICATIONS	Cardizem, ASA, NTG prn.

ELCA Procedure 6/5/90
Left Circumflex Bifurcation

CASS SEGMENT	GUIDE CATHETER	GUIDEWIRE	LASER CATHETER	ENERGY DENSITY	PULSES	BALLOON CATHETER	NUMBER OF INFLATIONS
21	—	0.018"	2.0 mm	45 mJ/mm^2	420	Not done	—

Discussion: The presence of a lesion at a true bifurcation is now known to be a contraindication for ELCA. Figure 7.13 demonstrates the lesion

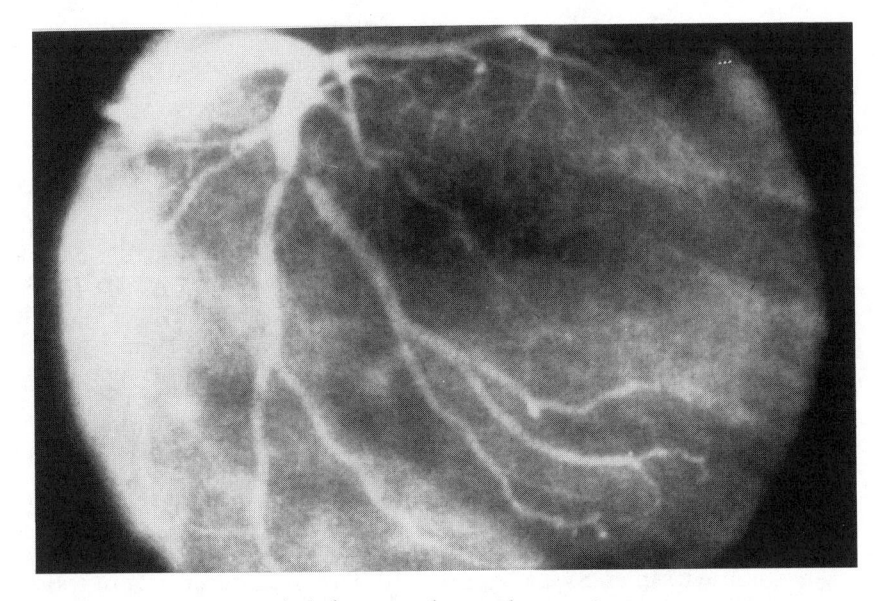

Figure 7.13. Example of a bifurcation lesion that resulted in a coronary perforation.

in this case. The laser perforated at the "carina." A bifurcation is differentiated from a lesion at a branch point in that the trajectory of the laser catheter changes as it goes through a bifurcation. The patient developed cardiac tamponade, which was treated by inflation of a balloon at the lesion and pericardiocentesis followed by emergency CABG. The patient did well following CABG and was discharged at 1 week.

Case 14: 3-Month-Old Circumflex Graft
J. H., 56-year-old black male

HISTORY	August 1979	Coronary artery bypass graft—six-vessel.
	September 1990	Non-Q-wave MI; repeat CABG—left internal thoracic artery graft to LAD; aortocoronary saphenous vein grafts to diagonal, obtuse marginal circumflex, and RPDA; autocoronary cryopreserved vein homograft to RPLS.
	January 1991	Unstable angina for 2 weeks with chest pain or exertion and at rest (CCSF class 4); mild CHF.
PAST HISTORY		Noncontributory.
MEDICATIONS		Cardizem, ASA.

ELCA Procedure 1/21/91
Vein graft to circumflex

CASS SEGMENT	GUIDE CATHETER	GUIDE WIRE	LASER CATHETER	ENERGY DENSITY	PULSES	BALLOON CATHETER	NUMBER OF INFLATIONS
18	—	0.018" ACS	2.0	50 mJ/mm^2	1540 (total)	Not done	—
19	—	0.018" ACS	2.0	50 mJ/mm^2		Not done	—

Discussion: This case represents the use of ELCA in an unfavorable lesion within an SVG. Figure 7.14A demonstrates a >2-cm lesion beginning at the ostium of a circumflex graft. Figure 7.14B shows the results following ELCA with a 2.0-mm catheter. If available, a 2.2-mm catheter

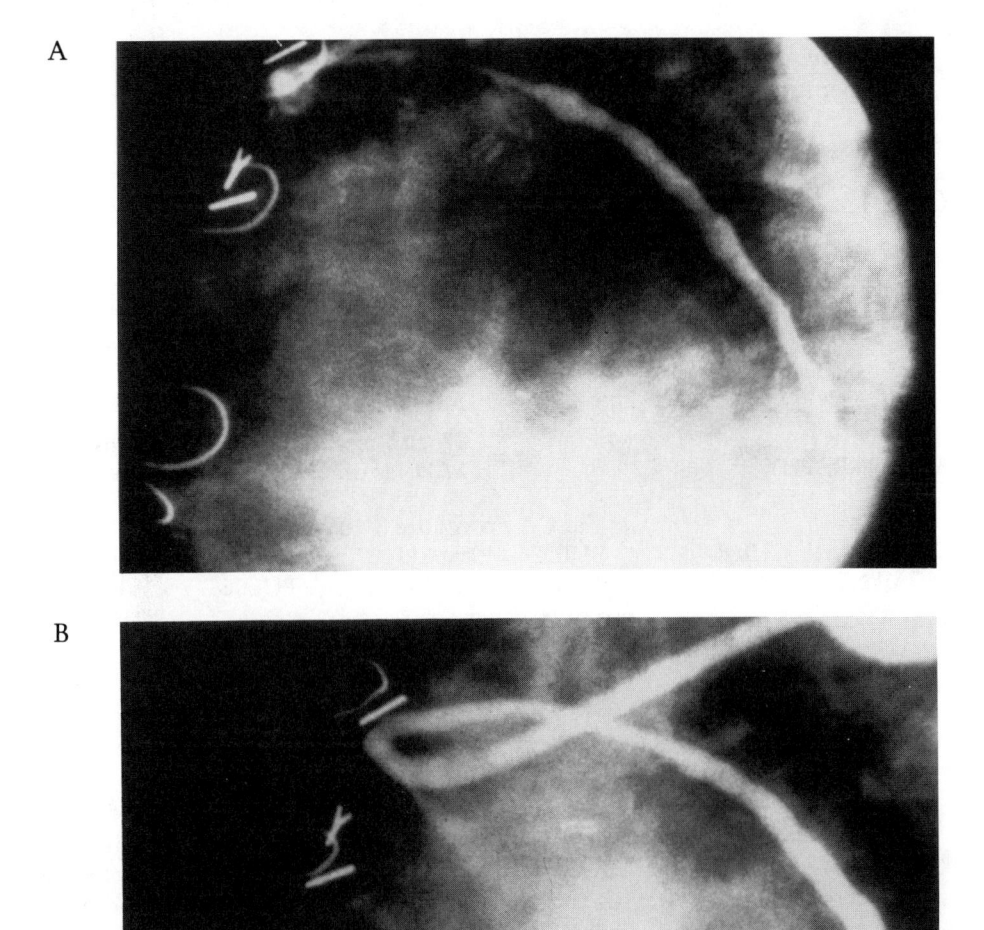

Figure 7.14. *(A)* Shows >2-cm lesion of SVG beginning at the ostium. *(B)* Shows results following ELCA at 50 mJ/mm^2 with the 2.0-mm catheter.

would have been optimal. The more recent cases (such as this one) are being performed at higher energy densities than were the earlier cases.

Case 15: Long LAD Lesion
H. B., 74-year-old male

HISTORY	June 1989	Unstable angina; LAD-PTCA with occlusion of diagonal branch.
	August 1989	Recurrent angina class III
MEDICATIONS		ASA, Diltiazem, Isordil
CORONARY ANGIOGRAPHY		17-cm long, critical stenosis of proximal LAD. No other significant disease.

ELCA Procedure 8/10/89

CASS SEGMENT	GUIDE CATHETER	GUIDE-WIRE	LASER CATHETER	PULSES	BALLOON CATHETER
12	8 Fr. Schneider SL-4	0.018" ACS laser wire	1.6 mm at 45 mJ/mm^2	680	—

Discussion: This represents an ideal ELCA lesion (Fig. 7.15A) classified as ACC/AHA type B by virtue of length. This case is typically simple and effective with ELCA. The small vessel diameter allowed "stand alone" laser even with the 1.6-mm catheter (Fig. 7.15B). More current technique would dictate beginning with an energy density of 50 mJ/mm^2. This patient had a 6-month angiogram without restenosis. He remains symptom-free at 14 months.

Case 16: Delayed Complication
L. J., 68-year-old white male

HISTORY	January, 1991	Routine treadmill on day of admission provoked dizziness, bradycardia at 30 beats/minute with sinus arrest. ST depression >2 mm was also noted (inferior/lateral).

Excimer Laser Coronary Angioplasty 165

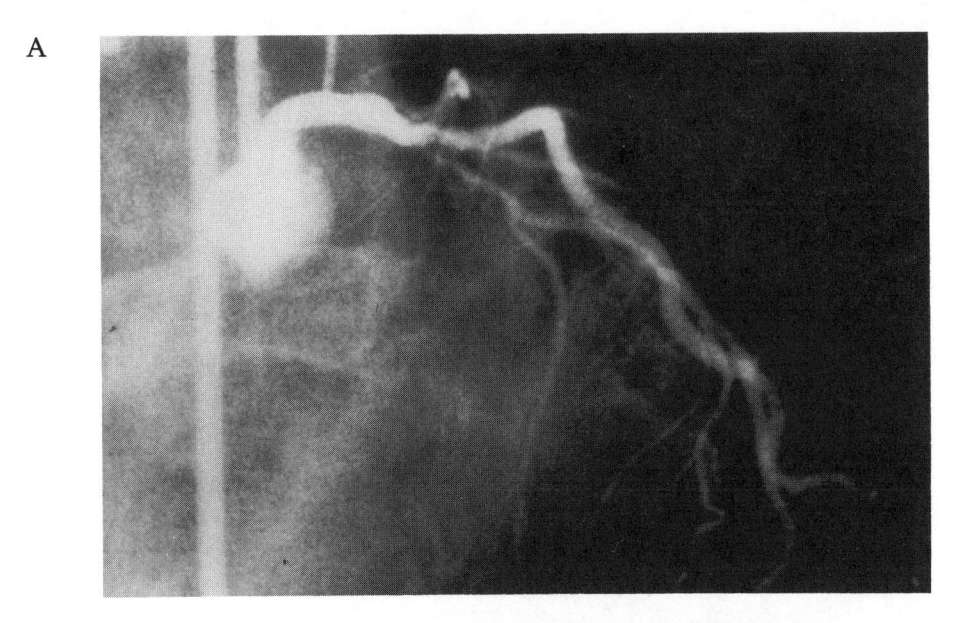

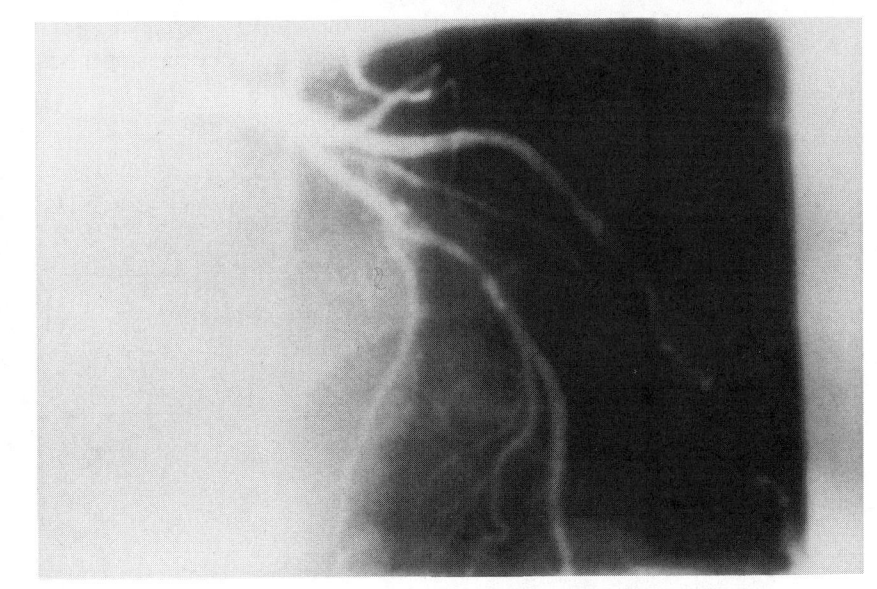

Figure 7.15. *(A)* Shows a 17-cm-long critical LAD stenosis. *(B)* Following ELCA with the 1.6-mm catheter, an excellent final result is seen.

166   Coronary Laser Angioplasty

PAST HISTORY   History of smoking in past; stopped 18 years ago. No history of HTN, hypercholesterolemia, heart disease, or diabetes.

MEDICATIONS   ASA.

ELCA Procedure 1/23/91
Ostial right coronary

CASS SEGMENT	GUIDE CATHETER	GUIDEWIRE	LASER CATHETER	ENERGY DENSITY	PULSES	BALLOON CATHETER	NUMBER OF INFLATIONS
1	—	0.018" ACS	1.3 mm	50 mJ/mm^2	1640 (total)	3.5-mm ACS-Stack	1
			1.6 mm	50 mJ/mm^2			
			2.2 mm	55 mJ/mm^2			

Discussion: This case shows the use of ELCA in a critical right coronary aorto-ostial stenosis (Fig. 7.16A). Using a sequential approach, a good

A

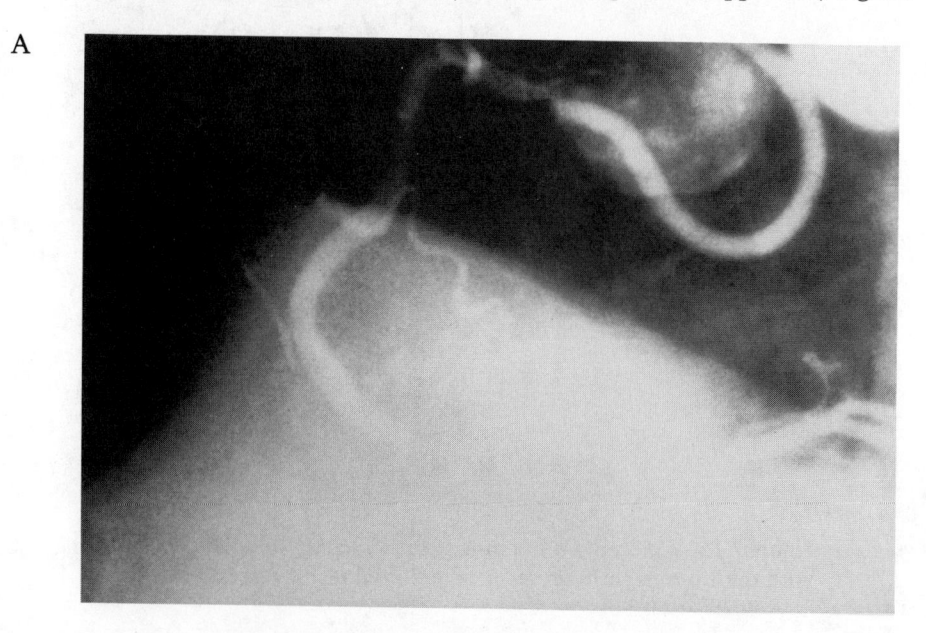

Figure 7.16. *(A)* Shows an RCA ostial stenosis.

Excimer Laser Coronary Angioplasty 167

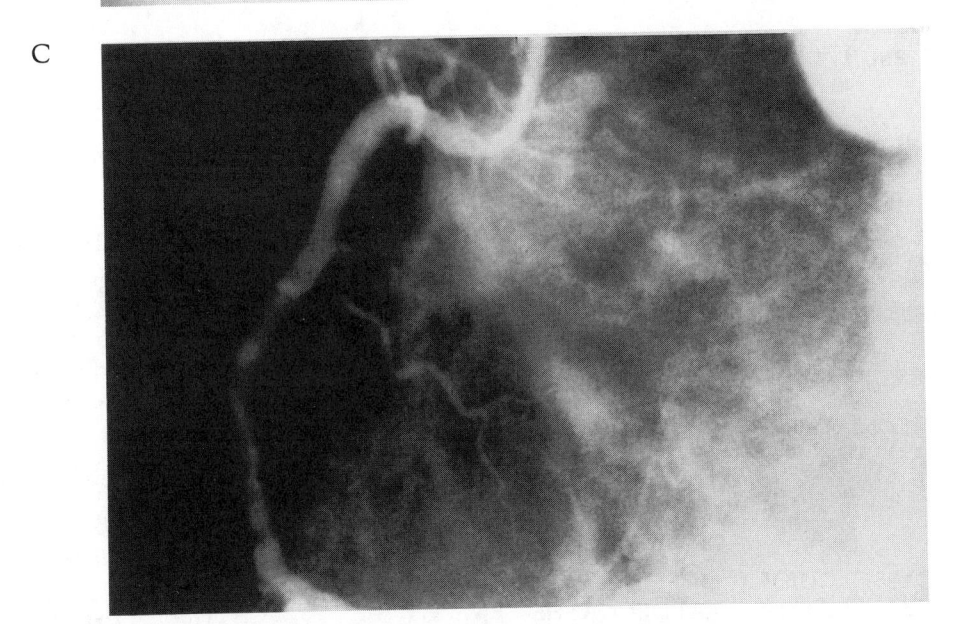

Figure 7.16. *(B)* Following 2.2-mm ELCA. A delayed ischemic response probably secondary to microemboli occurred leading to a non-Q MI. *(C)* Shows the results post-PTCA—performed to optimize the lumen.

result following ELCA with a 2.2-mm catheter was obtained (Fig. 7.16*B*). Ten minutes after being removed from the table, the patient developed ST elevation and chest pain. Repeat angiography revealed a widely patent ostium with excellent flow. There was no response to nitroglycerine. The pain persisted and adjunctive PTCA was performed to maximize the lumen, yielding an excellent result (Fig. 7.16*C*). The chest pain and ST elevation persisted for 2 hours. The CPK reached 500 U. There were no Q waves. The patient did well and had a negative stress test at 4 weeks. We believe this case demonstrates delayed microemboli. Embolus has occurred in approximately 1 percent of ELCA cases—this is the first delayed case we have seen. When this occurs, it is usually best treated conservatively, and the clinical course generally stabilizes as long as a macroembolus has not occurred. Macroemboli may require emergency CABG. At 6-month angiographic follow-up there was no restenosis.

Case 17: Long Recanalized Total Occlusion
J. L., 50-year-old white male

HISTORY	December 1990	History of progressively increasing exertional chest pain, CCSF classification 3. Recent thallium showed very large inferolateral and apical defects.
PAST HISTORY		Coronary artery disease first diagnosed approximately 5 years ago. Medical management effective until progression of symptoms over the last year. History of obesity and hypercholesterolemia.
MEDICATIONS		ASA, Cardizem, nitroglycerine.

ELCA Procedure 12/12/90
Right coronary

CASS SEGMENT	GUIDE CATHETER	GUIDEWIRE	LASER CATHETER	ENERGY DENSITY	PULSES	BALLOON CATHETER	NUMBER OF INFLATIONS
1,2	8 Fr. AL2	0.16	1.3 mm	60 mJ/mm^2	1280	2.5-mm	4
			1.6 mm	55 mJ/mm^2		Medtronics	—

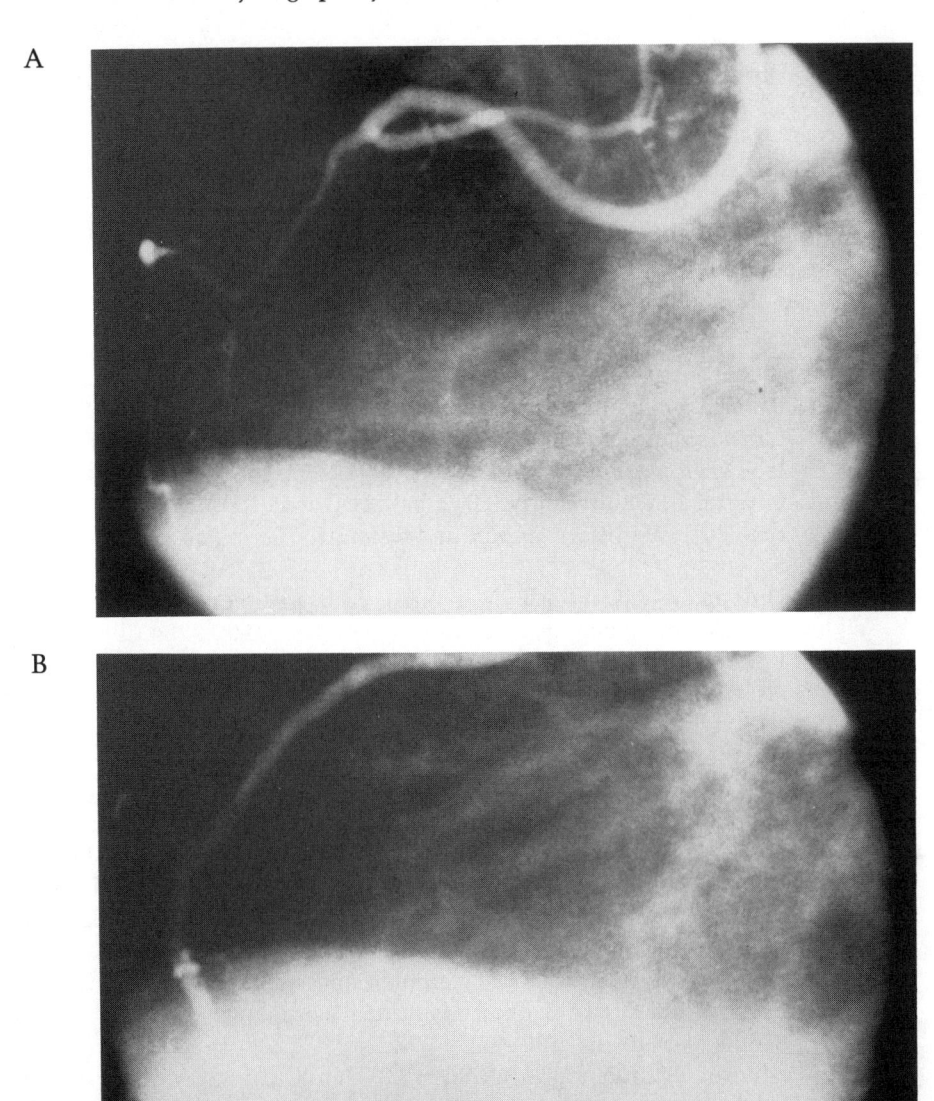

Figure 7.17. *(A)* Shows a chronically occluded, diffusely dissected RCA. *(B)* Following ELCA with the 1.3-mm and 1.6-mm catheters and adjunctive PTCA.

Discussion: An excellent example of ELCA and adjunctive PTCA to treat a chronically occluded, diffusely diseased RCA (Fig. 7.17A). The wire was a 0.16-inch USCI standard. Debulking was performed with the 1.3-mm and 1.6-mm catheters. Adjunctive PTCA at 4 ATM further enhanced the lumen (Fig. 7.17B). The combination of ELCA and PTCA in these lesions often yields outstanding angiographic results. At 6-month angiographic follow-up there was no restenosis.

References

1. Cook SL, Eigler L, Shefer A, Goldenberg T, Forrester J, Litvack F. Percutaneous excimer laser coronary angioplasty of lesions not ideal for balloon angioplasty. *Circulation* 1991;84(2):632–643.
2. Ghazzal Z, Weintraub WS, Ba'albaki HA, et al. PTCA of lesions longer than 20 mm: initial outcome and restenosis. *Circulation* 1990;82(4):III-5.
3. Untereker W, Litvack F, Margolis J, et al. Excimer laser coronary angioplasty of saphenous vein grafts. *Circulation* 1990;82(4):III-680.
4. Ryan TJ, Faxon DP, Gunnar RM, and the ACC/AHA Task Force on Assessment of Diagnostic and Therapeutic Procedures (Subcommittee on Percutaneous Transluminal Coronary Angioplasty). Guidelines for percutaneous transluminal coronary angioplasty. *Circulation* 1988;78:486–502.
5. Eigler N, Cook S, Kent K, et al. Excimer laser angioplasty of ostial coronary stenosis: results of multicenter study. *Circulation* 1990;82(4):III-1.
6. Ellis SG, Vandormeel MG, Cowley MJ, et al. Coronary morphologic and clinical determinants of procedural outcome with angioplasty for multivessel coronary disease. *Circulation* 1990;82:1193–1202.
7. Holmes DR, Vlietstra RE. Complex and multivessel dilatation. In: Topol EJ, ed. Textbook of interventional cardiology. Philadelphia: W.B. Saunders, 1990:223–239.
8. Ishinger T, Gruentzig AR, Meier B, Galan K. Coronary dissection and total coronary occlusion associated with percutaneous transluminal coronary angioplasty: significance of initial angiographic morphology of coronary stenoses. *Circulation* 1986;74:1371–1378.
9. Ellis SG, Roubin GS, King SB, et al. Angiographic and clinical predictors of acute closure after native vessel coronary angioplasty. *Circulation* 1988;77:372–379.
10. Ryan TJ, Klocke FJ, Reynolds WA. Clinical competence in percutaneous transluminal coronary angioplasty. *Circulation* 1990;81:2041–2046.

11. Pinkerton CA, Slack JD, Orr CM, Vantassel JW, Smith ML. Percutaneous transluminal coronary angioplasty in patients with prior myocardial vascular surgery. *Am J Cardiol* 1988;61:15G–22G.
12. Topol EJ, Ellis SG, Fishman J, et al. Multicenter study of percutaneous transluminal coronary angioplasty for right coronary ostial stenosis. *J Am Coll Cardiol* 1987;10:246–252.
13. Holmes Dr, Vlietstra RE, Reeder GS, et al. Angioplasty in total coronary occlusion. *J Am Coll Cardiol* 1984;3:845–849.
14. Kereiakes DJ, Selmon MR, McAuley BJ, McAuley DB, Sheehan DJ, Simpson JB. Angioplasty in total coronary occlusion: experience in 76 consecutive patients. *J Am Coll Cardiol* 1985;6:526–533.

CHAPTER 8

Other Pulsed Lasers for Angioplasty Including Solid-State Lasers

---

TIMOTHY J. GARRAND
LAWRENCE I. DECKELBAUM

CORONARY balloon angioplasty was first performed by Andreas Gruntzig in 1977, and has become an increasingly utilized nonsurgical intervention for obstructive coronary artery disease (1). Despite the rapid growth and refinement of balloon angioplasty over the past decade, balloon angioplasty remains limited by a 30–40 percent rate of restenosis and an inability to adequately treat diffuse disease or chronic total occlusions (2,3). Laser vaporization of atherosclerotic plaque has been proposed as a means to overcome these limitations (4–6). This chapter reviews the current application of pulsed lasers for angioplasty, specifically focusing on nonexcimer lasers.

Lasers can operate in either continuous wave or pulsed mode, depending on their construction and method of lasing. Continuous wave lasers have a constant power output when turned on, and the peak power is the same as the average power. Pulsed lasers operate by storing energy and suddenly releasing the energy in a short burst, or pulse. The advantage of a pulsed laser over a continuous wave laser is that the energy stored between pulses allows higher peak power to be achieved. The ability to achieve high peak power in pulsed delivery of laser energy, as will be discussed later in this chapter, is advantageous in diminishing

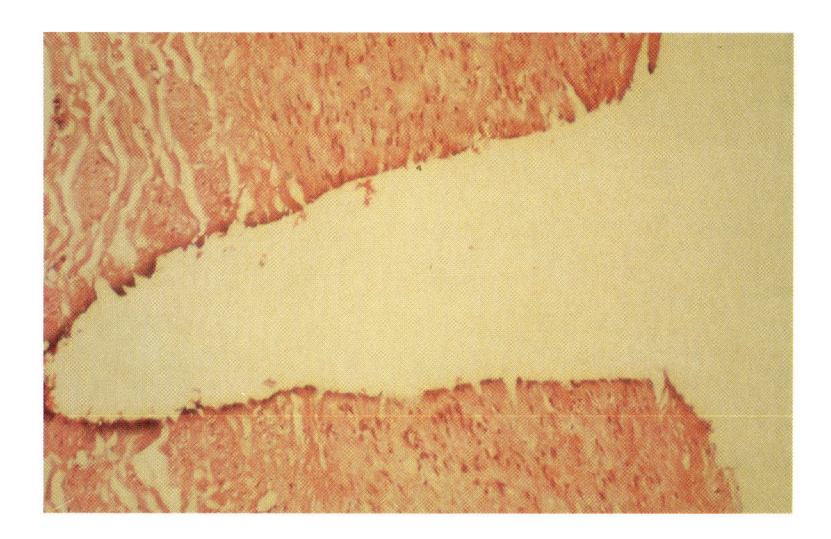

Plate I. This 2 mm–deep 0.8 mm–wide crater is the result of ablation of atherosclerotic aortic tissue at 350 mJ/mm² from a 200 microsecond–pulsed erbium:YAG laser delivered via a 400-micron zirconium fluoride fiber. The effects of shock wave and rapid gas expansion can be seen in the lower left portion of the photograph.

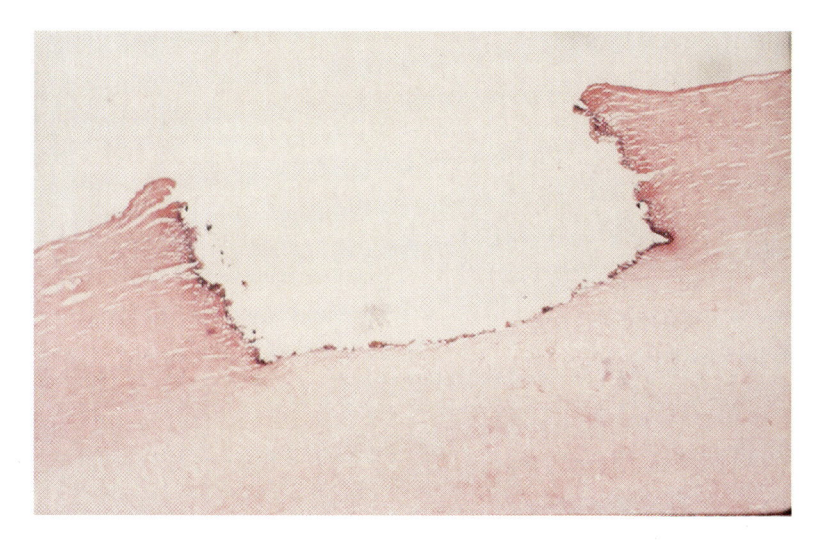

Plate II. This photomicrograph shows a representative section of human atherosclerotic aorta after ablation with a 2.1 micron holmium:YAG laser operating at 550 mJ/mm² delivered to the tissue via a 400-micron low-OH silica fiber. Energy density at the fiber output was 790 mJ/mm² with a pulse duration of 200 microseconds. Three pulses produced this crater 650 microns in diameter. However, an additional 10 pulses resulted in no further ablation of the underlying atheroma. Note the zone of thermal damage 100 microns in width and the vacuolization prominent at the crater margins.

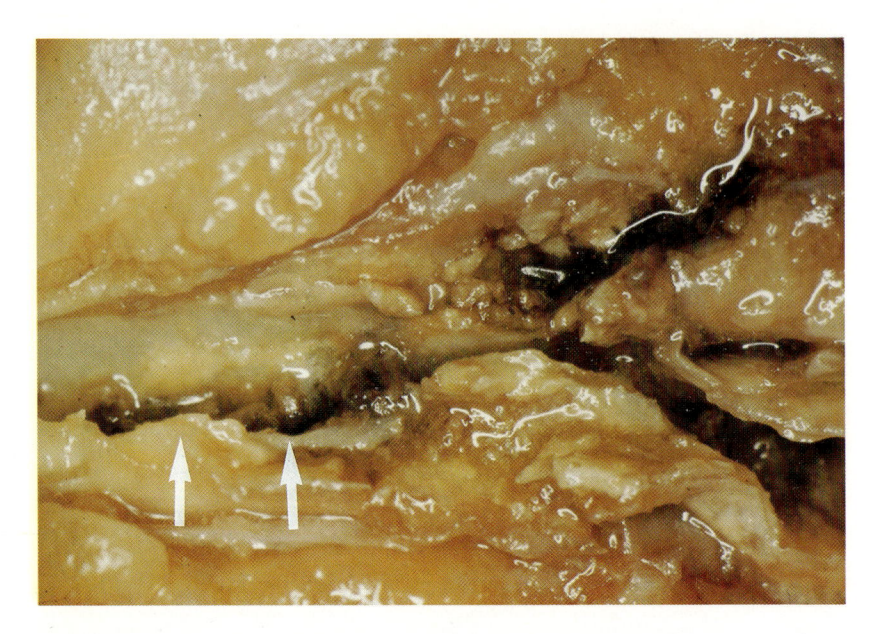

Plate III. Gross macroscopic specimen of the left anterior descending artery. The area of laser ablation in the proximal part of the lesion prior to the origin of the second diagonal branch shows some discoloration *(arrows)*, but the lumen is patent without signs of severe tissue injury.

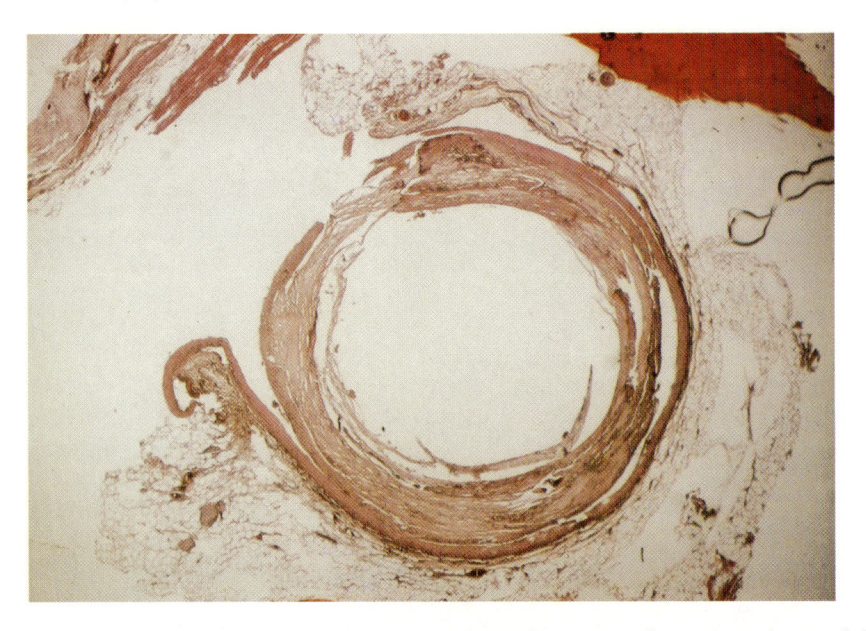

Plate IV. Histologic cross-section of the area of laser ablation in the proximal part of the lesion of the left anterior descending artery (Plate III, *arrows*) illustrating a relatively smooth-walled central lumen with minimal charring and thermal injury induced by the excimer laser. (Hematoxylin-eosin stain; original magnification ×10.)

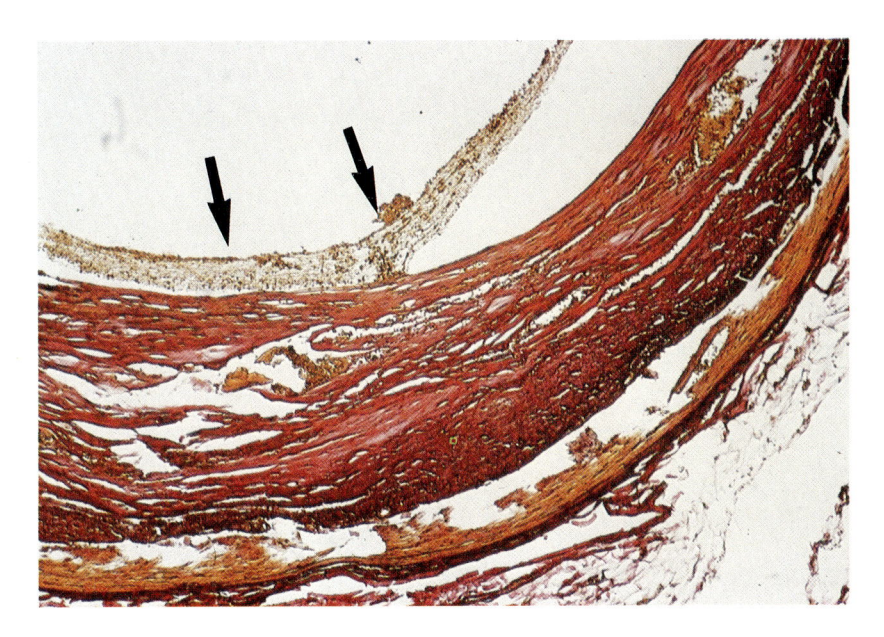

Plate V. Portion of a cross-section of Plate III with fibrin formation and platelet deposition *(arrows)* on the intimal layer. Again, no signs of thermal injury are noted. (Elastica-von-Gieson stain; original magnification ×40.)

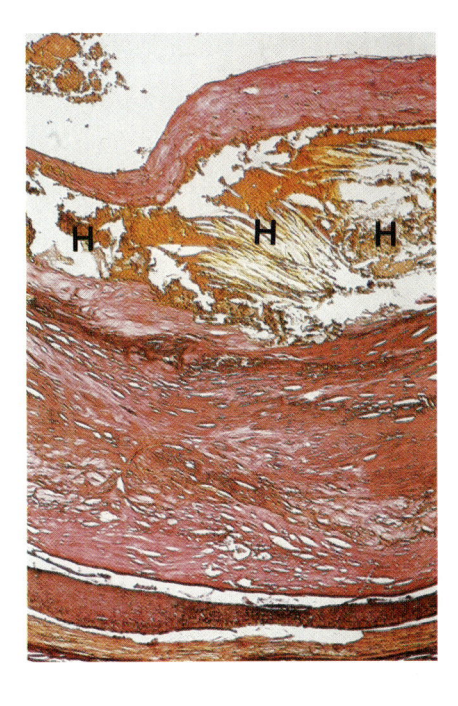

Plate VI. Portion of a cross-section of the distal segment of the left anterior descending artery where balloon angioplasty was performed. There was approximately 75 percent narrowing of luminal cross-sectional area. The section shows laceration with severe hemorrhage *(H)* and a disrupted plaque without signs of thermal injury. (Elastica-von-Gieson stain; original magnification ×68).

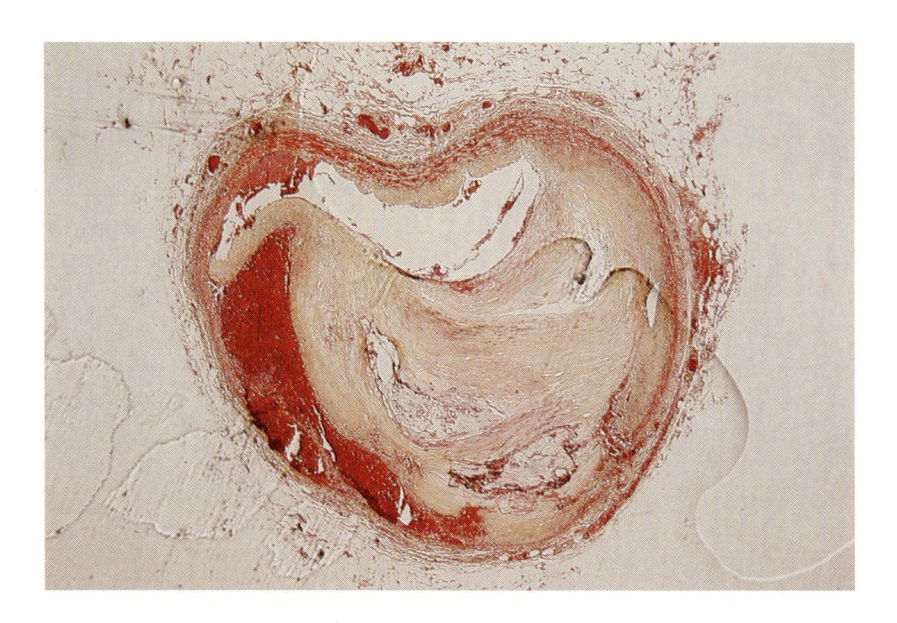

Plate VII. Segment of a coronary artery from a patient who died 48 hours after PTCA. The balloon angioplasty site shows separation of atheroma from adjacent normal arterial wall with dissection of blood through disrupted media (Hematoxylin-eosin stain, × 25). (Reproduced with permission from Potkin et al. Am J Cardiol 1988;62:40–41.)

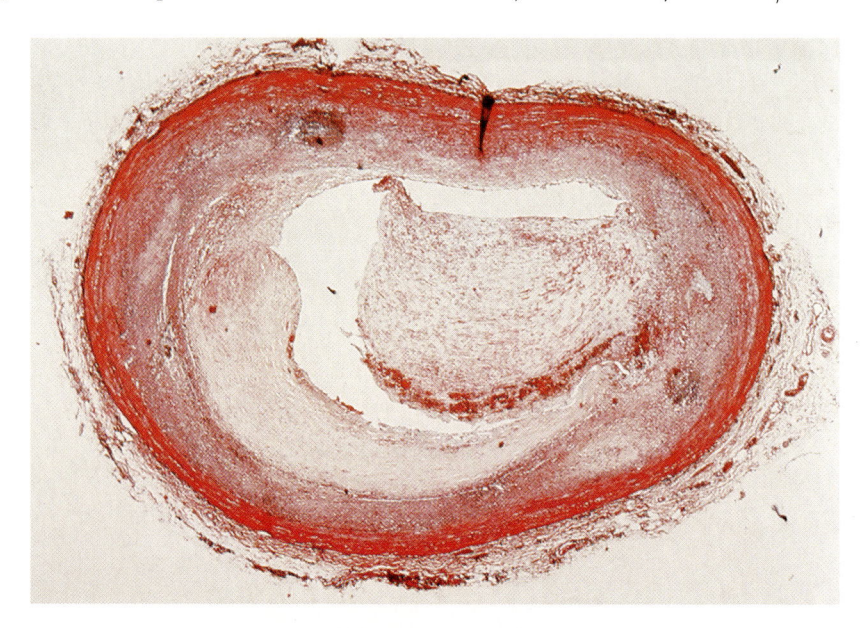

Plate VIII. The histologic effect of balloon angioplasty. Severe dilatation most commonly produces three effects: stretching of the normal segment, dissection at the junction of the normal and atheromatous segment, and hemorrhage in the dissection plane. The direct effect on the atheroma is minimal.

thermal tissue damage during laser vaporization and enabling ablation of calcified atherosclerotic plaque.

Methods of Laser Pulse Generation

Four methods are commonly used to generate pulsed laser output: pulsing the energy source, Q-switching the cavity, cavity dumping, and mode-locking the cavity. Continuous wave lasers can be converted to pulsed output by mechanically interrupting, or "chopping," the beam. However, chopped-wave lasers do not benefit from the ability to achieve high peak power, as energy is not stored within the laser between pulses.

The typical laser cavity consists of a resonator cavity containing the lasing medium positioned between two parallel mirrors, as depicted in Figure 8.1 (7). The lasing medium can be a gas (as in the argon, excimer, or carbon dioxide lasers), a solid (as in the neodymium:YAG, holmium:YAG, or alexandrite lasers), or a liquid (as in the dye laser). Lasing is initiated by exciting the lasing medium with an energy source, such

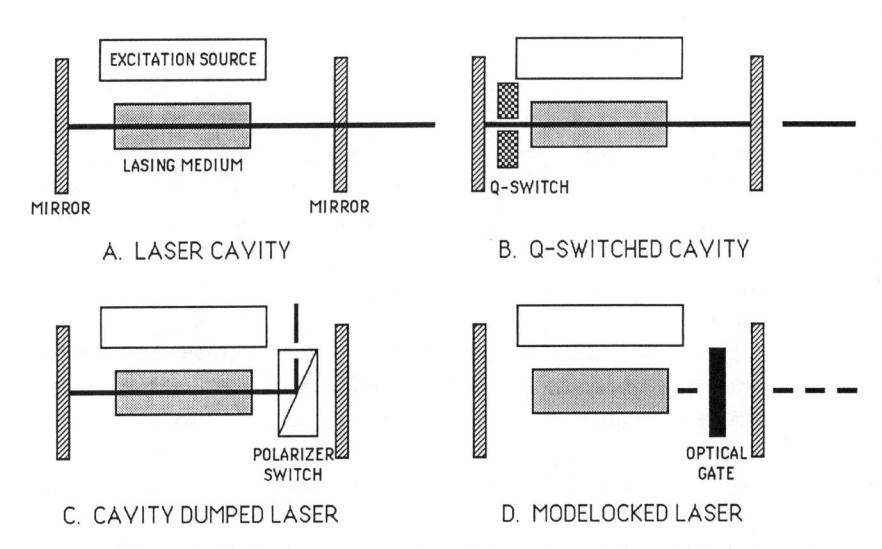

Figure 8.1. Methods for generating pulsed laser energy. Panel (A) shows a laser cavity with the lasing medium aligned between two mirrors. Pulsed output can be obtained by pulsing the excitation source. The other panels (B–D) illustrate three laser cavity modifications capable of producing pulsed laser output.

as a flashlamp or radio frequency generator. The energy excites the electrons of the atoms within the lasing medium to a higher energy level. As the electrons return to lower energy levels, photons are released and resonate back and forth between the mirrors of the laser cavity, stimulating other atoms to release photons, resulting in the cascade effect of light amplification by stimulated emission of radiation. Laser light is emitted when photons are able to exit the laser cavity. This can occur if one of the mirrors is partially reflective to allow transmission of laser light (as in Fig. 8.1A), or if the laser light is redirected out of the cavity by a reflector (as in Fig. 8.1C).

Pulsed laser emissions can be produced by pulsing the exciting energy source. The flashlamp-excited lasers, such as the neodymium:YAG, holmium:YAG, and dye lasers, can emit pulsed laser energy by cycling the input energy source. This method of pulsed energy generation is known as the "free-running" or normal-spiking mode, and produces microsecond (10^{-6} sec) laser pulses.

Q-switching interrupts the lasing process by altering the resonator characteristics of the cavity. The "Q" refers to the "quality" of the cavity to act as a photon resonator. The laser cavity is switched between a high- and low-quality resonator to store laser energy (as depicted in Fig. 8.1B). When the low-quality reflector is present, lasing is interrupted and excitation energy is stored within the lasing medium. Return to a high-quality reflector allows lasing to occur and the stored energy is released from the cavity. The laser pulse duration depends on the time required for the stored energy to be released and is in the nanosecond (10^{-9} sec) range. The first Q-switch employed rotating mirrors, but current Q-switches are more complex and use acousto-optic, electro-optic, or dye switches to alter the laser resonator. Q-switching has been employed in solid-state and liquid-state lasers to increase pulsed peak power.

Cavity dumping is a method of pulse generation by periodically diverting, or "dumping," some or all of the laser energy out of the laser cavity. The laser cavity is similar to the one depicted in Figure 8.1A, but the mirrors are both reflective and do not allow laser light to exit the cavity. Instead, a polarizer switch periodically reflects the laser energy out of the cavity, as shown in Figure 8.1C. Some ionized gas lasers employ cavity-dumping to generate nanosecond pulsed output.

Another technique for generating laser pulses is mode-locking. A mode-locked laser uses a fast optical gating switch to restrict laser energy within the cavity to a short pulse, as depicted in Figure 8.1D. The optical gate is open while the pulse is traveling through and closed the rest of the time. The only light allowed to circulate in the laser cavity is in the short pulse. Mode-locked lasers can generate very short pulses, in the picosecond (10^{-12} sec) range. The disadvantage of mode-locked lasers is an inability to achieve high peak power because of generation of very short pulses that are released rapidly without sufficient time for energy storage. Low peak power results in performance similar to continuous wave lasers and limits the applicability of mode-locked lasers to angioplasty.

Effect of Laser Profile and Wavelength on Laser Ablation

Laser radiation can be delivered in a time-varying fashion that is characterized by the laser power profile. Figure 8.2 shows the power output over time for continuous wave and pulsed lasers. Continuous wave lasers have power output that is constant over time. In contrast, pulsed lasers deliver energy in brief pulses, each of which is separated by an emission-free interval. Pulsed lasers can have very high peak powers that exceed the average power by several orders of magnitude.

Using continuous wave lasers, plaque ablation is characterized by thermal injury to the surrounding tissue (8–10). There is a zone of coagulation necrosis at the periphery of the vaporized crater and a deeper zone of polymorphous lacunae. Thermal damage occurs due to the progressive heating of tissue with continuous wave irradiation. To avoid thermal damage it is necessary to pulse the laser energy so that heat dissipation can occur between pulses (10–13).

The ability of the laser to ablate tissue while minimizing thermal injury to the surrounding tissue depends on careful selection of pulsed laser parameters. Optimization of heat dissipation during tissue vaporization can occur with short pulse duration, low repetition rate, and large pulse energy (10–20). Elimination of thermal damage during tissue ablation using short laser pulse duration may result from a thermal process with enhanced dissipation of heat. Thermal damage depends on the thermal relaxation time of the tissue, or the characteristic time for first-order temperature dissipation (21,22). The interval between pulses must be long enough, and pulse duration must be short enough, to allow time for heat dissipation. If either factor is exceeded, thermal damage to the surrounding tissue occurs. The pulse duration must be much less than the thermal relaxation time of the irradiated tissue to minimize

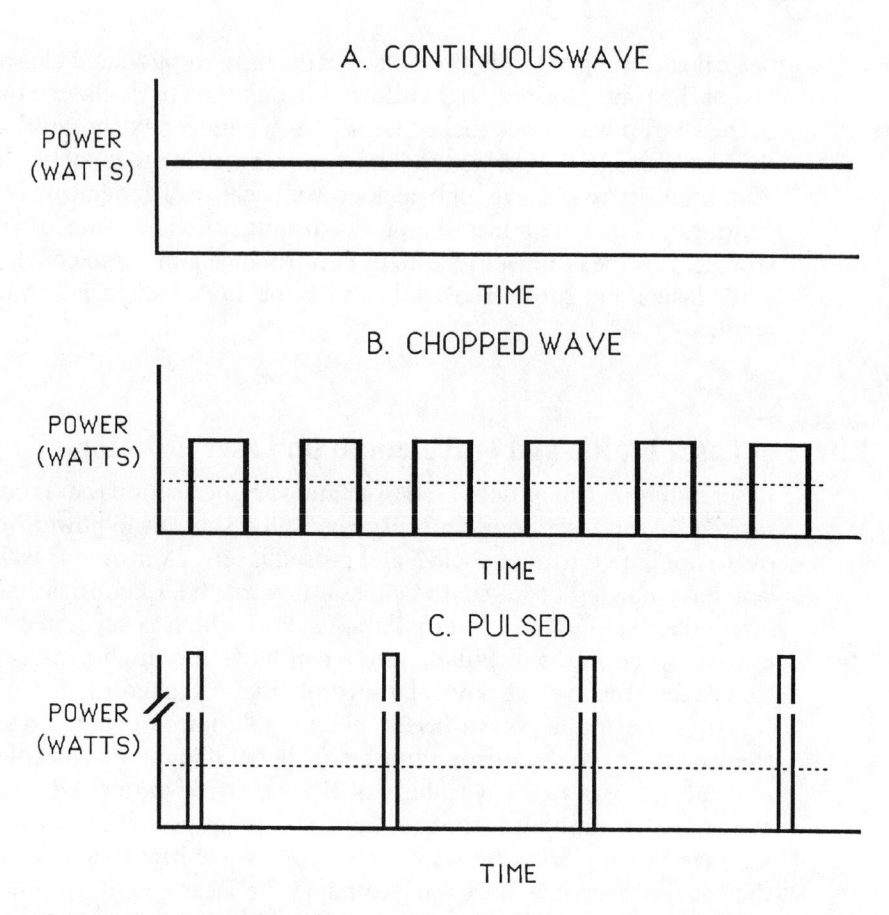

Figure 8.2. (A) A continuous-wave laser has a constant power output with the average power equal to the peak power. (B) Chopping the laser output results in periods of no power output and reduces the average power (dotted line) below the peak power. (C) True pulsed laser output can result in dramatic increases in peak power (note the break in the ordinate) with long radiation-free intervals while maintaining average power.

heat diffusion during each laser pulse. A low repetition rate is also important, as a trail of pulses too closely spaced in time may not allow dissipation of residual thermal energy, resulting in heat accumulation and thermal injury to the surrounding tissue.

To minimize thermal damage, each individual laser pulse must also have a large enough fluence, or energy density, to completely vaporize the irradiated tissue volume. This rapid vaporization dispells hot gases and particulate matter and leaves little heat to be conducted to the adjacent tissue. As a result, thermal diffusion to the boundary tissue is minimized. Alternatively, the high peak power resulting from short pulse duration may ablate tissue by a nonthermal mechanism. Nonthermal ablative mechanisms, such as photochemical decomposition, could remove tissue without requiring heating to boiling-point temperatures.

For a pulsed laser system, there is a peak power, or pulse energy, threshold above which one can achieve "clean" ablation or ablation without thermal damage. This threshold is wavelength-dependent and is lowest for the wavelengths most strongly absorbed by tissue. Strong absorption results in confinement of laser energy to the surface of the tissue, allowing for "clean" tissue vaporization at lower pulse fluences.

Choice of wavelength for laser ablation affects tissue vaporization due to the depth of absorption (23–25). Arterial tissue absorbs laser energy most strongly in the midinfrared and ultraviolet wavelengths, due to strong absorption by tissue water and proteins, respectively (25). Output from lasers emitting near the absorption peaks of water, for example, is deposited within several microns of the tissue surface, whereas poorly absorbed wavelengths are deposited within several millimeters of the tissue surface. Because of their strong wavelength absorption, ultraviolet and infrared lasers have the lowest peak power threshold for ablation with minimal thermal damage.

Ablation Lasers

Based upon the above energy and wavelength considerations, the best laser for angioplasty should be a pulsed laser operating at a wavelength strongly absorbed by atherosclerotic plaque. The laser should be able to achieve high peak power for "clean" ablation at a repetition rate that enables heat dissipation yet results in a reasonable rate of ablation. The laser energy must also be able to be transmitted through a flexible optical fiber to allow transcatheter intraarterial delivery of ablative energy.

Several lasers are currently available with potential application for laser angioplasty. Table 8.1 lists the lasers that have been evaluated for angioplasty, along with their respective wavelengths, absorption coefficients, and penetration depths. These lasers emit in the infrared, visible, or ultraviolet range. The advantages and disadvantages of each laser type will be briefly reviewed.

Infrared lasers include the carbon dioxide, erbium:YAG, hol-

Table 8.1. Characteristics of Lasers Evaluated for Angioplasty

LASER	WAVELENGTH (NM)	α (CM⁻¹)[a]	PENETRATION DEPTH (μ)	PROFILE
CO_2	10,600	600	17	CW, pulsed
Erbium:YAG	2940	10,000	1	Pulsed
Holmium	2060	35	286	Pulsed
Thulium	1950	85	120	Pulsed
Nd:YAG	1060	4	2500	CW, pulsed
Dye laser	750–400	4–30	2500–333	Pulsed
Argon	515	14	714	CW
	488	20	500	CW
Alexandrite (fd)	378	35	285	Pulsed
Excimer	351	40	250	Pulsed
	308	200	50	Pulsed
	248	600	17	Pulsed

α = the estimated tissue absorption coefficient.
CW = continuous wave; fd = frequency doubled.
[a]Modified from L. Esterowitz (24) with permission.

mium:YAG or YSGG, thulium:YAG, and neodymium:YAG lasers. The carbon dioxide laser is a gas laser that emits in the far infrared region at 10.6 microns and can operate in a continuous wave or pulsed mode. The carbon dioxide wavelength is strongly absorbed by water, as noted in Table 8–1. Tissue penetration is 17 microns at this wavelength, resulting in high surface absorption. Continuous wave or chopped-wave irradiation results in thermal damage (12,15). However, Abela et al. noted that ablation of atherosclerotic plaque in saline reduced the amount of thermal damage during ablation (9). The use of shorter pulse durations of carbon dioxide irradiation also decreases the extent of tissue thermal damage. Walsh et al. reported a reduction of thermal damage to 50 microns as compared to 750 microns when 2-microsecond versus 50-millisecond pulses from a carbon dioxide laser were used to ablate guinea pig aorta in air (18). Deckelbaum et al. demonstrated that a high-peak-power carbon dioxide laser emitting 1-microsecond pulses can ablate myocardial tissue with minimal residual histologic thermal damage (12).

Strong absorption of mid- and far-infrared wavelengths by silica has prevented the transmission of carbon dioxide laser energy by silica fiber optics. Successful transmission of infrared wavelengths by use of hollow metal and glass "fiber" wave guides, as well as novel materials, has been reported (26,27). Hollow wave guides use air as the wave guiding medium and rely on transmission of wavelengths by total internal reflection from their internal walls. Their limitations include decreased flexibility (because of the need for larger fiber diameters) and bend-sensitive losses that occur when the fiber is subjected to multiple bends.

Bulk-fiber materials for transmitting infrared radiation include glass and crystalline materials. The former category comprises heavy-metal halide glasses, such as zirconium fluoride and chalcogenide (e.g., arsenide selenium fibers) (28). Crystalline infrared-transmitting materials include silver halide, thallium halide, and sapphire fibers. Generally, halide and chalcogenide fibers tend to be environmentally sensitive. In contrast to silica-based fibers, they are expensive, toxic, fragile, hygroscopic, and subject to low damage thresholds that limit their biomedical applications. Nevertheless, carbon dioxide laser angioplasty has been performed experimentally in vivo with silver halide fibers (29).

Water absorption peaks are present at 2.9 and 1.9 microns (30). The erbium:YAG laser is a solid-state laser that emits pulsed energy near one of these peaks, at a wavelength of 2.94 microns. Of the currently available infrared lasers, the erbium:YAG wavelength has the strongest absorption by water and has a tissue depth penetration of 1 micron (31,32). High absorption of this wavelength by tissue water allows ablation with the least thermal damage of the infrared lasers (33–35). Pulsed output has been obtained in normal spiking (free-running) mode or with Q-switching (17). Ablation of aorta with 200-microsecond (normal spiking mode) or 90-nanosecond (Q-switched) pulses resulted in minimal thermal damage with either laser mode. However, the extent of thermal damage was halved using the shorter-duration, Q-switched pulses (5–10 microns compared to 10–20 microns). Nuss et al. demonstrated the pulsed erbium:YAG laser to be the most efficient infrared laser for vaporization of bone and to be capable of ablation of calcified plaque with a minimum of thermal damage (35). Despite the excellent ablation characteristics of the erbium:YAG laser, in-vivo application is limited by the inability to transmit the energy by silica fiber optics. The energy from an erbium:YAG laser has, however, been transmitted by zirconium fluoride fibers for atherosclerotic plaque vaporization in vitro (36–38).

The holmium:YAG and holmium:YSGG lasers represent a compromise between performance and fiber-optic transmission. The holmium laser is a solid-state laser and emits at a wavelength of 2.1 microns. This wavelength has good water absorption due to its proximity to the 1.9-

micron water absorption peak, and is capable of being transmitted through low hydroxyl silica fibers (39,40). The holmium laser can ablate plaque without substantial thermal damage, but the 2.1-micron wavelength has a higher ablation threshold and causes more thermal damage compared to the 2.94-micron wavelength of the erbium:YAG laser (35). The laser is capable of pulsed output in normal spiking or Q-switched modes. Pulse duration in the Q-switched mode is 200 nanoseconds, as compared to 250 microseconds in normal spiking mode (40,41). The use of Q-switched pulses can reduce the extent of thermal damage to 0–20 microns, as compared to 50–60 microns in the normal spiking mode. Acoustic shock-wave damage to pericrater tissue has been noted at high-peak-power densities (40).

The holmium:YAG laser has been used in vitro to recanalize totally occluded, noncalcified tibial arteries (42). In-vitro ablation of calcified plaque by the holmium:YAG laser has been reported at energy levels compatible with fiber transmission. Kopchok et al. reported the ability to ablate calcified plaque with a holmium:YAG laser through a silica fiber (40). The threshold laser pulse energy required for the ablation of calcified plaque was approximately two to seven times that required for the ablation of noncalcified plaque. Ablation of calcified plaque by the holmium:YAG laser, as well as by other pulsed lasers, appears to be accompanied by plasma emission (35,43).

Preliminary studies with the thulium:YAG laser have evaluated laser ablation using a wavelength closer to the 1.9-micron absorption peak of water (44). The thulium:YAG laser emits at a wavelength of 2.0 microns and has a lower ablation threshold than the holmium lasers, due to better water absorption (24). Energy from this solid-state laser can be transmitted via silica fiber optics.

The neodymium:YAG laser can operate in a continuous wave or pulsed mode and emits in the near-infrared at a fundamental frequency of 1064 nm. Visible and ultraviolet wavelengths of 532, 355, and 266 nm can be obtained if the laser is operated in a frequency-doubled, -tripled, or -quadrupled mode, respectively. The 1064-nm wavelength is not well absorbed by tissue water, allowing deep tissue penetration of laser light (approximately 2.5 mm) and subsequent thermal damage due to heating of deep tissue layers during ablation. Ablation at this wavelength can be enhanced by irradiating arterial tissue in the presence of substances, such as blood, that have greater absorption for 1064-nm light (45,46). Abela et al. demonstrated enhanced ablation at 1064 nm when atherosclerotic plaque was pretreated with sudan black in vitro (9). As with other ablation lasers, use of shorter pulse durations can reduce thermal damage during ablation. Geschwind et al. used a continuous wave neodymium:YAG laser emitting at 1064 nm to compare the effect of short versus long exposure times of 2–50 seconds on atherosclerotic plaque ablation (45,46). Thermal damage was more notable during long exposure times. Deckelbaum et al. reported that clean ablation could not be achieved at a pulse duration of 200 microseconds, but could be achieved with a Q-switched pulse of 10–20 nanoseconds (10,19). However, these high peak powers were near the damage threshold of silica and could not be transmitted by small-diameter fibers.

The next class of lasers emits light in the visible wavelength range, and includes the dye, argon, and frequency-doubled neodymium:YAG lasers. This class of lasers is not well absorbed by water, but may be well absorbed by specific chromophores.

The dye laser is a tunable device, able to emit pulsed laser energy in the 400- to 750-nm wavelength range by using various dyes such as coumarin, diphenylstilbene, or rhodamine as lasing media. Laser output can be transmitted by silica fiber optics. Evaluation of this laser in vitro has been predominantly for the selective ablation of atherosclerotic plaque. This approach is based on the premise that a wavelength might be chosen that will selectively ablate atherosclerotic plaque without damaging normal tissue. Prince et al. noted enhanced absorption of yellow plaque at 420–530 nm as compared to normal tissue in vitro (47,48). Enhanced absorption of yellow plaque over this wavelength range was due to the high concentration of carotenoids. As a result, enhanced ablation (e.g., lower ablation threshold) of atherosclerotic as compared to normal tissue was observed using a flashlamp-excited dye laser. Prince et al. also reported a lower ablation threshold and greater ablation efficiency of calcified plaque compared to normal artery at an ablation wavelength of 482 or 658 nm (49). However, the magnitude of the difference in absorption between atherosclerotic and normal tissue in the above studies is probably not of sufficient magnitude to result in absolute selectivity of ablation during intraarterial laser irradiation; energy fluences needed for plaque ablation still damage normal arterial tissue.

The argon laser is an ionized gas laser that emits blue-green continuous wave or pulsed energy at 488 or 515 nm. Output from this laser can be transmitted via silica fiber optics. As can be seen in Table 8.1, the argon laser wavelengths are not strongly absorbed by water when compared to the infrared and ultraviolet lasers. This decreased absorption causes a higher ablation threshold and a larger zone of thermal damage

(9,20). Use of short pulse durations in the 35- to 63-millisecond range have been reported to decrease thermal injury with chopped-wave argon lasers (13). Ablation with a mode-locked argon laser was reported to cause an amount of thermal damage similar to continuous wave laser ablation, due to high repetition rate (256 × 106 Hz) and low peak power (10). The argon laser has been reported to ablate mild to moderately calcified tissue, but is ineffective in ablating heavily calcified tissue (50,51).

The frequency-doubled neodymium:YAG laser emits at a wavelength of 532 nm. This wavelength was reported by Grundfest et al. to cause tissue fissuring from acoustic shock-wave damage during ablation and was ineffective in ablating calcified tissue (20). Furthermore, Litvack et al. were unable to transmit nanosecond 532-nm pulses by fiber optics at energies used for ablation (25).

The last class of clinical lasers are the ultraviolet lasers, consisting of the frequency-doubled alexandrite, excimer, and frequency-tripled or -quadrupled neodymium:YAG lasers.

The alexandrite laser can operate in a continuous wave or pulsed mode and is able to emit at multiple wavelengths. This solid-state laser has a fundamental wavelength in the 700–800-nm visible range, but frequency doubling with 350–400-nm output is possible. The tissue absorption coefficient and depth of penetration at 378 nm are equivalent to that at 2.1 microns, the wavelength of the holmium laser (see Table 8.1). The frequency-doubled alexandrite laser operating in a Q-switched mode with pulse duration of 60 nanoseconds can achieve tissue ablation with gross and histologic effects similar to those of a 355-nm excimer laser (52,53). Pulse width in the Q-switched mode is variable from 60–250 nanoseconds, facilitating transmission of the 378-nm wavelength by silica fiber optics (53,54).

The excimer laser is a pulsed ionized gas laser capable of emitting at wavelengths of 355, 308, 248, and 193 nm. These wavelengths are well absorbed by tissue, and absorption is best at the shorter wavelengths, as shown in Table 8.1. The lowest threshold energy required for ablation would be expected at 248 and 193 nm, and the highest ablation threshold at 355 nm. Isner et al. and Grundfest et al. reported the ability of the excimer laser to ablate aorta with minimal thermal damage at 355 and 308 nm, but the thermal damage was less with 308-nm irradiation as compared to 355-nm irradiation (11,20,55). The excimer laser pulse durations can be prolonged to greater than 100 nanoseconds, enabling ready transmission by silica fiber optics (25). However, the lower ultraviolet wavelengths, such as 266 and 193 nm, are not readily transmitted by conventional silica fibers. Experimental and clinical studies are discussed in more detail in Chapters 4–7 of this book.

Ablation of calcified tissue with a Q-switched, frequency-tripled (355 nm) or -quadrupled (266 nm) neodymium:YAG laser has been reported (10,25). The histologic effects of frequency-tripled neodymium:YAG laser ablation were similar to those of 355-nm excimer ablation. Fiber transmission at these short pulse durations may be difficult.

Laser Operation Considerations

The lasers discussed in this chapter are solid-state, liquid, or ionized gas lasers. Solid-state lasers tend to be more reliable, smaller, and cheaper to operate compared to gas or dye lasers. For example, in a 1985 review, the cost required to purchase and maintain the excimer laser was calculated at $410–468 per hour for a 100–200-watt excimer laser over a 5-year or 10,000-hour span of operation (56). The dye lasers require replenishment of the dyes and can be cumbersome to operate. Solid-state lasers tend to be reliable with stable output energies, but may require periodic replacement of the rod or excitation unit. Therefore, solid-state lasers have a much lower hourly maintenance cost when compared to the gas or dye lasers.

Clinical Development of Laser Angioplasty

McGuff et al. used pulsed energy from a ruby laser to ablate atherosclerotic plaque in 1963, only 3 years after the first laser was developed (57). However, the concept of laser angioplasty had to await the development of balloon angioplasty before renewed interest led to clinical application. In 1984, Ginsburg et al. described the first clinical laser ablation of atherosclerotic plaque using a continuous wave argon laser coupled to a bare optical fiber to recanalize an occluded peripheral artery (58). Since that time, several pulsed lasers have been used in clinical trials of laser angioplasty. In general, except for the excimer laser, all reported clinical trials to date have studied a limited number of patients and provide incomplete data on the potential for pulsed laser angioplasty.

The argon laser has been used in clinical laser angioplasty trials in peripheral and coronary arteries. A fiber optic coupled to an argon laser was used by Ginsburg et al. and Nordstrom et al. to cross occluded or stenosed vessels in the peripheral vasculature (59,60). The laser in both studies was a continuous wave argon laser operated in a chopped mode and coupled to a single optical fiber. Ginsburg was able to cross 15 of 16 lesions, but was unable to cross a calcified lesion. Two laser-induced perforations were noted. Nordstrom crossed 33 of 36 total or high-grade stenoses in the peripheral vasculature, and one laser-induced perforation was reported. Both studies required balloon angioplasty to enlarge the neolumen created by laser angioplasty.

Several studies have been conducted in the coronary arteries using a chopped-wave argon laser. Choy et al. performed laser angioplasty of a right coronary artery intraoperatively using a chopped argon laser (61). Success was noted in reducing the stenosis, but the vessel was totally occluded on follow-up angiography. A 20-fiber, 1.5-mm-diameter catheter coupled to an argon laser was used intraoperatively by Bott-Silverman et al. to recanalize coronary arteries in six patients (62). Six arteries were partially recanalized and perforation occurred in one patient. Percutaneous argon laser angioplasty of the coronary arteries has been reported by Cote et al., Foschi et al., Nordstrom et al., and Mast et al. (63–66). These studies report an acute success rate of 56–100 percent in crossing noncalcified occlusions. Cote et al. used a four-fiber catheter over a guidewire to recanalize occluded coronary arteries. Foschi et al. and Nordstrom et al. used a balloon catheter containing a single 200-micron fiber with a diverging lens at the tip. Despite the use of a continuous wave laser, which is associated with thermal damage in vitro, the complication rates were low. This may have been due to the delivery of brief pulses of argon laser irradiation to minimize thermal damage. No perforations were noted in any of the three studies.

The carbon dioxide laser has had limited in-vivo use due to the difficulty in transmitting 10,600-nm radiation through reliable, flexible fiber optics. Intraoperative coronary endarterectomy using pulsed carbon dioxide laser energy was reported by Livesay and colleagues using a hand-held rigid wave guide (27,67). Five of six high-grade coronary stenoses were crossed without perforation. One lesion was not recanalized due to heavy calcification.

Neodymium:YAG laser angioplasty has been performed in peripheral vessels. Geschwind et al. were the first to report the clinical use in three patients of a pulsed neodymium:YAG laser to cross occluded femoropopliteal arteries without complication (46). Neodymium:YAG laser ablation followed by balloon angioplasty was used by Murray et al.

and Neubar et al. to recanalize ischemic limbs in 26 and 19 patients, respectively (68,69). Perforation occurred in one patient in the first study, and an inability to cross calcified plaque was noted in the second study.

The pulsed dye laser has been used in the peripheral and coronary arteries. Geschwind et al. and Leon et al. used a pulsed dye laser system to cross occluded femoropopliteal arteries (70,71). Their system incorporated a low-power helium-cadmium laser to induce arterial fluorescence to discriminate atherosclerotic from normal arterial sites prior to ablation. Both studies used the laser system coupled to a 200- or 500-micron fiber to cross occluded vessels. Further recanalization was then achieved by balloon angioplasty. The first study crossed occlusions in all 19 patients but noted one fiber-wire perforation and two dissections. These were attributed to mechanical factors related to the stiff optical fiber. The second study crossed 10 of 12 femoropopliteal occlusions and noted one mechanical perforation. The two lesions not crossed were heavily calcified.

Leon et al. used a fluorescence-guided dye or holmium system in the coronary arteries of patients with total occlusions, diffuse disease, or ostial lesions (72). The initial results from this study showed successful crossing of the coronary lesions in 11 of 12 patients. The procedure was complicated by abrupt closure, dissection, or side-branch occlusion in seven patients. These complications may have been precipitated by the tissue fissuring during in-vitro holmium laser ablation and attributed to shock-wave damage.

Summary

Laser angioplasty has the potential to improve upon the current success of conventional balloon angioplasty. The use of pulsed laser energy during laser angioplasty minimizes the extent of thermal damage to the surrounding tissue and permits calcified plaque ablation. The elimination of thermal damage may result in a more benign healing process, a less thrombogenic surface, and improved preservation of structural tissue integrity. These potential benefits, however, remain to be proven.

Several pulsed lasers have currently been evaluated for laser angioplasty. The selection of an appropriate laser depends on several factors, including power-output profile, ablation characteristics, transmission by flexible fiber-optic catheters, reliability, and cost. The best combination of the above has not been determined, and several different clinical laser angioplasty trials are currently underway. It is clear that even at this early stage of development, further clinical studies are warranted to more fully evaluate the potential of laser angioplasty using pulsed lasers.

References

1. Gruentzig AR, Senning A, Seigenthaler WE. Nonoperative dilatation of coronary-artery stenosis: percutaneous transluminal coronary angioplasty. *N Engl J Med* 1979;301:61–68.
2. Kent KM, Bentivoglio LG, Block PC, et al. Long-term efficacy of percutaneous transluminal coronary angioplasty (PTCA): report from the National Heart, Lung, and Blood Institute Registry. *Am J Cardiol* 1984; 53:27C–31C.
3. Holmes DR, Vlietstra RE, Smith HC, et al. Restenosis after percutaneous transluminal coronary angioplasty (PTCA): a report from the PTCA Registry of the National Heart, Lung, and Blood Institute. *Am J Cardiol* 1984;53:77C–81C.
4. Isner JM, Steg PG, Clarke RH. Current status of cardiovascular laser therapy. *IEEE J Quantum Elect* 1987;QE-23:1756–1771.
5. Litvack F, Grundfest W, Papaioannou T, Mohr F, Jakubowski AT, Forrester JS. Role of laser and thermal ablation devices in the treatment of vascular diseases. *Am J Cardiol* 1988;61:81G–86G.
6. Deckelbaum LI. Laser angioplasty. *Cardiol Clin* 1988;6(3):345–346.
7. Hitz CB. Understanding laser technology. Oklahoma: PennWell Publishing Co., 1985.
8. Cummins L, Navenberg M. Thermal effects of laser radiation in biological tissue. *Biophys J* 1983;42:99–102.
9. Abela GS, Normann S, Cohen D, Feldman RL, Geiser EA, Conti CR. Effects of carbon dioxide, Nd-YAG, and argon laser radiation on coronary atheromatous plaques. *Am J Cardiol* 1982;50:1199–1205.
10. Deckelbaum LI, Isner JM, Donaldson RF, et al. Reduction of laser-induced pathologic tissue injury using pulsed energy delivery. *Am J Cardiol* 1985;56:662–667.
11. Grundfest WS, Litvack IF, Goldenberg T, et al. Pulsed ultraviolet lasers and the potential for safe laser angioplasty. *Am J Surg* 1985;150:220–226.
12. Deckelbaum LI, Isner JM, Donaldson RF, Laliberte SM, Clarke RH, Salem D. Use of pulsed energy delivery to minimize tissue injury result-

ing from carbon dioxide laser irradiation of cardiovascular tissue. *J Am Coll Cardiol* 1986;7:898–908.
13. Kramer JR, Bott-Silverman C, Ratliff NB, et al. Removal of atherosclerotic plaque using multiple short exposures of argon ion laser light. *Am Heart J* 1987;113:1038–1040.
14. Puliafito CA, Steinert RF. Short-pulsed Nd:YAG laser microsurgery of the eye: biophysical considerations. *IEEE J Quantum Elect* 1984;QE-20:1442–1448.
15. Eldar M, Battler A, Gal D, et al. The effects of varying lengths and powers of CO_2 laser pulses transmitted through an optical fiber on atherosclerotic plaques. *Clin Cardiol* 1986;9:89–91.
16. Zweig AD, Weber HP. Mechanical and thermal parameters in pulsed laser cutting of tissue. *IEEE J Quantum Elect* 1987;QE-23:1787–1793.
17. Walsh JT, Flotte TJ, Deutsch TF. Er:YAG laser ablation of tissue: effect of pulse duration and tissue type on thermal damage. *Lasers Surg Med* 1989;9:314–326.
18. Walsh JT, Flotte TJ, Anderson RR, Deutsch T. Pulsed CO_2 laser tissue ablation: effect of tissue type and pulse duration on thermal damage. *Lasers Surg Med* 1988;8:108–118.
19. Deckelbaum LI, Lam JK, Clubb S, Cabin HS. Pulse duration is the major determinant of thermal damage during pulsed laser tissue ablation (abstr.). *J Am Coll Cardiol* 1985;7:238A.
20. Grundfest WS, Litvack F, Forrester JS, et al. Laser ablation of human atherosclerotic plaque without adjacent tissue injury. *J Am Coll Cardiol* 1985;5:929–933.
21. Welch AJ. The thermal response of laser irradiated tissue. *IEEE J Quantum Elect* 1984;QE-12:1471–1481.
22. Anderson RR, Parrish JA. Selective photothermolysis: precise microsurgery by selective absorption of pulsed radiation. *Science* 1983;220:524–527.
23. Esenaliev RO, Oraevsky AA, Letokhov VS. Laser ablation of atherosclerotic blood vessel tissue under various irradiation conditions. *IEEE Trans Biomed Eng* 1989;36:1188–1194.
24. Esterowitz L, Hoffman C. A comparison of the erbium mid-IR laser and the short-wavelength UV excimer lasers for medical applications. Proceedings of the International Conference on Lasers 1986;536–539.
25. Litvack F, Grundfest WS, Goldenberg T, et al. Pulsed laser angioplasty: wavelength power and energy dependencies relevant to clinical application. *Lasers Surg Med* 1988;8:60–65.
26. Scheggi Am, Falciai R, Gironi G. Characterization of oxide glasses for hollow-core middle IR fibers. *Appl Opt* 1985;24:4392–4394.

27. Livesay JJ, Colloey DA. Laser coronary endarterectomy: proposed treatment for diffuse coronary atherosclerosis. *Tex Heart Inst J* 1984;11:276–279.
28. Miyashita T, Manabe T. Infrared optical fibers. *IEEE J Quantum Electronics* 1982;QE18:1432–1450.
29. Eldar M, Battler A, Neufeld HN, et al. Transluminal carbon dioxide-laser catheter angioplasty for dissolution of atherosclerotic plaques. *J Am Coll Cardiol* 1984;3:135–137.
30. Curcio JA, Petty CP. The near-infrared absorption spectrum of liquid water. *J Opt Soc Am* 1951;14:302–305.
31. Esterowitz L, Hoffman CA, Tran DC, et al. Angioplasty with a laser and fiber optic at 2.94 microns. *Proc Soc Photo-Opt Instrum Eng* 1986;605:32–35.
32. Walsh JT, Deutsch TF. Er:YAG laser ablation of tissue: measurement of ablation rates. *Lasers Surg Med* 1989;9:327–337.
33. Kaufmann R, Hibst R. Pulsed Er:YAG and 308-nm UV-excimer laser: an in-vitro and in-vivo study of skin-ablative effects. *Lasers Surg Med* 1989;9:132–140.
34. Nelson JS, Yow L, Liaw LH, et al. Ablation of bone and methacrylate by a prototype mid-infrared erbium:YAG laser. *Lasers Surg Med* 1988;8:494–500.
35. Nuss RC, Fabian RL, Sarkar R, Puliafito CA. Infrared laser bone ablation. *Lasers Surg Med* 1988;8:381–391.
36. Bonner RF, Smith PD, Leon MB, Tran SD, Esterowitz L. A new erbium laser and infrared fiber system for laser angioplasty (abstr.). *Circulation* (suppl II) 1986;74:II-360.
37. Wolbarsht ML, Esterowitz L, Tran D, Levin K, Storm M. A mid-infrared (2.94 micron) surgical laser with an optical fiber delivery system (abstr.). *Am Soc Laser Med Surg* 1986;6:257.
38. Bonner RF, Smith PD, Leon ML, et al. Quantification of tissue effects due to pulsed Er:YAG laser at 2.9 microns with beam delivery in a wet field via zirconium fluoride fibers. *Proc SPIE* 1987;713:2–5.
39. Stein E, Sedlacek T, Fabian RL, Nishioka NS. Acute and chronic effects of bone ablation with pulsed holmium laser. *Lasers Surg Med* 1990;10:384–388.
40. Kopchok GE, White RA, Tabbara M, Saadatmanesh V, Peng SK. Holmium:YAG laser ablation of vascular tissue. *Lasers Surg Med* 1990;10:405–413.
41. Nishioka NS, Domankevitz Y. Reflectance during pulsed holmium laser irradiation of tissue. *Lasers Surg Med* 1989;9:375–381.
42. Garrand TJ, Stetz ML, O'Brien KL, Gindi G, Sumpio BE, Deckelbaum

LI. Design and evaluation of a fiber-optic fluorescence-guided laser recanalization system. *Lasers Surg Med* 1991;11:106–116.
43. Deckelbaum LI, Scott JJ, Stetz ML, O'Brien KL, Baker G. Detection of calcified atherosclerotic plaque by laser-induced plasma emission (abstr.). *Circulation* (suppl III) 1990;82:III-105.
44. Bonner RF, Bartorelli A, Almagor Y, Keren G, Hansch E, Leon MB. Cardiac pacing by shock waves during pulsed laser angioplasty (abstr.). *J Am Coll Cardiol* 1990;15:56A.
45. Geschwind HJ, Teisseire B, Boussignac G, Vieilledent C. Transluminal laser angioplasty in man. *Semin Intervent Radiol* 1986;3:69–74.
46. Geschwind HJ, Boussignac G, Teisseire B, Benhaiem, Bittoun R, Laurent D. Conditions for effective Nd-YAG laser angioplasty. *Br Heart J* 1984;52:484–489.
47. Prince MR, Deutsch TF, Mathews-Roth MM, Margolis R, Parrish JA, Oseroff AR. Preferential light absorption in atheromas in vitro: implications for laser angioplasty. *J Clin Invest* 1986;78:295–302.
48. Prince MR, Deutsch TF, Shapiro AH, et al. Selective ablation of atheromas using a flashlamp-excited dye laser at 465 nm. *Proc Natl Acad Sci* 1986;83:7064–7068.
49. Prince MR, LaMuraglia GM, Teng T, Deutsch TF. Preferential ablation of calcified arterial plaque with laser-induced plasmas. *IEEE J Quantum Electronics* 1987;QE-23:1783–1786.
50. Lawrence PF, Dries DJ, Moatamed F, Dixon J. Acute effects of argon laser on human atherosclerotic plaque. *J Vasc Surg* 1984;1:852–859.
51. Abela GS, Seeger JM, Barbiere E, et al. Laser angioplasty with angioscopic guidance in humans. *J Am Coll Cardiol* 1986;8:184–192.
52. Kuper JW, Langert WE, Baker MC, et al. Medical applications of alexandrite laser systems. Topical Meeting on Tunable Solid State Lasers 1987;183–184. Oct. 26-28, 1987, Williamsburg, Virginia: Optical Society of America.
53. Deckelbaum LI, Stetz M, Cutruzzola FW, Kuper JW, Baker MC, Barrett JJ. A pulsed ultraviolet alexandrite laser for angioplasty: evaluation of tissue ablation and fiberoptic conduction (abstr.). *J Am Coll Cardiol* 1987;9:188A.
54. Sam CL, Walling JC, Jenssen HP, Morris RC, O'Dell EW. Characteristics of alexandrite lasers in Q-switched and tuned operations. *SPIE Advances in Laser Engineering and Applications* 1980;247:130–136.
55. Isner JM, Donaldson RF, Deckelbaum LI, et al. The excimer laser: gross, light microscopic and ultrastructural analysis of potential advantages for use in laser therapy of cardiovascular disease. *J Am Coll Cardiol* 1985;6:1102–1109.

56. Klauminzer GK. Cost considerations for industrial excimer lasers. *Laser Focus/Electro-Optics* 1985:108–111.
57. McGuff PE, Bushnell D, Soroff HS, Deterling RA. Studies of the surgical applications of laser (light amplification by stimulated emission of radiation). *Surg Forum* 1963;14:143–145.
58. Ginsburg R, Kim DS, Guthaner D, Toth J, Mitchell RS. Salvage of an ischemic limb by laser angioplasty: description of a new technique. *Clin Cardiol* 1984;7:54–58.
59. Ginsburg R, Wexler L, Mitchell RS, Profitt D. Percutaneous transluminal laser angioplasty for treatment of peripheral vascular disease: clinical experience with 16 patients. *Radiology* 1985;156:619–624.
60. Nordstrom LA, Castaneda-Zuniga WR, Young EG, Von Seggern KB. Direct argon laser exposure for recanalization of peripheral arteries: early results. *Radiology* 1988;168:359–364.
61. Choy DSJ, Stertzer RH, Myler RK, Fournial G. Human coronary laser recanalization. *Clin Cardiol* 1984;7:377–381.
62. Bott-Silverman C, Cothren R, Hayes G, Kramer J, Loop F, Feld M. In vivo intraoperative coronary laser angiosurgery (abstr.). *Lasers Surg Med* 1988;8:8.
63. Cote G, Smith A, Andrus S, Lane J, Dumont M, Madden M. Immediate results of percutaneous argon laser coronary angioplasty (abstr.). *Circulation* (suppl II) 1989;80:II-477.
64. Foschi AE, Myers GE, Flamm MD. Laser-enhanced coronary angioplasty via direct argon laser exposures: early clinical results in totally occluded native arteries (abstr.). *Circulation* (suppl II)1989;80:II-478.
65. Nordstrom LA, Haughland JM, Strauss GS, Peterson CR, Monson BK, Dyrud P. Direct laser angioplasty: clinical results of 53 consecutive human peripheral and 5 coronary cases (abstr.). *Lasers Surg Med* 1988;8:7.
66. Mast G, Plokker T, Ernst S, Bal E, Gin MTJ, Ascoop C. Argon-laser angioplasty for chronic total coronary occlusions: first European experience (abstr.). *Circulation* (suppl III) 1990;82:III-677.
67. Livesay JJ, Leachman DR, Hogan PJ, et al. Preliminary report on laser coronary endarterectomy in patients (abstr.). *Circulation* (suppl III) 1985;72:III-302.
68. Murray A, Wood RFM, Mitchell DC, Edwards DH, Grasty M, Basu R. Peripheral laser angioplasty with pulsed dye laser and ball-tipped optical fibres. *Lancet* 1989;1:1471–1474.
69. Neubar T, Klepzig M, Heintzen MP, Richter EI, Zettler E, Strauer BE. Peripheral percutaneous transluminal laser angioplasty in humans: in

vitro investigations and clinical results with a novel laser catheter system. *Clin Cardiol* 1989;12:313–320.
70. Geschwind HJ, Dubois-Rande JL, Shafton E, Boussignac G, Wexman M. Percutaneous pulsed laser-assisted balloon angioplasty guided by spectroscopy. *Am Heart J* 1989;117:1147–1152.
71. Leon MB, Almagor Y, Bartorelli AL, et al. Fluorescence-guided laser-assisted balloon angioplasty in patients with femoropopliteal occlusions. *Circulation* 1990;81:143–155.
72. Leon MB, Keren G, Bartorelli AL, et al. Fluorescence-guided laser coronary angioplasty: a clinical status report (abstr.). *Circulation* (suppl III) 1990;82:III-496.

CHAPTER **9**

Laser Balloon Angioplasty: Evolving Technology

J. Richard Spears

Background

THERMAL energy at subvaporization thresholds has been used for many decades in clinical medicine. High-frequency electrocautery, the first common means for applying thermal energy, has proved useful during surgical control of bleeding since thermal shrinkage of vessels and coagulation of blood by this technique is effective, structural integrity of tissues is maintained, and long-term tissue reactions are relatively benign. As an extension of this procedure, Sigel et al. (1,2) demonstrated in the 1960s that electrocautery could be used to create portocaval anastomoses and to close linear incisions in arteries and veins in dogs. During the same period, other investigators used incoherent, broad-band light from a xenon arc lamp to seal retinal tears. Within a few years, however, coherent light from lasers—initially ruby (3) and subsequently argon and krypton ion lasers—developed during this era superseded the use of incoherent light in ophthalmologic applications, principally treatment of diabetic retinopathy and closure of retinal tears, because of the precision with which coherent light can be focused and because of the more suitable match between laser wavelength and tissue absorption of light.

Surgical anastomosis of small tubular soft-tissue structures with conventional suture technique is time-consuming and often associated with inflammatory cell reactions that may interfere with the long-term success of such procedures. In 1966, Yahr et al. (4) were the first to report the potential utility of laser energy for anastomosis of blood vessels, while in 1978 Klink et al. (5) and von Klitzing et al. (6) investigated the experimental feasibility of the use of a CO_2 laser to induce end-to-end fallopian-tube anastomoses. Shortly thereafter, Jain and Gorisch (7) demonstrated that energy from a Nd:YAG laser (1.06 μm) could be used to repair linear incisions in small vessels experimentally. Jain later demonstrated that "sutureless" microvascular anastomoses could be achieved with the same laser, both in animals and in man (8,9). A similar application of laser energy was subsequently described for a variety of other tissues, including large vessels, nerves, ileum, and vas deferens (10–14). Compared to the use of electrocautery, the application of lasers to thermally coagulate tissues was attractive for several reasons. Laser energy can be applied in a noncontact manner, allowing the operator to visually monitor the degree of coagulation, which is usually evident as a color change such as blanching (or darkening when free blood is present at the anastomotic site) and shrinkage of tissue. In addition, the depth of thermal penetration can theoretically be controlled with the use of laser radiation by simply matching the thickness and type of tissue with an appropriate wavelength of laser energy. For example, 10.6-μm energy from a CO_2 laser is absorbed within the first 100 microns and may be useful for anastomosis of thin-walled structures, while energy from an argon-ion laser penetrates into arterial tissue several hundred microns and is more suitable for anastomosis of large vessels. Tissue heating results from both absorption of laser energy and thermal diffusion from superficial to deep layers of tissue. By contrast, heating occurs solely by thermal diffusion when an electrocautery device is used, and the relatively slow rate of thermal diffusion through most soft tissues then translates into large thermal gradients within the tissue. As Sigel et al. noted (1), excessive coagulation of superficial tissues with an electrocautery device, which can easily occur in an attempt to adequately heat deeper layers, is associated with disruption of connective tissue elements and poor bonding between tissues.

Fortunately, the biologic responses such as inflammatory cell infiltration that are associated with laser-induced anastomoses have been found, in general, to compare favorably with those associated with conventional suture technique. In fact, White et al. (12) demonstrated with the use of radioactive proline that the deposition of collagen in an experimental model was markedly reduced at the site of laser-induced anastomoses 1 week after treatment, compared to that associated with sutured tissues. Although the strength of the thermal bonds is initially weaker than that achieved with sutures, properly applied it is greater than the force applied by physiologic arterial pressure, and it increases over time to the same level as that associated with sutures. Most reports have shown that the thermal coagulation necrosis is not associated with a loss of mural integrity or a potential for occasional aneurysm formation, which very probably represents the result of either inadequate or excessive tissue heating. Interestingly, laser-anastomosed arteries in growing swine have been shown to retain a capacity for commensurate normal growth, unlike arteries anastomosed with conventional suture technique (15).

Laser Balloon Angioplasty: Experimental Studies

During laser balloon angioplasty (LBA), heat provided by absorption of Nd:YAG laser energy (1.06 μm) by arterial tissues surrounding an inflated balloon, along with simultaneously applied tissue pressure, is used to remodel the arterial lumen (16–19). Two important tissue effects result acutely: fusion of tissues separated during prior conventional balloon inflation and reduction of arterial recoil. A third acute tissue effect, which was discovered only after clinical experience was gained, is dessication and remodeling of thrombus. In addition, LBA may favorably alter adverse responses to arterial injury caused by angioplasty in two ways: 1) an appropriate level of protein denaturation might reduce the thrombogenicity of tissues at the luminal surface, and 2) thermal induction of adherence of a water-insoluble drug carrier to the luminal surface and to deeper layers of the arterial wall might provide persistent activity of a suitable drug.

From the previous discussion, it is apparent that only one potentially useful tissue effect sought during LBA—thermal fusion of juxtaposed tissues—had been studied in the past. At the time we initiated in-vitro studies of human postmortem atheromatous plaque-media separations, it was unknown, however, whether laser energy could be used to fuse tissue layers together at a plane relatively deep below the irradiated surface of the tissue. I noted in 1983 that, by simple immersion of arterial tissue layers, held together with a hemostat under saline at 90–100° C for less than a minute, a firm bond between tissues was created and that it should be possible to use heat to seal balloon angioplasty–induced arterial dissections. In contrast, heating the tissue layers by contact on only one side with a hot surface, such as the wall of a glass beaker heated to as high as 150° C, was unsuccessful in bonding the tissues together. The reason for lack of success of the latter approach was that thermal diffusion was relatively slow, the nonheated surface acted as a heat sink, and the severe temperature gradient over a depth on the order of 1–2 mm resulted in differential contraction of the superficially heated plaque and the inadequately heated adjacent media. It was apparent that, in vivo, a means would have to be found to achieve more uniform heating to a similar depth when the source of energy is from one side of the tissue. Not surprisingly, we found that CW CO_2 and argon ion laser radiation were inadequate in bonding separated arterial tissue layers. The relatively deeply penetrating nature of Nd:YAG laser energy at 1.06 μm through most soft tissues, however, made it possible to fuse separated layers of human postmortem atheromatous aortas to a depth of approximately 2 mm.

In attempts to bond separated tissue layers under simple in-vitro conditions with 1.06-μm radiation, we were not successful until firm tissue pressure was applied simultaneously by use of a transparent glass slide. The necessity for tissue pressure had not been described in studies of laser-induced anastomoses, but had been described by Sigel in experimental studies of thermal coaptive closure of vessels with electrocautery. The need for simultaneous application of heat and pressure was fortuitous, since application of tissue pressure is the basis of conventional balloon angioplasty and, perhaps more importantly, the other two acute tissue effects of LBA—reduction of arterial recoil and remodeling of thrombus—also require a combination of the two modalities.

Unlike previous applications of photocoagulation technology, tissue fusion during LBA has to be performed without visual assessment of the onset and degree of coagulation. Fluoroscopic monitoring provides an excellent means for controlling the amount of distending balloon pressure but yields no useful information related to the heat required to additionally remodel the arterial lumen. Prior to a clinical application, we therefore needed to define the relationship between the laser dose and the efficacy of tissue bonding, so that a laser dose could be administered in a relatively "blind" manner with the expectation of clinical efficacy. From a technical viewpoint, it is considerably easier to study the effect of modifications of laser exposure parameters on sections of atheromatous aortas on the resultant bond strength, compared to circumferentially intact arteries. In addition, technical obstacles at the time of our initial laser dosimetry studies precluded the availability of a multidose LBA catheter until after completion of an FDA Phase I clinical study. Considering that the geometry of a laser exposure would drastically alter the tissue response, thus making laser dosimetry studies of aortic sections irrelevant to optimizing dosimetry for a cylindrical exposure, we needed to study the relationship among the temperature history of tissue, the fundamental tissue effect of laser exposure, and the adequacy of fusion of separated tissue layers. Once the optimal temperature history for bonding tissue layers was defined, the laser dose could be adjusted for the specific pattern of laser exposure desired.

Virtually no information related to the temperature history of tissues and the efficacy of laser and thermal fusion of any type of juxtaposed tissues was available prior to our in-vitro studies. An important reason for the lack of such information is that accurate measurement of tissue temperature during laser exposure is quite difficult. Thermographic imaging, properly performed, can provide accurate temperature measurements of an irradiated surface, but an interface between air and tissue is required, thereby altering the thermal boundary conditions compared to in-vivo conditions, and the technique cannot be used to measure temperature below the tissue surface such as at the plane of a plaque-media separation. Thermisters or thermocouples are widely employed to measure tissue temperature, but the metal components of these devices result in excessive self-heating during a laser exposure, so that an artifactually high temperature reading may be observed. To some extent, we circumvented problems associated with the use of a thermister by positioning the thermister on the adventitial surface during laser exposure of the intimal surface, that is, at least 1 mm below the irradiated surface, reducing the effect of self-absorption of radiation, which would have exceeded that of soft tissue had the latter been normally present [20]. In addition, the size of the thermister, 5 mm, was similar to the estimated size of the zone of irradiation at the plane of tissue separation, allowing the thermister to provide an average temperature of the entire zone of irradiation. Measurements were made of the thermister temperature response as a function of the thickness of tissue irradiated, so that an estimate of the actual temperature at the plane of tissue separation, usually 0.3 to 0.5 mm superficial to the thermister, could be made. In general, the temperature at the plane of tissue separation was estimated to be 10–15° C higher than the thermister readings at the adventitial surface. Although there may have been a slightly greater temperature rise within relatively thin (< 1 mm) tissue sections as a result of the presence of the thermister, compared to normal in-vivo thermal boundary conditions, the measurements accurately reflected the actual temperatures achieved at the plane of tissue separation, and a correlation could then be made between the temperature history of tissue and the resultant bond strength of the tissues.

We anticipated that, clinically, it would be desirable to reduce the period of laser exposure to a minimum to reduce the period of balloon occlusion of a coronary artery. Moreover, the interpretation of the results of studies of tissue temperature is facilitated by adjusting the laser exposure so that a single plateau temperature results. A decremental power format was therefore devised to achieve a target tissue temperature within 5 seconds of the onset of laser exposure by starting with a relatively high laser power, and to maintain a relatively constant temperature thereafter for the remainder of a 20–30-second exposure by stepwise reduction of the laser power (20,21). Fortuitously, it was found that in comparison with a constant power format, the decremental power format was more energy efficient in achieving a given target temperature, and for the same peak temperature achieved, it also was associated with a greater weld strength of the juxtaposed tissue layers. The reason for the former observation probably lies in the fact that a rapid rise in tissue temperature allows less time for thermal diffusion to adjacent nontargeted tissues, so less energy is required to heat targeted tissues with the use of the decremental power format. A subsequent in-vitro study (22) also demonstrated that CW Nd:YAG laser energy transmission through the arterial wall is reduced during exposure, very probably as a result of thermal breakage of noncovalent bonds and increased efficiency of radiation scattering; rapid tissue heating would allow this effect to occur quickly, reducing the amount of energy required to achieve a target tissue temperature compared to a constant power format. One can only speculate why the decremental format was associated with a greater weld strength of arterial tissue layers, but the possibility exists that relatively rapid heating of collagen is more effective in denaturation of this molecule, as suggested by an in-vitro study. Schober et al. (23) demonstrated by electron microscopy that interdigitation of fibrillary substructures of collagen is at least partly responsible for laser and thermal fusion of juxtaposed tissues in a murine model of vascular anastomosis. Transient breakage of the noncovalent bonds of collagen during laser exposure may free the fibrillary substructures, thereby allowing interdigitation to occur between adjacent collagen molecules across the plane of separation of juxtaposed tissues upon reformation of noncovalent bonds during tissue cooling.

With the use of a 20-second CW Nd:YAG decremental power format, a threshold plateau adventitial temperature of approximately 80° C was required to induce any measurable tissue bond between intima-media pairs. The actual corresponding threshold temperature at the plane of tissue separation was therefore approximately 90° C. The weld strength of tissues was found to be linearly related to the plateau temperature achieved over an 80–150° C adventitial temperature range. At higher temperatures, rapid dessication of tissues at the intimal surface occurred with the potential for initiation of vaporization of the solid components of the tissue. As Welch et al. (24) pointed out, vaporization of arterial tissue occurs at a threshold temperature of approximately 180° C. Temperatures greater than 100° C result in the liberation of steam and somewhat higher temperatures are required to produce steam for tissue under pressure. Due to the heat loss of evaporation of water, the temperature of tissue under pressure plateaus at 100–120° C during dessication, despite continued laser exposure, which helps to provide a measure of safety in terms of avoiding actual tissue vaporization during attempts to thermally bond tissues together.

The thermal profile of the atheromatous arterial wall as a function of tissue thickness changes from a fairly linear relationship at relatively low laser doses to one that is flat to a depth of 1.5 mm with a rapid taper thereafter at relatively high laser doses. Very probably, at relatively high doses, when superficial tissue temperatures exceed the threshold for the phase change of water, much of the additional absorbed laser energy is simply lost in the heat of evaporation of water and superficial temperatures do not rise further until complete dessication occurs. Our findings related to the depth of thermal penetration are similar to those of Marchisini et al. (25), who found that, for gastric mucosa, the maximum depth of coagulation necrosis was approximately 2 mm. Beyond 2 mm, relatively long exposures at a high dose, a dose that would result in significant dessication at the tissue surface, would be required to achieve a tissue temperature great enough to fuse separated tissue layers.

When laser exposure durations over a 5- to 30-second range were studied in terms of strength of welds of human postmortem atherosclerotic aortic intima-media pairs, a minimum duration of 5 seconds, corresponding to the time required to reach temperatures >90° C, was found necessary to produce any measurable tissue fusion. Tissue bonding was fairly predictable only for durations of > 10 seconds. The improvement in weld strength over a 5–20-second exposure duration appeared linear irrespective of the peak temperature achieved, while further improvements in weld strength tended to plateau for longer exposure durations.

Arterial Recoil

Following balloon angioplasty, arterial recoil reduces the magnitude of the minimum luminal diameter achieved. Within 30 minutes after coronary balloon angioplasty, vasomotor tone increases and may at least in part explain Nobuyoshi et al.'s (26) observation that the mean minimum luminal diameter of a large group of patients was found to be 10 percent smaller 1 day after the procedure, but that by 1 month the minimum luminal diameter approached the acute post-PTCA result. Considering that the mean minimum luminal diameter immediately after initially successful angioplasty is approximately 30 percent smaller than the diameter of the inflated balloon in most studies, it is likely that passive viscoelastic recoil may be even more important than an increase in vasomotor tone as a component of arterial recoil following PTCA. In addition, unlike an increase in vasomotor tone, the loss of luminal diameter from passive recoil is permanent.

In 1984, we initiated studies to examine the potential safety of circumferential heating of the arterial wall during balloon inflation of the normal dog carotid artery (17). We had yet not used a Nd:YAG laser to fuse separated layers of the arterial wall due to lack of the laser. We were nonetheless able to test with an argon ion laser (principal lines 488 and 515 nm) the hypothesis that full-thickness thermal injury, at a tissue temperature of approximately 90° C, around the circumference of the normal dog carotid artery would not be associated with any significant adverse effects on the arterial lumen. Via a distal side branch, a compliant Silastic balloon was placed into the common carotid artery and inflated to 2 atm, which produced a similar tissue pressure because of the balloon compliance, with a resultant 20 percent increase in diameter above baseline values. This was done with and without laser-thermal energy application on control and treatment sides, respectively. By use of a chromophore dissolved within the fluid used to inflate the balloon, strong absorption of the argon ion laser radiation from the distal end of a flat-cleaved silica fiber optic positioned in the midportion of the 2-cm-long, 5-mm-diameter balloon resulted in effective local heating of the fluid in the balloon and the adjacent arterial wall with the delivery of only 3 watts for 1–2 minutes. Angiography was repeated at multiple time intervals (1 day, 1 week, 1 month, 6 months, 1 year) for each dog after the procedure, and one dog was sacrificed at each time interval for histologic examination.

The surprising angiographic finding was that not only was there no evidence of an adverse effect on the arterial lumen, such as loss of mural integrity, aneurysm formation, or stricture, but also the luminal diameter of the thermally treated arterial wall was larger acutely and at each time period after treatment than the lumen of the contralateral control artery, which had been treated with the same balloon but without delivery of thermal energy. Gorisch et al. (27) demonstrated experimentally that when rabbit mesenteric arteries and veins are heated to at least 70–75° C, shrinkage of the tissue, attributed to thermal contraction of collagen fibers, reduced vessel caliber by approximately 20 percent. During LBA, in contrast, the inflated balloon, filled with incompressible fluid, prevents such thermal shrinkage during laser exposure. In fact, application of isometric tension during heating appears to be an effective means for reshaping arterial tissue and for reducing the passive viscoelastic recoil upon release of isometric tension. The results of the application of LBA vs. conventional angioplasty of the normal rabbit iliac artery provide additional strong support for this concept (28). In 36 New Zealand White male rabbits, LBA was applied with a homemade balloon catheter to one iliac artery, and conventional balloon angioplasty was applied to the contralateral iliac artery. Conventional balloon angioplasty produced no significant increase in luminal diameter despite the application of approximately 2 atm tissue pressure with a highly compliant Silastic balloon, the diameter of which was approximately 20 percent greater than baseline values of the artery. LBA with the same catheter produced a significant acute mean increase of approximately 0.4 mm. Either 176 or 300 joules of CW Nd:YAG laser energy were delivered over a 20-second exposure duration from the distal flat-cleaved end of a 400-μm silica fiber optic. Although no diffusing tip terminated the fiber optic, a roughly cylindrical pattern of radiation emitted from the balloon was achieved with the use of a perfluorochemical emulsion, the particle size of which was similar to the laser wavelength, thereby providing efficient scattering. The minimal absorption of 1.06-μm radiation by the perfluorochemical emulsion permitted the delivery of >15 watts without raising fluid temperature within the balloon to >100° C. Parenthetically, the current clinically used, analogous perfluorochemical emulsion, Fluosol-DA 20 percent, cannot be used effectively in this manner because the mean particle size was reduced to a value too small (265 nm) to scatter 1.06-μm radiation efficiently.

When a prototype LBA catheter with a fiber-optic diffusing tip became available from the USCI Division of C. R. Bard, Inc., similar studies of the effect of CW Nd:YAG laser irradiation on the dog coronary arterial lumen and wall were performed (29). A 3-mm balloon was used to deliver 20-sec laser exposures of 20 to 35 watts from a roughly 5-mm-long diffusing tip that had a Gaussian axial distribution and a 2:1 ratio of azimuthal asymmetry of radiation emission over the midportion of the balloon. Despite the nonuniform pattern of laser energy exposure from this catheter, which therefore had a "hot spot" near the proximal end of the diffusing tip, the catheter appeared effective in increasing luminal diameter over most of the length of the 20-mm-long balloon. Ergonovine provocation failed to induce vasoconstriction of laser-irradiated coronary segments, unlike control adjacent segments, at the time of a subacute follow-up, consistent with irreversible damage to medial smooth muscle cells and associated loss of vasoconstrictor potential.

Minimal loss of luminal diameter over a period of 1 year follow-up by computerized analysis of digitized angiographic images was found in the dog carotid and coronary artery studies. In fact, dogs subjected to seven to ten repetitive CW 1.06-μm laser doses of approximately 400 joules per dose delivered over a 3-cm-long segment of the circumflex coronary artery demonstrated lumina that were completely normal in appearance by angiography 1 year after the procedure. In contrast, the normal rabbit iliac artery demonstrated a mean loss of approximately 0.6 mm over a period of 1 month after LBA at a laser dose associated with a peak tissue temperature of approximately 115° C. At a somewhat lower laser dose, the mean loss of the initial gain in diameter was significantly less. Peak temperatures of tissue in the dog coronary artery study were similar at the higher laser doses, but over time a commensurate loss of luminal diameter, compared to that of the high-dose rabbit study, was not found. The reason for the difference in chronic response of luminal dimensions between the two species is unknown, but as discussed below, the results of clinical studies suggest that the normal rabbit iliac artery model may be more predictive of luminal responses in man than the dog model.

Acutely in all models, evidence of pathology at the light-microscopic level is remarkably lacking when the peak temperature achieved is less than approximately 100° C. Dvorak et al. (30) have shown that microwave-induced hyperthermia can be used to "fix" various soft tissues for ultrastructural examination in a manner analogous to the effects of glutaraldehyde. Although estimated peak temperatures were considerably lower than those associated with LBA, they are sufficiently high that, if applied to tissues in vivo, a loss of cell viability could be expected. Thus, standard histologic techniques are inadequate for assessing not only the degree of acute thermal injury at temperatures < 100° C, but also the mere presence of an acute loss of cell viability cannot be detected at these temperatures. Thomsen et al. (31) have recently demonstrated that polarized light microscopy may be useful in this regard by detecting changes in the birefringence of certain types of collagen subjected to in-vivo laser-thermal injury.

When the peak tissue temperature exceeds 100–110° C, overt evidence of thermal injury can be found in both in-vivo tissues and in-vitro human atheromatous aortic sections. Prominent is homogenization of tissues with a loss of structural detail, along with tissue shrinkage from dessication and more intense eosinophilic staining of sections examined under hemotoxylin and eosin staining. At slightly higher temperatures, pleiomorphic lacunae are found, which almost certainly represent the rapid local formation of steam.

By 24 hours after LBA, laser-thermal injury associated with a peak tissue temperature of approximately >70° C produces evidence of a loss of tissue viability as noted by the appearance of cell nuclei that are pale staining by hemotoxylin and eosin. An inflammatory cell infiltrate can be seen several days to approximately a week after thermal injury in both the rabbit and dog models, with replacement of the original smooth muscle cells with fibroblasts over a 1-week to 1-month period. Collagen deposition by Masson's trichrome stain is prominent by 1 month after thermal injury; additional collagen deposition over the remainder of 6 to 12-month follow-up studies appears to be small relative to that found at 1 month.

LBA Catheter Development

Construction of a clinically usable LBA catheter and laser delivery system was technically demanding for several reasons. To make a balloon

Laser Balloon Angioplasty: Evolving Technology 203

catheter that would have mechanical properties, including deflated balloon profile, flexibility, and trackability, similar to those of a conventional balloon catheter, the size of the fiber optic used to deliver laser radiation was limited to approximately 100 μm or less. With the use of a relatively narrow Nd:YAG rod within the laser cavity and collimation of the output, a laser beam with a relatively narrow diameter was produced. A series of lenses, developed initially by E. Sinofsky (USCI Division, C. R. Bard, Inc.), could then be used to couple up to 50 watts of output to the proximal end of a silica fiber optic with 85–90 percent coupling efficiency. Since little radiation impinged on the fiber-optic cladding, no damage to the fiber optic occurred during prolonged (>1 min) exposures at 50 watts, and there was no need to use a specialized cooling mechanism at the input end of the fiber optic.

The most technically limiting problem in the fabrication of an LBA catheter was the development of a suitable diffusing tip at the distal end of the fiber optic. Ideally, to improve the predictability of tissue temperature responses, one would need to start with a nearly cylindrical pattern of energy emitted by the diffusing tip. The azimuthal distribution of photon density should be uniform. The axial distribution, however, would actually have to be slightly "saddle-shaped" to reduce the greater effect of thermal diffusion within tissues adjacent to the midportion of the irradiated field (with associated greater temperature rises) compared to the proximal and distal ends (if a truly cylindrically uniform pattern of radiation were employed for a balloon having a typical length of 20 mm). On the other hand, adequate treatment of most discrete lesions in the coronary artery with laser-thermal energy probably does not require a diffusing tip longer than approximately 10 mm. At the time the initial LBA clinical studies were performed, however, such subtle variations in the pattern of laser radiation were not possible as a result of the manner in which the diffusing tip was constructed. In fact, simply providing a means for transforming the longitudinal direction of laser energy propagation along the fiber optic to a radial one, without immediately damaging diffusing tip and catheter shaft materials adjacent to the exit point of the radiation, was quite difficult.

When 30 watts of Nd:YAG laser power are transmitted by a 100-μm silica fiber optic, the power density at all points is approximately 3820 watts/mm.^{2} This power density is more than sufficient to melt most metals, including gold, despite the high reflectivity of the latter at 1.06 μm (approximately 99%). It also destroys most high-temperature ceramic materials, including relatively transparent ones, if the output at the distal end of the fiber optic were coupled to a diffusing tip fabricated from such materials. Yet an important prerequisite in the design of a diffusing tip was that its presence should not reduce the normal flexibility of the deflated balloon; any material or materials used to construct a diffusing tip therefore had to perform better than any metal, glass, or ceramic, and nevertheless also be flexible.

As mentioned earlier, we had used a perfluorochemical emulsion within a balloon in our early rabbit studies to scatter laser radiation emitted from the distal end of a 400-μm core fiber optic. The relative lack of absorption by water, the perfluorochemicals (perfluorodecalin and perfluorotripropylamine), or the emulsifiers during scattering permitted the use of the emulsion as a diffusing tip. However, when a smaller fiber optic is used to deliver approximately 30 watts or more, the emulsion near the output end of the fiber optic quickly boils and shortly thereafter carbonizes, resulting in severe damage to the fiber optic and a sudden fall in power output from the balloon. To our knowledge, no other fluid that theoretically could be used in a clinical coronary application (e.g., Intralipid) is as effective in scattering 1.06-μm radiation with minimal absorption occurring.

During extensive empiric testing of a wide variety of materials, I discovered a flexible polymer that could be used to terminate or to reclad a silica fiber optic and that would not be damaged by prolonged exposure to the high power density mentioned above. Although the material has a threshold of only approximately 150° C to thermal damage, the high transparency (>99%) of thin sections of the material accounts for the lack of thermal damage during laser exposure in a water environment. The polymer can be fabricated in the form of a fiber optic, but is considerably more flexible than a silica fiber optic; it was therefore possible to fabricate the polymer in the shape of a helix, several turns of which could be wound about the central shaft of a conventional balloon catheter within a 20-mm-long balloon. Transmission of light along the polymer, when the latter was used as an extension of a silica fiber-optic, is poor relative to that of a fiber-optic, resulting in the desired effect of lateral radiation loss. However, the magnitude of the loss is insufficient when the polymer "fiber" is relatively straight. An important advantage of the helical design, therefore, lay in the fact that a small radius of curvature did not allow the usual internal reflection at the boundary of two materials having a different index of refraction (a high index of refraction for the polymer and a relatively low index of refraction for water) to occur. The helical design thus provided an adequately "lossy" fiber; in addition, from a mechanical viewpoint, axial flexion of a helix is associated with less resistance than flexion of the same material as a straight fiber. A final component of this early prototype diffusing tip consisted of a thin sleeve of polyethylene terephthalate material that both covered the polymer fiber for structural support and joined the silica and polymer fibers together.

The initial clinical LBA studies were conducted with a catheter having a diffusing tip fabricated in an analogous manner. Some difficulty in translating prototype specifications to a manufacturing production line resulted in a diffusing tip that was relatively short, approximately 5 mm, and had a 2:1 variation in power density azimuthally. However, the degree of uniformity of radiation emitted from the diffusing tip needed to achieve the desired tissue responses was and remains incompletely studied. Radiation penetration through arterial tissues at 1.06 μm is dominated by scattering rather than by absorption. Reflection and backscattered radiation produce an "integrating sphere" effect within an irradiated cylindrical artery as described by Cheong and Welch (32), thereby reducing inhomogeneities in power density that would otherwise occur with the use of a nonuniform diffusing tip, within the tissue in both axial and azimuthal directions.

An important additional problem with the first clinically available LBA catheters was that the durability of the diffusing tip was limited to only several laser exposures of 300–400 joules/dose. In view of the limited supply of the devices, extensive studies relating laser dosimetry to tissue temperature responses could not be performed prior to the Phase I trial. When a somewhat more durable catheter did become available, laser dosimetry studies demonstrated that the laser dose needed to initiate thermal fusion of tissues was slightly lower than the doses employed during the Phase I trial. Therefore, in subsequent trials, the laser dose was reduced somewhat.

Engineers at USCI recognized that an improved diffusing tip could be made if the silica cladding of the silica fiber optic were etched (for example, in hydrofluoric acid with a precision of several microns) and if the fiber optic were appropriately recladded. Independent techniques developed by USCI engineers and myself achieved the necessary precision. As a result, the current LBA diffusing tip has a much-improved axial and azimuthal distribution of light intensity and is mechanically a much more rugged device. An additional feature developed by Sinofsky consists of a thin layer (< 50 angstroms) of gold deposited on the proximal and distal cones of the balloon to reflect radiation, particularly at the latter location, so that the potential for irradiation of undiluted blood within the lumen of the artery adjacent to these locations would be minimal.

Until a smaller fiber optic is used that would permit a greater number of turns of the helix around the central shaft of the balloon catheter, some deviation from an ideal pattern of emitted laser radiation will be present with the current design. Moreover, the current design does not protect the guidewire within the central channel of the catheter from laser exposure. Simple flushing of the central channel with normal saline at a rate of about 0.25 cc/sec is sufficient to prevent excessive heating of the guidewire and to avoid the resultant potential for bonding of a heated wire and the central channel.

Further improvements will no doubt become available in the future. For example, I have demonstrated the feasibility of fabricating a diffusing tip in the form of a sleeve surrounding the central shaft. Azimuthal light distribution is quite uniform with this design, and the central channel is protected from excessive laser exposure, obviating the need for saline perfusion and even permitting perfusion of blood if desired.

The currently used LBA balloon is highly transparent to Nd:YAG laser radiation at 1.06 μm, so that tissue heating occurs solely as a result of absorption of the radiation by the tissue. The first clinical LBA catheter incorporated the use of deuterium oxide ("heavy water"), a nontoxic isotope of water (33), as the fluid to inflate the balloon because the lower absorption by this fluid compared to ordinary water reduced the thermal challenge to the diffusing tip and adjacent materials. As the diffusing tip improved, the use of deuterium oxide was found to be no longer necessary, and any of a variety of ordinary contrast-medium preparations have subsequently been used to inflate the LBA balloon. The peak rise in temperature of the fluid within the balloon during a relatively high clinical laser dose has been found to be only approximately 5° C, when the balloon is placed in a breaker of saline, since none of the components of the diffusing tip and adjacent catheter materials absorb the radiation (i.e., the balloon and its contents are quite transparent to 1.06-μm energy). In contrast, when the balloon is in contact with the arterial wall in vitro under simulated in-vivo thermal boundary conditions, the average peak temperature of fluid within the balloon rises to approximately 70° C when the peak temperature within tissue is 90–100° C.

Thus, the fluid within the balloon is heated primarily by thermal diffusion from the adjacent arterial wall.

Nd:YAG laser radiation at 1.06 μm was chosen for clinical use because the depth of penetration into the atheromatous wall adequate to seal mural dissections is approximately 2.5 mm. Many clinically important coronary lesions are eccentric, so that when plaque is sheared off a 3-mm vessel during PTCA, it may be important to be able to fuse tissue to this depth. We have been unable to fuse human atheromatous postmortem separated layers of neointima and media, when the former exceeds 0.5 mm in thickness, with either argon ion (488, 515 nm) laser radiation, CW Nd:YAG laser radiation at 1.32 μm, indirect heating by contact with a hot object, or use of a radio-frequency probe at 600 kHz. Temperatures of >80° C are required for thermal fusion of separated arterial tissue layers, so that, in view of the thermal properties of the atheromatous arterial wall, temperatures at the luminal surface must exceed approximately 130° C when superficial heating techniques are used to attempt to fuse neointima thicker than 0.5 mm to the underlying media.

A potentially useful advantage in the use of 1.06-μm radiation is that, because of internal redistributive scattering, it is possible to heat tissue layers below the luminal surface to a greater extent than the surface itself; contact with the fluid-filled balloon that is not heated by the radiation could increase this effect further. A continuous turnover of cold fluid in the balloon via the inflation and deflation channels (without changing distending balloon pressure or volume) could be used to enhance cooling of the luminal surface while heating subsurface tissues to higher temperatures during attempts to seal a dissection. At present the optimal temperature of tissue at the luminal surface, in terms of adverse biologic reactivity, is not well studied, so it would be premature to design such a system.

Other than tissue penetration, the most important reason that 1.06-μm radiation has clinical utility is the fact that absorption of energy at this wavelength by thrombus is considerably greater than for thrombus-free arterial tissues. In fact, Motamedi et al. (unpublished observation) have found that the absorption coefficient of thrombus at 1.06 μm is approximately an order of magnitude greater than that of the arterial wall; as a result, a laser dose sufficient to fuse separated tissue layers together will result in the rapid dessication of thrombus with effective remodeling of the residue into a thin, nonobstructive film that remains adherent to the luminal surface. Thus, the use of radiation at this wavelength during LBA automatically discriminates between thrombus and thrombus-free tissues, with an appropriately more aggressive thermal response occurring in thrombus.

A potential disadvantage inherent in the use of 1.06-μm laser radiation to directly heat the arterial wall is that temperature responses could theoretically be less predictable than the use of any energy source to heat the fluid in the balloon which would provide a truly "hot balloon" for heating tissue indirectly by thermal diffusion. This laser is heterogeneous in pathology and therefore potentially heterogeneous in absorption coefficients between various types of thrombus-free tissues. To evaluate the variability in temperature response of tissue during LBA as currently performed with direct exposure of tissue to Nd:YAG laser radiation, R. Crilly in our laboratory irradiated the luminal surface of both normal porcine (n = 4) and postmortem human atherosclerotic aortas (n = 12) with an expanded, collimated 2-cm-diameter laser beam (1.06 μm), the intensity of which was uniform to within 20 percent over a central region of 8 mm, and thermographic imaging was used to record the temperatures achieved during a 20-sec laser exposure. A power level was adjusted to 43 watts to raise porcine aortic temperature to a peak of 100°C, while using a spatial resolution of approximately 1 mm. Each aorta was placed on a 2-mm-thick high-density polyethylene plate during laser exposure. The composition of human atheromatous aortas varied from advanced white fibrotic plaque (n = 4) to dark yellow plaques (n = 3), early lipid plaque (n = 1), minimal to advanced fibrotic plaque stained with hemoglobin (n = 3), and an ulcerated, necrotic lesion (n = 1).

Both the rate of rise and the peak temperature (spatially and temporally) achieved within the irradiated region demonstrated remarkably little variation between mean values for the two species (< 10°C) and between various types of human atheromatous lesions (S.D. < 10°C) over a fully inclusive response range of 92° to 114°C (Fig. 9.1). By contrast, when a 1-mm layer of thrombus was allowed to form on the luminal surface of porcine aorta, a peak temperature at 150°C was achieved at the surface of the thrombus under the same conditions, producing marked dessication. Since selective dessication of thrombus appears to be a desirable tissue effect clinically, direct laser exposure of lesions with 1.06-μm radiation appears to have the potential to automatically discriminate between thrombus and all other lesions commonly encountered and to produce appropriate temperature elevations within both thrombus and thrombus-free tissues. It should be noted that the

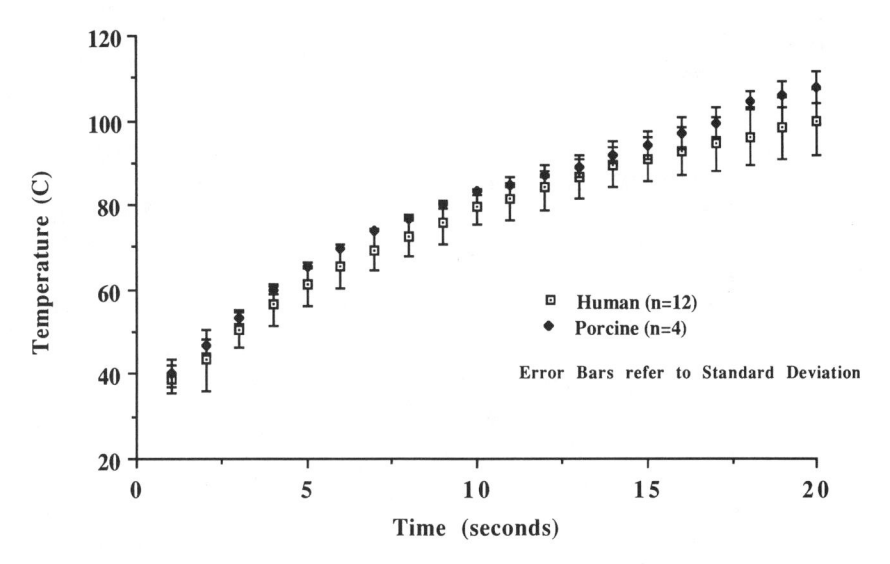

Laser Balloon Angioplasty: Evolving Technology 209

Figure 9.1. Peak temperature rise, as recorded with a thermographic camera, at the luminal surface of a wide variety of different types of human postmortem atherosclerotic aortic lesions as well as of normal porcine aortas. The same Nd:YAG laser power, exposure duration, and spot size were used for each exposure. Despite the heterogeneity in tissue type, the thermal response of each type was similar. In contrast, the peak surface temperature of thrombus (not shown) subjected to the same laser exposure is approximately 40° C higher as a result of the much greater absorption coefficient of this tissue, and selective, rapid dessication of thrombus therefore occurs when a laser dose sufficient to seal a dissection or reduce arterial recoil is given in vivo.

air-tissue interface used in this study would be expected to exaggerate any heterogeneity in temperature responses, compared to in-vivo conditions, given the thermal insulating effect of air. The small variation in the temperature response of thrombus-free tissues is consistent with the notion that, in the absence of a relatively thick layer of a strongly absorbing chromophore, temperature rises during 1.06-μm radiation exposure occur primarily as a result of water absorption and scattering, and that perhaps the relatively large field and long exposures used help to reduce potential heterogeneities by the associated relatively large amount of scattered radiation produced and thermal diffusion. In addition, the cylindrical geometry during in-vivo LBA would be expected to further reduce any variations in temperature responses because of an "integrating sphere" effect as discussed above.

Clinical LBA Studies

Unlike virtually every other new angioplasty procedure, the first clinical application of LBA was in coronary rather than in peripheral arteries for at least two reasons. Because of the much-larger-sized balloon that would be needed for a peripheral application, a correspondingly greater laser dose would be required, necessitating the use of a larger fiber optic and a different type of diffusing tip; clinical experience with the latter would not have been directly extrapolatable to the coronary tree, which was our primary interest. Perhaps more importantly, the dog coronary artery study demonstrated no adverse reactions with LBA to the lumen either acutely or chronically, myocardial function was unaffected, and laser exposure did not appear to be arrhythmogenic.

Subsequent to completion of a Phase I trial initiated on March 10, 1988, approximately 350 patients have been treated in 12 investigational centers in several FDA- and Internal Review Board (IRB)-approved protocols. Common to each protocol has been the requirement that each patient initially be treated with conventional balloon angioplasty to the best of the operator's ability. LBA has subsequently been performed immediately after PTCA by using a balloon of the identical dimensions. For the first approximately 250 patients, the only LBA balloon size available was a 3.0-mm × 20-mm balloon. In 1990, 2.5-mm and 3.5-mm LBA balloon catheters have also been made available. The only difference in the mechanical performance between the conventional and LBA catheters has been that the distending pressure used for the latter has been restricted to 4 atm, since higher balloon pressures may compress the central shaft of the catheter within the balloon, with the potential associated risk of thermally bonding the guidewire to the central shaft. Given the latter constraint, the tissue pressure applied during initial conventional balloon inflation and subsequent LBA are similar. Each patient has therefore served as his or her own control in a comparison of the acute efficacy of LBA vs. PTCA.

The LBA procedure differs from the initial PTCA procedure in several other minor ways besides the laser exposure itself. A dose-response relationship appears to exist for each patient, with great variability between patients in the amount of discomfort experienced during laser exposure. As a result, at doses of approximately > 320 joules delivered over a 20-second laser exposure, some form of analgesia is usually recommended, such as fentanyl 50 to 100 μg i.v. Preliminary experimental studies in our laboratory suggest that 10–15 mg lidocaine, given directly into the coronary artery shortly before laser exposure, is quite effective in eliminating a hyperventilatory response to high-dose LBA in lightly anesthetized dogs. Aversano et al. (34) demonstrated clinically that the severity of angina during ischemia associated with conventional balloon angioplasty is cut in half by prior injection of intracoronary lidocaine, and it is likely that their approach will eventually find similar utility during LBA procedures.

Also unlike PTCA, normal saline is injected through the guide catheter during a LBA balloon inflation to hemodilute blood at the distal end of the balloon and within the proximal portions of side branches adjacent to the inflated balloon. Experimentally, we have found that CW Nd:YAG laser irradiation of blood at a normal hematocrit can result in the formation of microscopic particles, but that at a hematocrit of 12 percent or lower, such particles are not formed (unpublished observation); hemolysis of red blood cells does occur at relatively low hematocrits, but this effect should not be clinically important. Despite the potential for formation of microemboli when blood at a normal hematocrit is irradiated with CW Nd:YAG laser energy, we have not found any evidence experimentally or clinically of such potential emboli when blood was not hemodiluted by flushing normal saline through the guide catheter during balloon inflation. In addition, when hemodilution was not employed, there has been no evidence for side branch occlusion as a result of laser-thermal coagulation of blood at the origin of an angiographically visible side branch. This observation may not be surprising, since it is well known that obliteration of relatively large arterial branches (approximately 1 mm or greater) with any form of thermal energy, such as electrocautery, cannot be achieved without simultaneous firm coaptation of apposing walls of the vessel. However, the potential does exist that excessive heating of undiluted blood at the origin of a side branch, adjacent to the inflated LBA balloon, can result in a moderate thermal constriction of the lumen of the side branch. For this reason alone, when a prominent side branch lies within the laser-irradiated field, we have recommended at least some hemodilution prior to laser exposure.

The CW Nd:YAG laser system used clinically for LBA was developed by Quantronix, Inc. (Fig. 9.2). It consists of an air-cooled 50-watt unit, which incorporates a number of computer-controlled functions to ensure the safety of the procedure. The most important such function is the operation of a thermal cutoff switch that is activated by excessive heating of the fiber optic or diffusing tip at any axial location and results

A

B

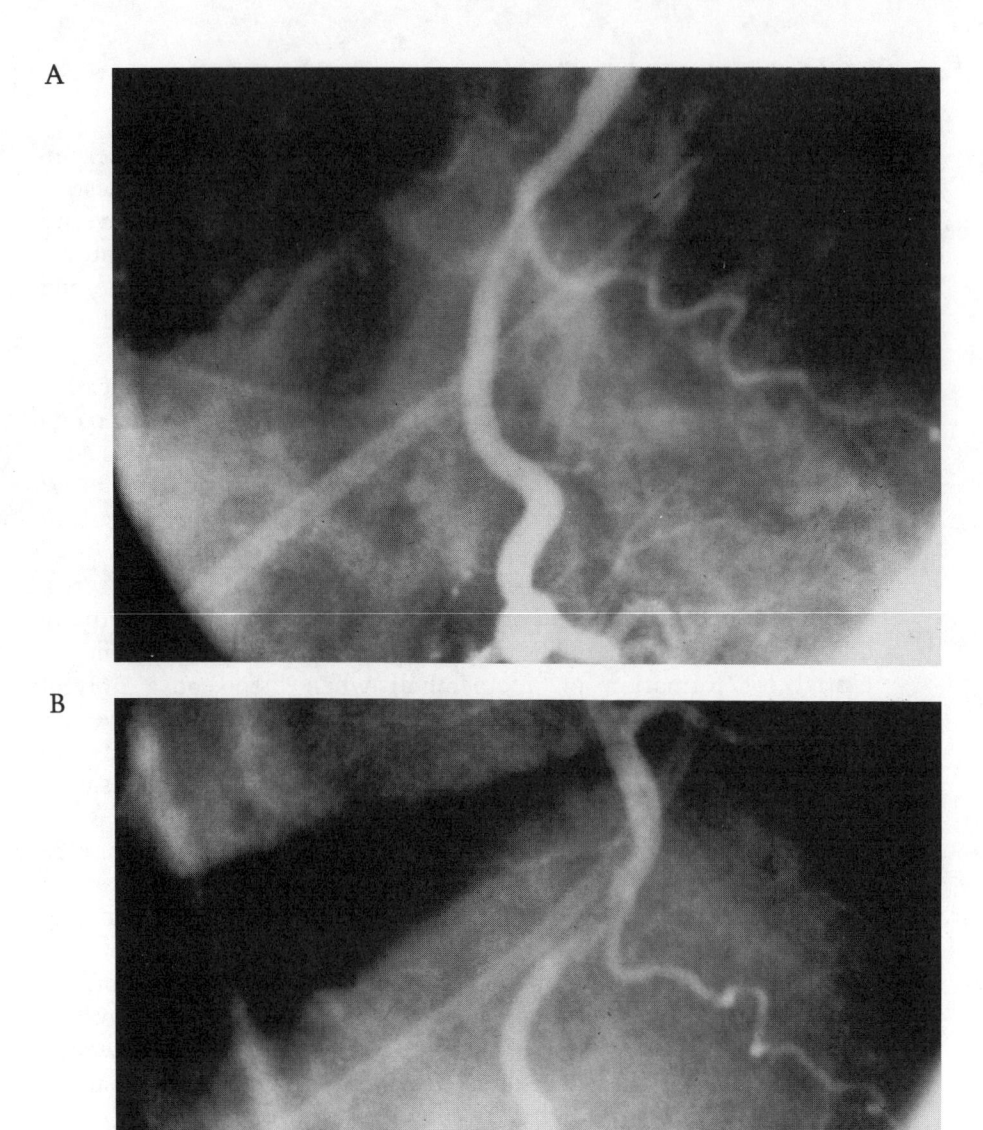

Figure 9.2. LBA treatment of PTCA-induced acute coronary closure from a dissection. A severe stenosis in the midportion of a dominant right coronary artery *(A)* progressed to acute closure during PTCA, which was successful only at temporarily maintaining vessel patency *(B)*.

Laser Balloon Angioplasty: Evolving Technology 213

C

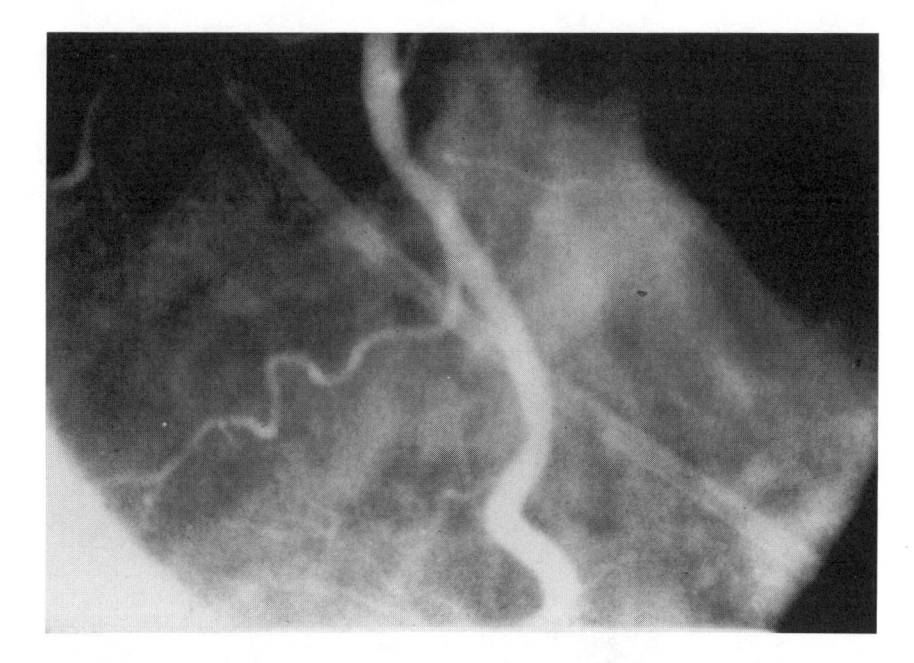

Figure 9.2. *(C)* LBA was successful in sealing the dissection, establishing vessel patency, and achieving a satisfactory angiographic result.

in an instantaneous termination of laser exposure in the event, for example, of fracture of the fiber optic. All laser functions are controlled via a small mobile unit, which is interfaced to the larger power supply and laser head so that laser dose selection, laser firing, etc., can be performed in close proximity to the sterile angioplasty field.

Two basic types of clinical LBA trials have been conducted to date. Approximately 230 patients have been treated electively with LBA after PTCA, while approximately 140 patients have been treated with LBA emergently for treatment of acute closure associated with PTCA. For both trials, the balloon size for LBA was the same as for the initial PTCA portion of the procedure.

A trial of LBA for treatment of acute closure was initiated because, in the first 55 patients treated electively, LBA was successful in the acute achievement of a residual stenosis of <50 percent in all cases, despite the fact that 14 (25%) of the patients had a >50 percent residual stenosis immediately after PTCA, as determined by computerized image processing of digitized cineangiographic frames (35). Three of the patients with an initial poor PTCA result had acute closure, which was reversed successfully with LBA.

No device-related acute complications have been noted in either type of LBA trial. Since adequate vessel patency was achieved in all of the first 55 patients, it may not be surprising that there were no in-hospital deaths, myocardial infarctions, or coronary bypass procedures in this group of patients.

Similarly, the incidence of major complications for the entire subsequent cohort in both types of LBA trials has been substantially lower than that reported in the NHLBI PTCA Registry. When LBA was used electively in 201 patients following PTCA (36), only 1 patient required coronary bypass surgery prior to hospital discharge to achieve a satisfactory clinical result. When used emergently for treatment of PTCA-induced acute closure, LBA obviated the need for surgical revascularization prior to hospital discharge in 85 percent of approximately 140 patients (Figs. 9.2, 9.3).

A

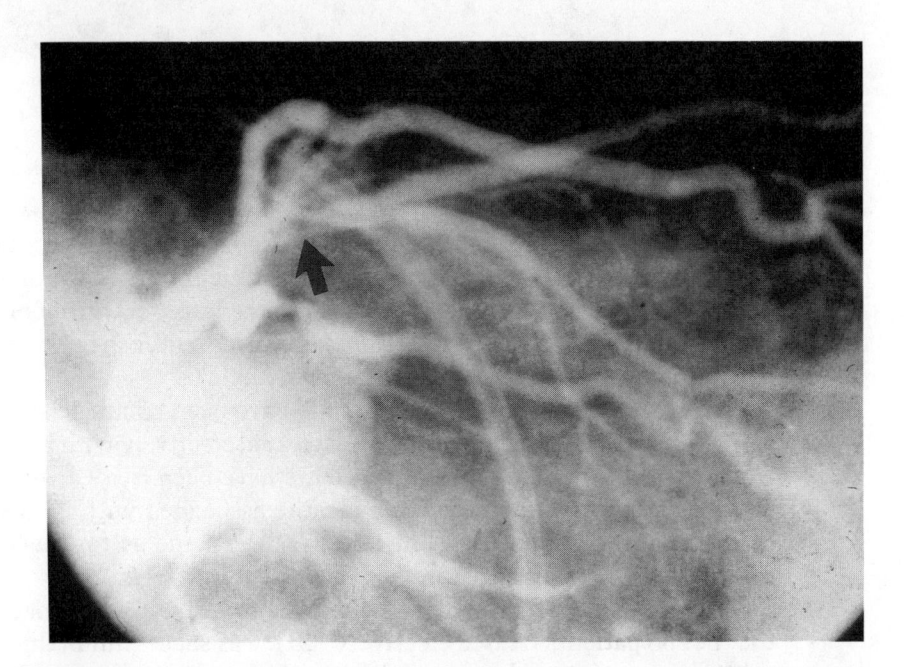

Figure 9.3. LBA treatment of PTCA-induced acute closure resulting from thrombus. One week after an anterior-wall myocardial infarction, the patient presented with recurrent chest pain, and angiography revealed a severe stenosis in the proximal segment of the left anterior descending coronary artery *(A)*.

B

C

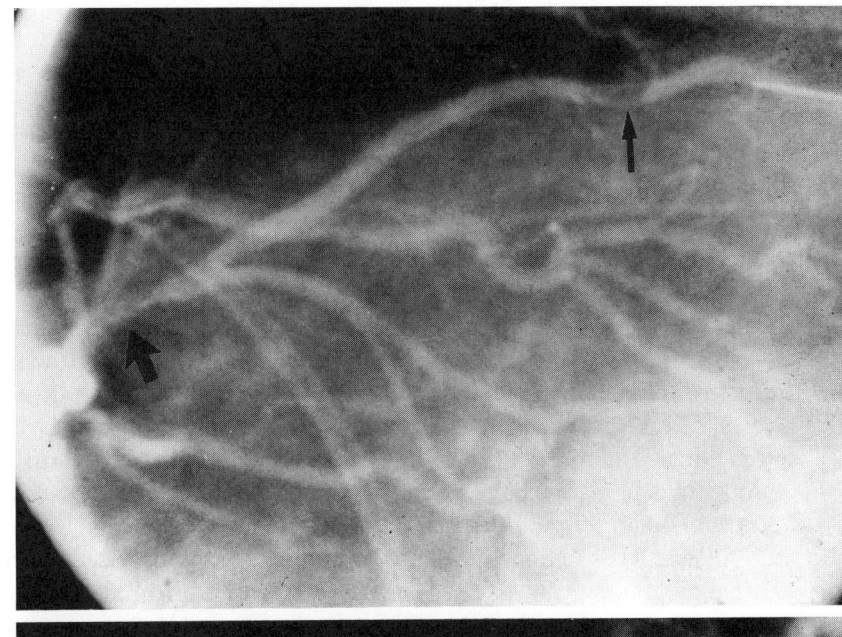

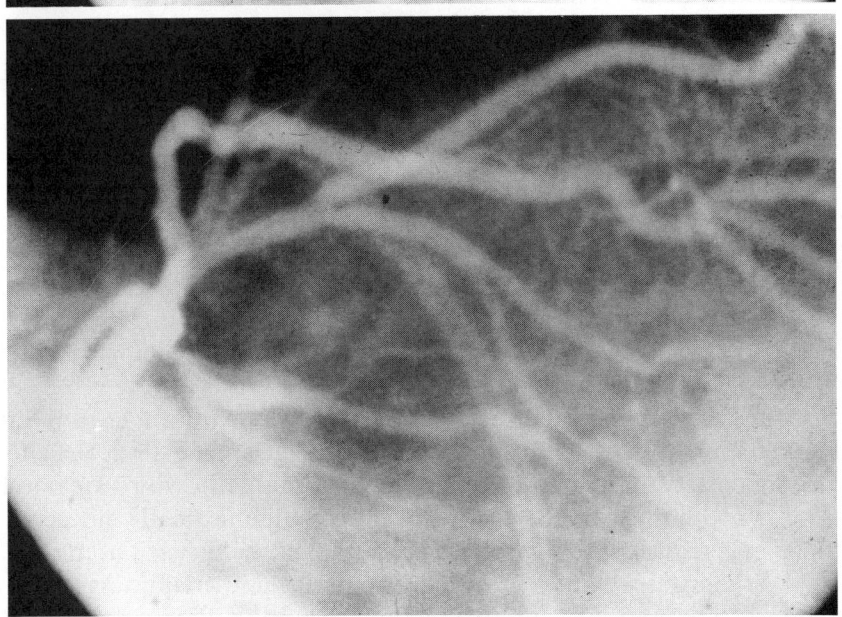

Figure 9.3. Following intracoronary administration of streptokinase and PTCA with prolonged balloon inflations *(B)*, the presence of thrombus at the site of the stenosis was evident *(large arrow)* along with an embolus *(small arrow)*, and severe ischemia resulted from the impending acute closure. No evidence of intraluminal thrombus was evident after LBA, which produced a satisfactory angiographic result *(C)*.

In the series of 201 patients treated electively with LBA, 51 of the patients (25%) had an unsuccessful result, defined as a > 50 percent residual diameter stenosis, immediately following the initial PTCA part of the procedure, despite the routine use of prolonged balloon inflations. The mean stenotic diameter by computerized image processing of cineangiograms from the 51 patients was 1.2 mm after unsuccessful PTCA or a 0.6-mm mean increase over the pre-PTCA mean value of 0.6 mm. Following subsequent LBA, however, the mean stenotic diameter was 2.0 mm, which was identical to the mean diameter following successful PTCA. The mean improvement of luminal diameter afforded by the application of LBA in the successful PTCA group, not surprisingly, was considerably less (0.3 mm) than that for the unsuccessful PTCA group. In general, we have found that the magnitude of improvement in luminal diameter provided by LBA is inversely proportional to the post-PTCA result. By 6 months after the procedure, computerized analysis of 102 angiograms demonstrated that the minimum luminal diameter was similar, approximately 1.5 mm, for both successful and unsuccessful PTCA groups, as a result of the application of LBA, and this long-term result was not significantly different from that of a small control PTCA group of 31 patients.

LBA Application of Bioprotective Materials

Irrespective of the degree of angiographic patency achieved with PTCA or any alternative angioplasty procedure, chronic restenosis will no doubt continue to be problematic unless adverse biologic reactivity of angioplastied tissues can be reduced.

Potential mechanisms of restenosis include thrombus formation, inflammatory cell infiltration, and proliferation of cells at the site of angioplasty injury. Proliferation of neointimal cells, which are fibroblasts, smooth muscle cells transformed from their normally quiescent state, or both, might result from the first two mechanisms or from a variety of other causes. (These include loss of the endothelial lining layer, which is associated with a loss of growth-regulating heparin sulphate and adhesion of a layer of platelets releasing [platelet-derived growth factor PDGF].) Alternatively, in many cases, the neointimal "proliferation" noted in restenosis lesions may simply represent organization of a mural thrombus by myofibroblasts.

It is likely that heparin, administered to an angioplastied lesion in sufficiently high doses for a prolonged period of time, could be used to reduce the incidence of restenosis, since it is a potent anticoagulant and a potent antiproliferative agent. At concentrations roughly an order of magnitude larger than those used clinically, it is also an effective inhibitor of thrombin bound to fibrin and could therefore at a high dose prevent the propagation of preexisting thrombus. However, prolonged i.v. administration of heparin is not practical and systemic high-dose therapy would be associated with an unacceptable risk of bleeding complications.

Local high-dose heparin therapy is feasible, however, with LBA by thermal induction of adherence of a suitable water-insoluble heparin carrier (37). Conceptually, the procedure could be performed by injecting a suspension of a heparin carrier into the lumen during inflation of the LBA balloon (Fig. 9.4). Tissue pressure provided by the inflated balloon would temporarily trap the heparin carrier at the luminal surface as well as between fracture planes and within vasa-vasorum and perivascular capillaries. The application of heat during LBA would then be used to bond the carrier to the tissues as a result of a transient phase change or formation of noncovalent bonds. Although a "perforated" balloon as described by Wolinsky et al. (38) can be used to inject heparin into the arterial wall, the drug does not persist at or near the luminal surface because of its solubility in water. In contrast, the use of a water-insoluble carrier of heparin would permit a longer period of drug retention.

We have been successful in the use of albumin microparticles, starch, and red blood cells as potential heparin carriers, which can be thermally bonded to the luminal surface and to deeper layers of the arterial wall in experimental studies. The anticoagulant activity of heparin is unaffected by exposure to temperatures as high as 150° C and remains pharmacologically active after attachment to a carrier. As a prototype carrier, heparin-albumin conjugates, wherein heparin is chemically bound to albumin in solution, were used to fabricate albumin microparticles in the presence of additional heparin. The physically entrapped heparin is released relatively quickly from the internal matrix of the microparticle, while the rate of disappearance of the chemically bound heparin fraction is governed by the rate of biodegradation of the albumin microparticles. The latter rate can be controlled by the degree of albumin cross-linking induced during the preparation of the microparticles. Biodegradation rates can be varied from periods of hours to months in this manner. We have tested the LBA-induced persistence of lightly and

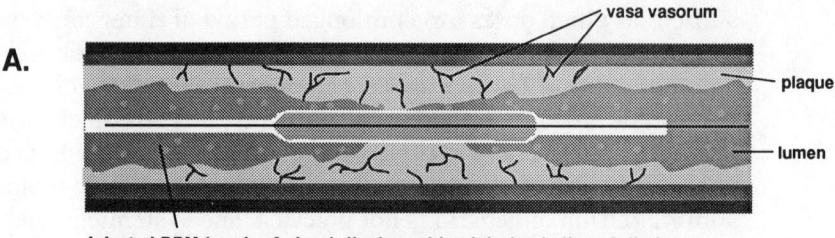

A. Injected BPM (carrier & drug) displaces blood during balloon inflation.

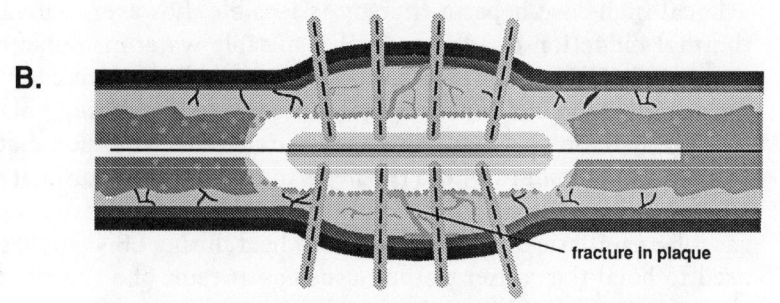

B. After physical trapping of BPM by balloon inflation, laser exposure performed.

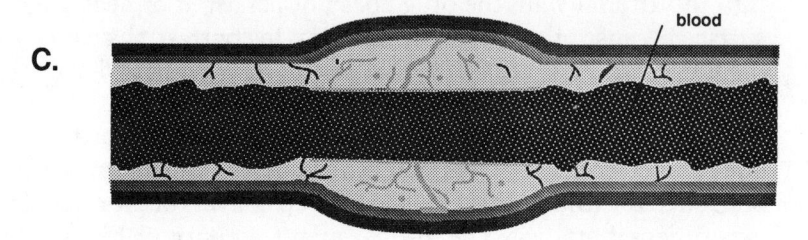

C. Adherence of BPM at luminal surface, within sealed fracture planes and vasa, results from laser/thermal exposure

Figure 9.4. Schematic representation of application of a drug carrier of "bioprotective material" at the luminal surface and within deeper layers with LBA.

moderately tightly cross-linked albumin microspheres prepared from albumin-heparin conjugates on the angioplastied luminal surface in dogs. Microparticles were noted at the luminal surface up to 1 week after application, and longer persistence has been noted within deeper tissue layers.

Fortunately, the laser dose required to induce adherence of each potentially useful carrier studied to date is similar to that used to remodel the arterial lumen. The potential therefore exists that application of a suitable drug carrier can be performed simultaneously during LBA treatment of the arterial lumen. Once an ideal carrier-drug combination has been identified and prepared, a great deal of work will be required, of course, to define the optimal drug concentration and persistence necessary to reduce adverse biologic reactivity associated with angioplasty. However, it is likely that LBA could be used to provide local high-dose drug therapy following not just balloon angioplasty, but also virtually any other alternative angioplasty procedure, including stent placement, mechanical atherectomy, and laser ablation angioplasty.

References

1. Sigel B, Dunn MR. The mechanism of blood vessel closure by high frequency electrocoagulation. *Surg Gyn and Obst* 1965;121:823.
2. Sigel B, Acevedo FJ. Electrocoaptive union of blood vessels: A preliminary experimental study. *J Surg Res* 1963; III:90.
3. Irvine A, Norton E. Photocoagulation for diabetic retinopathy. *Am J Ophthalmol* 1971;71:437.
4. Yahr WZ, Strully KJ, Hurwitt ES. Blood vessel anastomosis by laser and other biomedical applications. *J Assoc Adv Med Instrum* 1966;1:28.
5. Klink F, Grosspietzsch R, von Klitzing L, Endell W, Wolfdietrich H, Oberheurer F. Surgical refertilization by means of a laser technique. Animal in-vivo studies and in-vitro experiments with human tubes for end-to-end anastomotic operation by a CO_2 laser technique. *Fertil Steril* 1978;30:100.
6. von Klitzing L, Grosspietzsch R, Endell W, Wolfdietrich H, Oberheurer F. Surgical refertilization by means of a laser technique. Animal experiment study. *Fortschr Med* 1978;96:357.
7. Jain KK, Gorisch W. Repair of small blood vessels with the neodymium-YAG laser: A preliminary report. *Surgery* 1979;85:684.
8. Jain KK. Sutureless microvascular anastomosis using an Nd-YAG laser. *J Microsurg* 1980;1:436.
9. Jain KK. Sutureless extra-intracranial anantomosis by laser. Letter to the Editor. *Lancet* 1984;2:816.
10. Gomes OM, Macruz R, Armelin E, et al. Vascular anastomosis by argon laser beam. *Texas Heart Inst J* 1981;145.
11. White RA, Abergek RP, Lyons R, et al. Biological effects of laser welding on vascular healing. *Lasers Surg Med* 1986;6:137.

12. White RA, Kopchok G, Donayre C, et al. Comparison of laser-welded and sutured arteriotomies. *Arch Surg* 1986;121:1133.
13. Sauer JS, Rogers DW, and Hinshaw JR. Bursting pressures of CO_2 laser-welded rabbit ileum. *Lasers Surg Med* 1986;6:106.
14. Lynne C, Carter M, Morris J, Dew D, Thomsen S, Thomsen C. Laser-assisted vas anastomosis: A preliminary report. *Lasers Surg Med* 1983;3:261.
15. Frazier OH, Painvin A, Morris JR, Thomsen S, Neblett CR. Laser-assisted microvascular anastomoses: Angiographic and anatomopathologic studies on growing microvascular anastomoses. *Surgery* 1985; 97:585.
16. Spears JR. Method and apparatus for angioplasty. U.S. patent no. 4,799,479.
17. Serur JR, Sinclair IN, Spokojny AM, Paulin S, Spears JR. Laser balloon angioplasty (LBA): effect on the carotid lumen in the dog carotid artery (abstr.). *Circulation* 1985;72 (suppl III):III-457.
18. Hiehle JF, Bourgelais DBC, Shapshay S, Schoen FJ, Kim DS, Spears JR. Nd:YAG laser fusion of human atheromatous plaque-arterial wall separations in vitro. *Am J Cardiol* 1985;56:953–957.
19. Spears JR. PTCA restenosis: potential prevention with laser balloon angioplasty (LBA). *Am J Cardiol* 1987;60:61B–64B.
20. Jenkins RD, Sinclair IN, Anand RK, Spears JR. Laser balloon angioplasty: effect of constant temperature on weld strength of human postmortem intima-media separations. *Lasers Surg Med* 1988;8:30–39.
21. Anand RK, Sinclair IN, Jenkins RD, Hiehle JF Jr, James LM, Spears JR. Laser balloon angioplasty: effect of constant temperature vs. constant power on tissue weld strength. *Lasers Surg Med* 1988;8:40–44.
22. Spears JR, Leonard BM, Sinclair IN, Jenkins RD, James LM, Sinofsky EL. Reversible plaque optical property changes during repetitive CW Nd: YAG laser exposure. *Lasers Surg Med* 1988;8:477.
23. Schober R, Ulrich F, Sander T, Durselen H, Hessel S. Laser-induced alteration of collagen substructure allows microsurgical tissue welding. *Science* 1986;232:1421.
24. Welch AJ, Valvano JW, Pearce JA, Hayes LJ, Motamedi M. Effect of laser radiation on tissue during angioplasty. *Lasers Surg Med* 1985;5:251.
25. Marchesini R, Andreola S, Emanuelli H, et al. Temperature rise in biological tissue during Nd: YAG laser irradiation. *Lasers Surg Med* 1985;5:75.
26. Nobuyoshi M, Kimura T, Nosaka H, et al. Restenosis after successful percutaneous transluminal coronary angioplasty: serial angiographic follow-up of 229 patients. *J Am Coll Cardiol* 1988;12:616.

28. Jenkins RD, Sinclair IN, Leonard BM, Sandor T, Schoen FJ, Spears JR. Laser balloon angioplasty vs balloon angioplasty in normal rabbit iliac arteries. *Lasers Surg Med* 1989;9:237.
29. Spears JR, Sinclair IN, Jenkins RD. Laser balloon angioplasty; experimental in vivo and in vitro studies. In: Abela G, ed. Lasers in Cardiovascular Medicine & Surgery. Norwell, MA: Kluwer, 1990:167.
30. Login GR, Dvorak AM. Microwave energy fixation for electron microscopy. *Am J Pathol* 1985;120:230.
31. Thomsen S, Pearce JA, Cheong W-F. *IEEE Trans Biomed Eng* 1989; 36:1174.
32. Cheong WF, Welch AJ. A model for optical and thermal analysis of laser balloon angioplasty. *IEEE Trans Biomed Eng* 1989;36:1233.
33. Czajka DM, Finkel AJ, Fischer CS, Katz JJ. Physiological effect of deuterium on dogs. *Am J Physiol* 1961;201:357.
34. Aversano T, Weisman HF, Walford GD, et al. Regional intracoronary analgesia for PTCA. *Circulation* 80 (IV) 1989;Suppl II:172.
35. Spears JR, Reyes VP, Wynne J, et al. Percutaneous coronary laser balloon angioplasty: initial results of a multicenter experience. *J Am Coll Cardiol* 1990;16:293.
36. Reyes VP, Plokker HWT, Leatherman LL, et al. Laser balloon angioplasty effectively treats unsuccessful PTCA. *Circulation* 82 (IV) 1990;Suppl II:277.
37. Spears JR, Kundu SK, McMath LM. Laser balloon angioplasty: Potential for reduction of the thrombogenicity of the injured arterial wall and for local application of bioprotective materials. *J Am Coll Cardiol* 1991 (in press).
38. Wolinsky H, Thung SN. Use of a perforated balloon catheter to deliver concentrated heparin into the wall of the normal canine artery. *J Am Coll Cardiol* 1990;15:475.

CHAPTER **10**

Laser Safety and Regulatory Issues: FDA Perspective

LYNNE A. REAMER
RICHARD P. FELTEN

Introduction

THE Center for Devices and Radiological Health, a center within the Food and Drug Administration, is authorized by Congress to provide controls to ensure that medical devices are reasonably safe and effective when marketed or used on people. This chapter addresses these issues through two different mechanisms. The first section briefly discusses general hazards that may exist when laser devices are used in cardiovascular surgery. The safety issues presented and the suggested measures for safe use are essentially based on laser-tissue bioeffects. In some cases these issues are simply previously known concerns being reconsidered as a result of new data, for example, the current concern with laser plume safety. On the other hand, new safety issues are appearing as the result of either new treatment techniques such as photosensitizers to increase tissue absorption of optical radiation, or the development of new instruments such as the excimer laser. The second section of the chapter addresses patient safety during the clinical investigation and discusses the formal processes used in granting medical device approval. Specific guidance is provided with regard to patient numbers, posttreatment follow-up, appropriate data collection, and the correct mechanism for submitting this information to the FDA.

General Laser Safety Issues

The broad issues of general laser safety have been well documented in previous publications (1–3). Ensuring a safe physical environment for laser surgery encompasses both engineering and administrative controls. These areas are covered by federal regulations as well as by voluntary standards and safety recommendations. The Federal Laser Products Performance Standard (Federal Laser Standard) (4) applies to the manufacturers of laser products and mandates specific warning labels and engineering performance requirements intended to limit unintentional laser radiation exposure. A voluntary user standard published by the Laser Institute of America and developed in accordance with procedures approved by the American National Standards Institute (ANSI) is ANSI Z-136.1, "Safe Use of Lasers" (5), which provides recommendations on user-implemented administrative and engineering safety controls. This ANSI standard is complemented by ANSI Z-136.3, "Safe Use of Lasers in Health Care Facilities" (6). The latter document is specifically designed to provide guidance to health care personnel working with and around lasers. ANSI Z-136.1 provides detailed safety guidance for all general laser hazards, while Z-136.3 addresses hazard procedures specific to medical lasers.

In the past, the major safety issues facing the health care professional during laser surgery were related to the fact that most traditional lasers obtained their effects through thermal processes. Safety recommendations regarding this area are contained in a recent publication by Dr. George Abela (7), and are still very relevant. For surgical laser procedures performed by cardiovascular physicians, which include gross tissue cutting, vascular vessel coagulation, and tissue vaporization, the same safety techniques can be used as are used by any laser surgeon. It is while performing those procedures unique to cardiovascular surgery, such as catheterization, that the cardiovascular physician must be prepared to address potential safety concerns not normally encountered by other laser surgeons.

As mentioned above, the accepted methods of reducing potential hazards caused by thermal laser–tissue interactions have recently been detailed. These recommendations have not changed nor are they likely to change in the foreseeable future. What needs to be addressed and clarified are the newer concerns resulting from either advances in laser technology or simply from renewed awareness of previously known concerns.

Laser Plume

Since the first laser procedure in which tissue was cut or vaporized, it has been known that some type of debris is produced. Many considered this debris an annoyance that could be reduced or eliminated by some type of smoke evacuation system. However, because many of these evacuation systems were not easy to use, the extent of their use varied from place to place. Recently, several published reports addressing the issue of transferance of infectious material in this plume of debris (8,9) have suggested that this debris might be more dangerous than originally thought. In addition, preliminary in-vitro data have been reported documenting the chemical alteration of tissue by thermal laser–tissue interaction with subsequent generation of potentially hazardous materials (10). What does this mean for cardiovascular laser therapy?

For procedures involving open wound cutting, coagulation, or vaporization, the cardiovascular physician need do no more than is recommended for all laser physicians. The health care professional and the patient can be protected by using good smoke evacuation systems; covering noninvolved tissue sites; and wearing appropriate protective clothing such as gowns, gloves, masks, etc. These recommendations have been published in various forms in several journals (11,12). The use of good smoke evacuation techniques will have the greatest effect since removal of laser debris and smoke at the site will reduce, if not totally eliminate, the potential for inhalation or contact with this potentially hazardous material.

During intravascular laser surgery the answers are not so clear. We need to keep in mind that the above-mentioned potential laser-plume hazards have not been confirmed in any in-vivo model systems. A number of studies have reported on laser by-products (13–16), but no data have been reported on the consequences of these products following removal of arterial plaque by laser procedures. Again, this effort has been limited because the majority of treatments occur in the peripheral vessels and are mostly performed in conjunction with balloon angioplasty. It is therefore very important that posttreatment monitoring of patients be carefully performed and that research continue in this area to specifically identify the laser-tissue by-products and the final "destination-resolution" of the by-products.

Photosensitizers

Photosensitizer use in cardiovascular therapy has been of research interest for several years. Photosensitizing compounds are chemicals that absorb light and, subsequent to this absorption, undergo some type of alteration that can either directly or indirectly produce biological changes in surrounding tissue. Two types of such compounds are of interest in cardiovascular therapy. The first class of compounds involves the use of chemicals that, upon injection or ingestion, could be taken up by the plaque and make the plaque more sensitive to laser energy. The structure of these compounds could be such (e.g., hematoporphrin derivative) that it causes plaque to preferentially absorb specific wavelengths of nonthermal light and, through some photochemical mechanism, produce plaque breakdown so it can be easily removed (17). A second set of compounds could be those that act as thermal absorbers (e.g., tetracycline), and these compounds could enhance the thermal destruction of plaque (18). In either case, the introduction of such photosensitizers presents the possibility that normal blood vessel tissue will also be damaged. The by-products might sequester elsewhere in the body and continue to be photosensitive, thus producing increased or unwanted photosensitive effects to other internal tissues. In addition, these exogenous photosensitive compounds might become located in the skin, making the patient totally light-sensitive for some extended period following treatment. Since human trials using these compounds are still extremely limited, a final decision on whether this area of research will actually prove beneficial is far from clear. Likewise, it is unclear if the use of these compounds in the cardiovascular system will result in any hazards uniquely different from those associated with the general use of photosensitizers in other parts of the body.

New Technology

Development of new lasers and laser systems for cardiovascular use continues. Besides the addition of the excimer laser to the list of lasers already being investigated for cardiovascular use, development continues in the area of laser fiber optics specifically designed for cardiovascular use. As these advances continue, the potential for new safety concerns for both the user and the patient also grows.

The excimer laser is a gas laser that produces unique ultraviolet (UV) wavelengths depending on the gas mixture excited. These UV wavelengths, as well as those produced through the use of doubling crystals, appear to have some unique advantages for plaque removal. For some UV wavelengths, nonthermal ablation appears to be the mode of action; for others, the absorption characteristics of the plaque are maximum for the particular wavelength (19). A growing body of in-vitro data reports mutagenic effects of UV wavelengths from the vaccuum UV to near UV (150–400 nm) (20–25). Although a few in-vivo studies have used chronic, high-exposure doses to mice (26,27), no in-vivo studies have been reported using the types of exposures that will be used in plaque removal. Performing such in-vivo studies to assess possible long-term sequelae from these low-UV exposures is difficult. Therefore, surgeons wishing to use these UV wavelengths will need to assess the proposed treatment site, the characteristics of surrounding normal tissues that might receive scattered UV laser energy, the survival of the directly exposed cells to UV, and the sensitivity of these surviving cells to mutation. It will be important for those studying this new area to determine the exposure parameters that will give the most efficient therapeutic effect with minimum risk of mutagenesis.

Besides the possible hazards of UV to the patient, excimer lasers and other UV laser systems can potentially present similar hazards to the user. While most studies using these devices are limited to intravessel use, care must always be taken that inadvertent exposure of operating room personnel does not occur. As improved UV-emitting fiber optics are developed, the increased possibility of inadvertent exposure via broken fibers, laser firing while the fiber is outside the vessel, etc., cannot be ruled out. It is therefore important that safety practices such as proper eyewear, correct handling of fibers, and standard operating procedures for firing of the laser be in place from the beginning.

In addition, excimer lasers present some unique workplace hazards that must be considered. The gases used in these lasers are highly toxic. Although the laser cavity should not need to be filled during patient treatment, gas leaks during use cannot be ruled out. It is therefore important that a sensitive warning monitor be in place in case such a leak occurs. Obviously, if the present efforts to develop UV-transmitting fibers are successful, this potential hazard could be greatly reduced by placing the laser in a separate room and delivering the energy via the fiber optic.

Advances in fiber-optic technology, for example, commercially available UV and infrared (IR) fibers, could also affect laser safety in cardiovascular surgery. The ability to use surgical fibers always carries the potential for inadvertent laser exposure via broken fibers. In addition to this common hazard, the advances in fiber technology have resulted in multifiber systems for cardiovascular use as well as combination fiber-metal systems. Each of these presents unique concerns. For example, the combination fiber-metal system allows actual laser energy to be directed at tissue or plaque, again presenting the need for care that vessel perforation or normal tissue damage does not occur as a result of direct laser energy interactions.

The advances in multifiber systems with the concomitant development of highly sensitive optical detection systems have resulted in advances in efforts to develop reliable systems for fluorescence differentiation of plaque and normal tissue. Here again, depending on the excitation wavelength chosen, care will be needed to avoid unacceptable damage to normal tissue. If these excitation wavelengths are in the UV region, the potential for mutational events again exists, even though the energies being used are considerably lower than those used in ablation. Since these lower levels are nonablative, all exposed cells can be expected to survive, whereas for ablative exposures the potential exists that many fewer cells will survive treatment. It is therefore possible that the use of UV wavelengths for fluorescent excitation might be a more serious risk than the use of these same wavelengths for plaque ablation.

If the use of UV wavelengths for ablation and fluorescence detection proves successful, then the need for research in this area becomes even greater. Clearly, it is possible to ensure that the health care provider is protected from inadvertent UV exposures even during these initial studies. What remains to be determined is whether exposing the patient to such UV is really a hazard.

Summary of Safety Issues

The expanded use and specific development of laser devices for cardiovascular surgery presents a double-edged sword to the cardiovascular physician. On one hand, these laser devices appear to have the potential to improve cardiovascular surgery. Simultaneously, they present a potential source of new hazards for the physician as well as the patient. Because of the uniqueness of the therapeutic procedures, the cardiovascular physician needs to know the common thermal and nonthermal hazards of laser surgery as well as those unique to the use of laser devices in cardiovascular surgery, such as blood-vessel-wall weakening or perforation due to thermal injury. Thus, the cardiovascular physician needs all of the skills common to this specialty area plus a thorough understanding of laser-tissue interactions to implement the appropriate safety measures during cardiovascular laser surgery.

As use of lasers in cardiovascular surgery continues and expands, and as new devices and techniques continue to be introduced, it will no longer be possible or desirable for the physician himself or herself to attempt to know all of the information needed. The skills and knowledge of the cardiovascular physician will, in many cases, now be augmented by a team of specialists who will interact to provide the best patient care possible. Pharmacists specializing in drug absorption and clearance will be needed if photosensitive compounds are to be used. Tissue optics specialists will be a valuable asset both in calculating proper light dose for sensitizers and also in detecting when fluorescence might be used to distinguish plaque from normal tissue. At the same time, trained laser safety personnel will be invaluable in understanding and implementing the necessary programs to ensure the safety of both patient and health care provider.

When looking at laser safety, it is important to remember that patient safety is related to patient therapy, and it is the interaction with tissue from the potentially hazardous insult (heat, UV) that provides the therapeutic benefit. This is not the case for the health care professional, however. The health care professional receives no benefit from exposure to any of these insults, and therefore all steps necessary should be taken to eliminate his or her exposure.

General Regulatory Issues

Before a laser device can be assessed for the treatment of atherosclerotic disease in a clinical population, very specific information must be obtained to completely characterize the laser device and its intended use. This information must be presented to the Food and Drug Administration (FDA) in the form of an investigational device exemptions (IDE) application, and must be approved by the FDA before any clinical investigation may begin. In addition, since the investigation involves a device subject to the Radiation Control for Health and Safety Act, the device must be certified and meet the Federal Performance Standard for Laser Products, 21 CFR 1040.10 and 1040.11 (4). Submission of an initial or model change report is required by 21 CFR 1002.10 or 1002.12 prior to the delivery of the laser device to an investigator. This report describes the laser device, its compliance with the requirements of the Federal Laser Standard, and the manufacturing and quality-control procedures and records utilized to ensure compliance.

Use of Lasers in the Treatment of Atherosclerotic Disease

The following information is a revised, up-to-date version of previously published guidance (7) for submitting an IDE application using laser devices to treat atherosclerotic disease. This information reflects changes in IDE application requirements that are the result of continued advances in the area of cardiovascular laser therapy. We do not discuss the general requirements of the IDE regulation contained in 21 CFR 812.20(b), 812.25, and 812.27 (4).

Reports of Prior Investigations

To completely characterize the laser device, all data, references, literature sources, or personal communications necessary to demonstrate that the proposed use of the laser device is safe for clinical use must be collected. The choice of laser output parameters—that is, wavelength, power density, cross-sectional area, temporal characteristics (continuous or pulsed), or fiber-optic tip temperature—must be shown to have been derived from careful consideration of factors such as 1) mode of tissue removal—cutting, vaporization, or coagulation; 2) the absorption characteristics of the target tissue; 3) thermal effects; and 4) healing characteristics. In-vitro and in-vivo testing must demonstrate that use of the laser device at its selected operating parameters will not perforate the blood vessel or cause excessive tissue damage. These data must be provided for each type of tissue to be treated—for example, clot or hard or soft plaque. Statements made regarding the ability of the laser device to perform its intended function must be substantiated by appropriate data from bench and animal testing. The data must show that the laser device can successfully be used as it is intended (e.g., in a dry or wet field, intraoperatively, percutaneously, with manual guidance, using a foot pedal, a flushing mechanism for debris, a fiber-tip temperature monitor). This supporting information must include theoretical considerations, laboratory tests, and results of animal and cadaver studies needed to justify the laser wavelength and energy characteristics being proposed for clinical use. The protocols for each prior study must be provided and must give a clear, concise description of the purpose of the study, how the protocol effectively addresses that purpose, and why the results support that purpose. The data must include the test medium; the animal species; site, type; and size of lesion; diameter of blood vessel; method of approach to the lesion; fate of debris; and the condition of the recanalized blood vessel compared to its pretreatment state versus posttreatment state. In addition, the data must include the specific laser treatment parameters used, such as diameter of laser beam or fiber tip; laser power; treatment procedures followed including exposure times, number of exposures, and time between exposures; fiber-tip temperature; how that tip temperature is monitored and measured and the accuracy of that measurement; and the dosimetric procedures followed that validate these laser parameters. Data from the work of others may be used if it can be shown that the target tissue, the beam quality, the fiber-tip temperature, and other operative and output parameters of the laser device used in these studies are equivalent to those in the proposed study. Careful correlations must be made by extracting the appropriate data from the studies. Simply providing summaries or copies of the publications from these studies is not sufficient.

It is helpful if the bibliography includes sufficient documentation to demonstrate the effective use of similar devices. Copies of the cited references must be provided, along with abstracts, personal communications, and unpublished reports. In-vivo animal data must include sufficient follow-up to demonstrate the healing characteristics of the lased blood vessel. The work of others may be used here if proper correlations are made.

If the laser device has the potential to produce toxic or mutagenic effects on tissue, it is necessary to evaluate this risk versus the patient risk from atherosclerotic disease. Studies must be initiated to investigate the extent or lack of toxicity or mutagenicity for the wavelength or wavelengths in question, but depending on this risk evaluation, the results of these studies might not be required prior to IDE approval. The data will be reviewed as they become available, either during the conduct of the clinical investigation or when a premarket approval application (PMA) is submitted. The FDA will seek advice from outside experts, including appropriate advisory panels, to evaluate these data.

If the laser device is radio-frequency (RF)-excited, the RF laser excitation frequency must be specified. Data must be presented to demonstrate that RF emissions from a laser device (RF-excited or electrical discharge) will not cause interference or other problems with pacemakers, electronic circuits used in monitoring, or computer instrumentation. Information must also be provided to show that the EMI from a laser device will not be sensed by a pacemaker's sensing circuitry and thus inhibit the pacemaker, leading to temporary cessation of pacing. In this instance, the FDA is concerned not about EMI-induced damage to the pacemaker itself, but about possible adverse effects on a patient or other exposed persons due to pacemaker inhibition caused by the temporal pattern of the laser-burst cycles during the surgical procedure. Results must be submitted of testing in which the laser device is held as close to the equipment as it is likely to be in the surgical suite. Comparisons must be made between the RF emissions from the laser device to those from other RF-emitting medical devices commonly used in the surgical suite. RF emission compliance with ANSI specifications must describe the means for ensuring that the E-fields reported are actually maximum; estimates of uncertainty and antenna-device distance for the various positions at which the RF data were obtained must be provided.

If direct-viewing during lasing is possible, an analysis of the data, and information to document that the physician will not be exposed to hazardous levels of laser energy, must be provided as required by the Federal Laser Standard.

Investigational Plan

The investigational plan must 1) include a clear statement of the objective of the proposed investigation, 2) provide a clear description of the intended use of the laser device (e.g., is use of the laser device meant to replace conventional bypass surgery, balloon angioplasty, atherectomy, or stent placement, or to be an adjunct to them?), and 3) specify the location of the blood vessels to be lased (peripheral or coronary). A definition of "success" must be provided, and the end points used to determine "success" must be identified. If more than one type of procedure (i.e., atherectomy, balloon angioplasty, or stent placement) is used in the same vessel, in the same lesion, or in different vessels or lesions, these data will have to be analyzed separately. This is of particular importance in establishing the indications for use of the device. Studies will be phased and initially limited to a single investigator and small numbers of patients. Follow-up data from the approved phase or phases must be reviewed by the FDA before the next phases can proceed. Under most circumstances, the investigation begins with one investigator and 10 to 20 patients. Follow-up data are collected and submitted to the FDA for review, and if the data are satisfactory, the next phase of the investigation may begin and patients and investigators are added to the investigation.

The proposed clinical protocol must completely describe all phases of the investigation. The methodology must include a step-by-step description of the laser procedure. The minimum and maximum laser operating parameters (power output, fiber-tip temperature, exposure time, time interval between exposures) and exact method of use (e.g., advancement-firing, withdrawal-firing, rate of advancement and withdrawal, expected number of pulses per type and length of lesion) must be clearly stated and the rationale explained. If marketed interventional devices or other investigational devices are also used on the study population, specific descriptions of each group must be provided along with the patient inclusion and exclusion criteria and the rationale (risk-benefit) for including or excluding that group. The protocol and reporting forms must clearly define and report the criteria by which a patient is selected for intervention by the investigational or marketed devices. "Intent to Treat" with your investigational device or an alternative must be established for each patient *prior to* intervention and this must be recorded so that true success rates can be determined. Examples of these groups could include laser first and only (sole therapy); laser first followed by balloon or atherectomy or stent or a combination of these (adjunct therapy—laser first); or balloon, atherectomy, or stent followed by laser (adjunct therapy—laser last).

Each time an adjunct procedure is used, the patient it is used on enters a separate category for analysis. This may require that the results of the study be divided among several patient groups depending on how the laser was used. The protocol must contain an analysis of how the investigation will provide the data to show that the laser procedure is safe and effective. Follow-up data must be collected immediately after the procedure and at postoperative intervals before discharge from the hospital. After hospital discharge, follow-up shall continue with repeat angiography at 6 months. If noninvasive evaluation is chosen, the noninvasive procedure must be validated to show correlation with invasive methods.

Patient report forms (PRFs) must be provided. The PRFs must reflect the type of data to be collected from each patient and must be consistent with the clinical protocol. The preoperative information must carefully document the patient's condition and include the results of all diagnostic tests. A diagram indicating the location of each lased blood vessel and lased site must be attached. The PRF for the actual laser procedure must include space to record the laser power or fiber-tip temperature before, during, and after the procedure to document the power or temperature actually delivered. Measurement of power or temperature after the procedure will be important in developing the laser operating parameters, particularly in the event of an unsuccessful attempt. In addition, the PRFs must document all medications given and any complications that occur during all stages of the patient's participation in the investigation. The form used at follow-up must also be provided.

If the lased blood vessel is to be excised and examined histologically, a description of the information to be provided from the histological examination and of how the excised lased segment will be evaluated for patency must be provided. If the knowledge obtained from the excised vessel is to be of value in understanding the effect of the procedure on atheromatous vessels, the examination of the excised segments must be described in detail on the PRFs to ensure consistency of the data.

The investigational plan must compare the risks and benefits of the laser procedure to those associated with the appropriate approved alternate procedure, for example, peripheral or coronary bypass graft surgery, balloon angioplasty, stents, or peripheral or coronary atherectomy. A discussion must be provided on the potential additional risks of plaque dislodgement; the fate of vaporized or charred material; heating and potential inflammatory response; fibrosis; mechanical or other perforation of the vessel wall; and the potential for delayed thrombosis, aneurysm formation, and restenosis. This discussion must explain how the risks will be minimized and must describe the benefits of using the laser device rather than an alternate procedure. In addition, if competitive flow will exist, an analysis of its effects on the lased blood vessel and the bypass graft must be provided.

Description of Device

The laser device typically consists of a laser power source and a fiber-optic catheter delivery system. The device description must be detailed and include not only the laser power source but also all the materials and dimensions of the delivery system. Clear drawings, diagrams, or photographs of the laser power source, the fiber-optic delivery system, and the optical path of the laser energy must be provided, including a technical description of the components (lenses, windows, etc.) in the optical path and their specifications (focal length, material type, thickness, etc.). If a bare laser fiber is used, the description must include beam divergence, beam diameter, spatial beam profile, and the procedures used to measure and map these parameters.

If the laser fiber optic will be capped with a metal tip, the material used to manufacture the metal tip must be identified, including how much of the fiber optic is covered and whether light can be reflected from the tip and out the side of the fiber. How long can the tip be heated before it deteriorates (tip useful life)? A description of the relative thermal profile along the length and at the tip must also be provided for the condition of maximum surface temperature at the end of the tip. How will the pulse rate and cooling rate keep the tip and plaque at optimal temperature? Does the tip gradually increase in temperature above an optimal procedural temperature? Is the cooling period sufficient to return the plaque to normal body temperatures between firings, or does the plaque gradually get hotter? If a pulsed system is used, will there be gradual increases in sideways heating over the period of treatment? Describe the preclinical testing performed, and include the results to demonstrate the correlation between input laser energy and average surface temperature.

In addition to a description of the laser device, diagrams or photographs must be provided for each important component of the laser system, such as the power supply, power monitor, laser-to-fiber-optic interface, fiber-optic connector, guide catheter, and angioscope. The principle of operation must describe how the laser device is activated and the specific procedure for calibration of laser power output prior to each use. If a separate power meter is used, how will the power meter detector be protected from damage when the laser device is calibrated?

How are power levels, temperature, and time intervals set before the laser device is activated? How are time intervals measured to ensure the accuracy of each exposure time? How is the laser power or fiber-tip temperature monitored during a procedure? For accurate data to be collected to establish laser operating parameters, the precise procedure must be described. All unique features of the system must be completely described; for example, will a saline or other type of flush be used, and where will it exit the lased vessel? The radiant power, fiber-tip temperature, pulse duration, number of pulses, and rate of advancement and withdrawal necessary to achieve the desired destruction of plaque must be described, as well as how the device will be manipulated in the blood vessel.

Manufacturing Information

Manufacturing information must be submitted for each component of the laser device and must include the identity of the supplier of each component. The information must be detailed enough to demonstrate that the laser device will be manufactured in such a way as to ensure its safe and effective use. A summary of tests performed and data to document the reliability and stability of the laser device must be provided. This must include tests and data on all critical components. All testing performed on the delivery system must be performed on devices sterilized by the intended method, for example, ethylene oxide, gamma radiation, or other means. If sterility is compromised before the device is to be used, how are these devices to be handled? Are they to be resterilized? If so, how many sterilizations can they withstand? What data are there to support resterilization?

Labeling

A draft of all laser device labeling must be submitted, not only that required by the IDE regulation, but also the labels required by the Federal Laser Standard (4). A draft of the instructions for use must be provided and must include indications, contraindications, warnings, precautions, and bibliography. The laser procedure itself must be explained in sufficient detail to provide the user with a description of the exact technique. The procedure will obviously be amended as experience is gained during actual clinical use.

Informed Consent Form

The informed consent form must include a summary description of the laser procedure and alternative procedures. Risks associated with the laser procedure must be clearly explained and compared to alternate methods of treatment. The form must also include an explanation of the follow-up studies to be performed and the time intervals involved. Acute complications must be discussed, as well as longer-term complications such as the potential for thrombosis or aneurysm formation and the possibility of restenosis. All other elements required by the IDE regulation must be contained in this form.

Other Information

Even though the investigation, in general, is initially limited to one investigator, a description of the training procedure for potential future investigators must be provided. In addition, the IDE must contain a summary of the intent of the investigation. This summary must be placed at the beginning of the application and must include a brief description of the device, the study design, and expected results, and must provide sufficient detail to describe the contents of the IDE. Each section of the application must be tabbed for ease of review.

If, at any time during the conduct of the clinical investigation, changes are made in the original protocol or the original laser device, these changes must be reported to the FDA in the form of a supplemental IDE application. The supplemental application must adequately address the precise change made and must be supported by all relevant data. Each change is unique to a particular investigation and is handled on a case-by-case basis. Examples of such changes can include the addition of a different patient group, use of an additional laser source, use of a laser device with a different power output, or use of a different laser delivery system.

Progress Reports

Throughout the course of the clinical investigation, progress reports shall be submitted and shall include the results from all patients entered into the study. Since these reports are submitted at regular intervals, apparent problems with the laser device or protocol can be detected before additional patients are subjected to unnecessary risk.

Premarket Approval Applications

Before a laser device can be marketed for use in the treatment of atherosclerotic disease, the manufacturer must submit a premarket approval (PMA) application to the FDA for approval. The FDA carefully reviews all the data to ensure that each indication for use of the laser device and each design is supported by data from a sufficient number of patients to draw scientifically valid conclusions. Currently, for a PMA for a laser device to be filed, enough patients must be enrolled so that at least 200 patients are treated with the laser as the first intervention. This number of patients is required to address the issues of acute complications and device failures. Additional patients will be required if the population differs significantly in patient group or lesion location, as would be the case 1) if sole therapy and adjunct therapy are the indications for use, 2) if infrapopliteal arteries were treated in addition to femoral and popliteal arteries, 3) for limb salvage candidates, 4) for bypass graft patients, or 5) if significant design changes are made to the laser during the course of the investigation. For investigations conducted in peripheral blood vessels, the 200-patient data base must contain data from a minimum of 50 successful procedures, with 6-month follow-up. For investigations conducted in coronary blood vessels, the 200-patient data base must contain data from a minimum of 75 successful procedures, with 6-month follow-up.

The FDA requires that the sponsor provide an update of the clinical data at least 4 weeks prior to an advisory panel review of the application. The clinical study must continue following the approved protocol until the laser device has been approved by the FDA for general marketing. All patients, successful or not, must be accounted for and reasons for discontinuing a patient must be provided. Since assessment of vessel patency at follow-up is crucial to the determination of device effectiveness, the physician must explain the need for follow-up to each patient entering the investigation and make every effort to obtain this data on all patients. Each patient in the investigation must be completely accounted for at all follow-up intervals. Postapproval requirements include additional follow-up on a selected group of patients to assess long-term complications and restenosis.

Prior to final PMA approval, the manufacturer must submit the proposed training manual that will be used to educate physicians in the use of the laser device. The commitment to train potential users is a condition of approval of the PMA.

Summary of Regulatory Issues

The safe use of laser devices in the treatment of atherosclerotic disease presents unique concerns not previously encountered by cardiovascular physicians. The FDA must be sure that these concerns are adequately addressed before a laser device can be approved for clinical investigation or marketing. As the FDA continues to review submitted data and as new information becomes available, the concerns discussed in this chapter may be modified. The FDA believes that every possible step must be taken to protect the patient from the potential unsafe design or use of laser devices.

References

1. Rockwell Associates, Inc. Laser safety training manual. 6th ed. Orlando, Fl.: Laser Institute of America, 1984.
2. Rockwell Associates, Inc., ed. Laser Safety in Surgery and Medicine. Orlando, Fl.: Laser Institute of America, 1983.
3. Sliney D, Wolbarsht M. Safety with lasers and other optical sources. New York: Plenum Press, 1980.
4. Title 21, code of federal regulations, parts 800 to 1299, revised as of April 1, 1990. Published by the Office of the Federal Register, National Archives and Records Service, General Services Administration, Superintendent of Documents, U.S. Government Printing Office, Washington, D.C. 20402.
5. American National Standards Institute, Inc. (ANSI). Safe use of lasers Z-136.1. Orlando, Fl.: Laser Institute of America, 1986.
6. American National Standards Institute, Inc. (ANSI). Safe use of lasers in health care facilities Z-136.3. Orlando, Fl.: Lasers Institute of America, 1988.
7. Abela GS, ed. Lasers in cardiovascular medicine and surgery: fundamentals and techniques. Boston: Kluwer Academic Publishers, 1990.
8. Garden JM, O'Banion KO, Shelnitz LS, et al. Papillomavirus in the

vapor of carbon dioxide laser–treated verrucae. *JAMA* 1988;259:1199–1202.
9. Sawchuk WS, Weber PJ, Lowy DR, Dzubow LM. Infectious papillomavirus in the vapor of warts treated with carbon dioxide laser or electrocoagulation: detection and protection. *J Am Acad Dermol* 1990;20:41–49.
10. Kokosa JM, Eugene J. Chemical composition of laser-tissue interaction smoke plume. *J Laser Appl* 1989;1(3):59–63.
11. Felten RP. Summary of laser plume effects and safety session. *J Laser Appl* 1989;1(2):4–5.
12. Garden JM. The hazards of laser plume: a mid-year committee report. Newsletter, American Society for Laser Medicine and Surgery 1989;3(1):6.
13. Isner JM, Clark RH. The current status of lasers in the treatment of cardiovascular disease. *IEEE J Quantum Elect* 1984;QE-20:1406–1420.
14. Choy DSJ. Vascular recanalization with the laser catheter. *IEEE J Quantum Elect* 1984;QE-20:1420–1426.
15. Case RB, Choy DSJ, Dwyer EM, Silvernail PJ. Absence of distal emboli during in vivo laser recanalization. *Lasers Surg Med* 1985;5:281–289.
16. Haller JD, Krokosky EM, Srinivasan R, et al. Ablation of human atherosclerotic plaque by 193 and 248 nm wavelength nanosecond-delivered laser energy. In: Proceedings of the ICALEO '85. Laser Institute of America 1985;49:11–16.
17. Moretti M. PDT takes a shot at atherosclerosis. *J Laser Appl* 1985;70.
18. McCarthy P. Laser on target: the future of an occlusion. *Am Health* 1986;12.
19. Rawls RL. Laser heart surgery teams chemistry and medicine. *CE News* 1984;62:14–15.
20. Jacobson ED, Krell K, Dempsey MJ. The wavelength dependence of ultraviolet light–induced cell killing and mutagenesis in L5178Y mouse lymphoma cells. *Photochem Photobiol* 1981;33:257–260.
21. Doniger J, Jacobson ED, Krell K, DiPaolo JA. Ultraviolet light action spectra for neoplastic transformation and lethality of Syrian hamster embryo cells correlated with spectrum of pyrimidine dimer formation in cellular DNA. *Proc Nat Acad Sci USA* 1981;78:2378–2382.
22. Coohill TP, Peak MJ, Peak JG. The effects of the ultraviolet wavelengths of radiation present in sunlight on human cells in vitro: yearly review. *Photochem Photobiol* 1987;46:1043–1050.
23. Muller D. Excimer lasers in medicine. *J Laser Appl* 1986;85–89.
24. Green H, Boll J, Parrish JA, et al. Cytotoxicity and mutagenicity of low intensity 248 and 193 nm excimer laser radiation in mammalian cells. *Cancer Res* 1987;47:410–413.

25. Mumakata N, Hieda K, Kobayashi K, et al. Action spectra in ultraviolet wavelengths (150–250 nm) for inactivation and mutagenesis of *Bacillus subtilis* spores obtained with synchrotron radiation. *Photochem Photobiol* 1986;44:385–390.
26. Cole C, Sambuco C, Davies RE, Forbes PD. Skin cancer action spectrum in hairless mice (abstr.). *Photochem Photobiol* 1984;39s:13s.
27. Kligman LH, Crosby MJ, Miller SA, Hitchins VM, Beer JZ. Skin cancer induction in hairless mice by long-wavelength UVA radiation (abstr.). *Photochem Photobiol* 1990;51s:18s–19s.

CHAPTER **11**

Restenosis: From Pathogenesis to Prevention

JAMES S. FORRESTER
BOJAN CERCEK
BEHROOZ SHARIFI
PETER BARATH
MICHAEL FISHBEIN
JAMES FAGIN

THERE are only a few widely practiced therapies in medicine with a 35 percent failure rate. Angioplasty is one. The Percutaneous Transluminal Coronary Angioplasty (PTCA) Registry of the National Heart, Lung, and Blood Institute and high-volume angioplasty centers report that the restenosis rate is 25–55 percent (1–5). Beyond loss of benefit to the patient, restenosis has major economic impact, since its treatment is often reangioplasty. At one of the nation's leading angioplasty centers, 37 percent of the PTCAs were repeat procedures (6). The number of projected angioplasties in 1992 is 300,000 (7). If one-third or 100,000 are repeat procedures and the cost of repeat angioplasty is $10,000, then the cost of restenosis to the health care system is one billion dollars per year.

Although the pathogenesis of restenosis is not yet established, there are now sufficient basic science data to allow us to make reasonable hypotheses. We will review these data from molecular and cell biology and show their relevance to the time course and the histopathology of restenosis. We will then develop a paradigm for the pathogenesis of restenosis and describe how this schema provides direction for developing preventive therapy in man.

Restenosis as Defined by Coronary Angiography

Coronary angiography is of relatively little value for predicting which lesions will restenose: only a few specific vascular morphologies such as long lesions, complete occlusions, and disrupted surfaces have a higher probability of restenosis (8). On the other hand, coronary angiography does define the time course of restenosis. Japanese investigators have performed serial coronary angiography in 229 patients at 1, 3, 6, and 12 months after successful PTCA (3). At 1 month the restenosis rate was 13 percent, at 3 months it was 43 percent, by 1 year it was 53 percent (Fig. 11.1). From these data we can conclude that restenosis most commonly develops between the first and third month post-PTCA. Serruys et al. have confirmed this conclusion in 342 patients in whom quantitative coronary angiography was performed at a single pre-

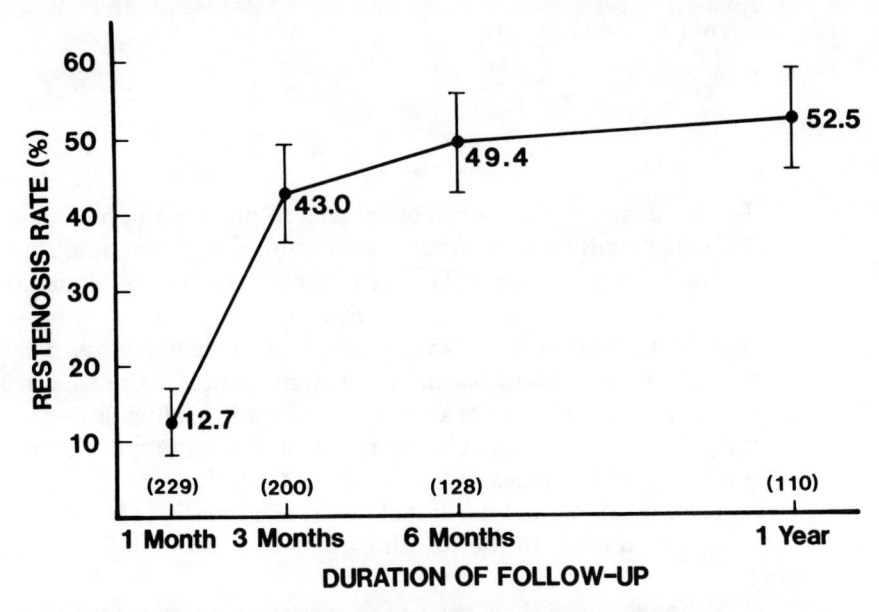

Figure 11.1. The restenosis rate following balloon angioplasty, as defined by serial angiography at 1, 3, 6, and 12 months after successful PTCA. At 1 month the restenosis rate was 13 percent, at 3 months it was 43 percent, by 1 year it was 53 percent. These data suggest that restenosis most commonly develops between the first and third months post-PTCA. (Data replotted from Nobuyoshi et al. J Am Coll Cardiol 1988; 12:616.)

determined follow-up time of 1, 2, 3, or 4 months (4). The most substantial change in lumen diameter occurred between the second and third months. Further, they found that almost all lesions show some evidence of narrowing by 120 days post-PTCA.

There is, however, a central limitation to understanding the pathogenesis of restenosis by analysis of angiographic images: as a method for detecting intimal injury, it is insensitive (9). In contrast, an excellent method for assessing damage to the vascular surface is coronary angioscopy. Used before, during, and after balloon angioplasty the dilatation sites that appear angiographically normal immediately after PTCA typically have angioscopic evidence of severe intimal trauma (10,11). The angioscopic data are supported by postmortem studies of patients dying within 30 days of PTCA. These studies consistently show that in both angiographically successful and failed angioplasty there is a high incidence of intimal dissection, hemorrhage, and thrombus formation (12–25). For instance, Potkin et al. found that 95 percent of angiographically successful angioplasties (Fig. 11.2) had evidence of extensive intimal damage (19; Plate VII).

In addition to damaging the vascular surface, PTCA also affects the vessel wall. Approximately 70 percent of coronary lesions are eccentric: seen in cross-section, the atherosclerotic vessel circumference consists of two segments: an atheroma and a normal vessel wall. When a balloon is inflated, its distending force creates three typical effects in the vessel wall. The atheroma is cracked and fissured. At the junction between the normal segment of the vessel and atheroma, these fissures often become long dissections (16–19; Plate VII). Finally, the normal segment of the vessel wall is substantially stretched (Fig. 11.3). When the segment can stretch no more, the balloon's distending force may tear apart the media (16).

These three effects (fissuring, dissection, stretching) each can increase the cross-sectional area of the vessel. When one examines a balloon-dilated atherosclerotic vessel by giant mount microscopy, however, the increase in cross-sectional area due to fissures and dissections appears to be minimal (19). Since postmortem fixation obscures the stretching effect of balloon dilation (the normal segment contracts during fixation) (26), the third in-vivo effect cannot be assessed. Nevertheless, there is an emerging belief that stretching of the normal vessel wall may be the most important contributor to the dramatic increase in vessel diameter commonly seen by angiography.

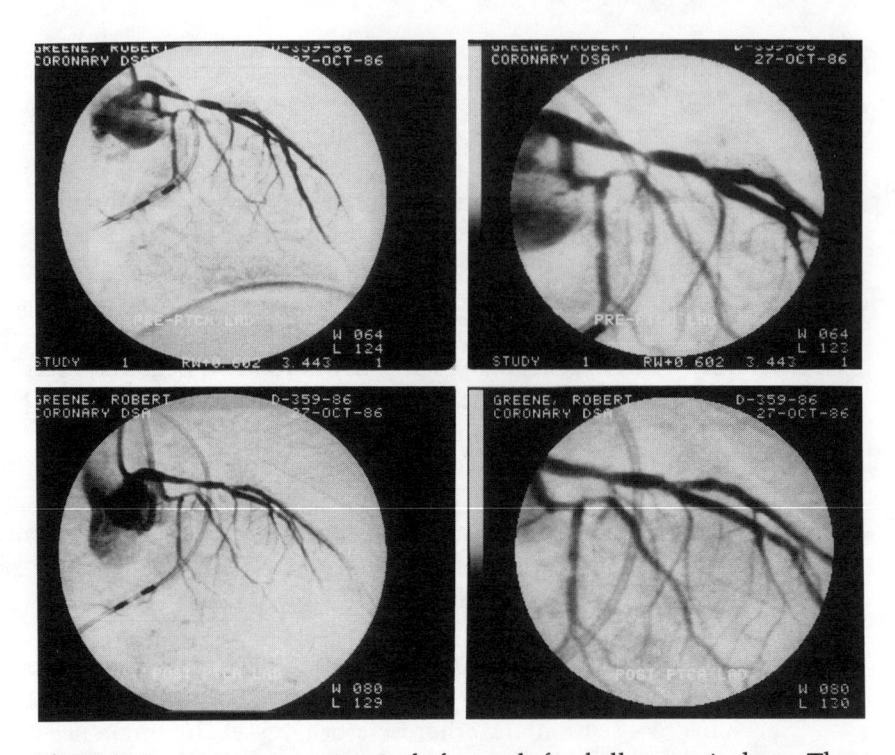

Figure 11.2. A coronary angiogram before and after balloon angioplasty. There is successful dilatation of the left anterior descending coronary artery; the patient was discharged without incident. Forty-eight hours following the procedure, the patient had a sudden cardiac arrest at home. Autopsy examination of the treated segment revealed histologic evidence of extensive intimal damage, a torn intimal surface, and dissection into the media. (Illustration kindly provided by Dr. Benjamin Potkin.)

The Relationship of Immediate Effect of PTCA to Late Restenosis: A Hypothesis

We believe that these three mechanisms of angioplasty-induced increase in arterial diameter are also the cause of restenosis. This hypothesis derives from correlating information from disparate sources. First, angiographic restenosis develops 1–3 months after PTCA. Second, both denuding (27,28) and stretching injury (29,30) are potent stimuli to intimal hyperplasia in normal animal vessels. Third, the histologic appearance of human restenosis in man is exuberant intimal hyperplasia

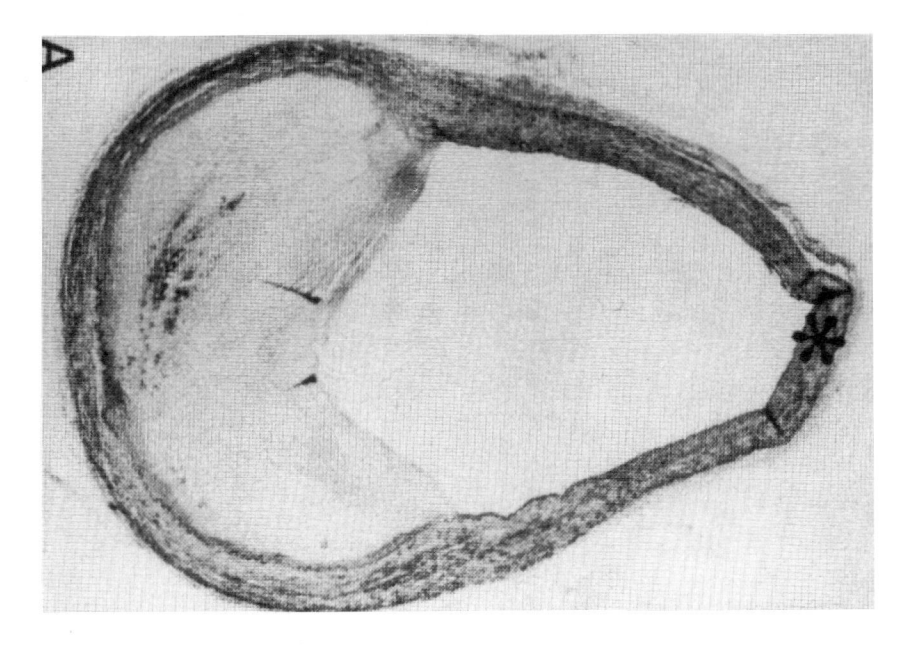

Restenosis: From Pathogenesis to Prevention 245

Figure 11.3. Stretching of the normal segment of a coronary artery following balloon inflation and laser-thermal radiation, which prevents postmortem retraction. Note that the atheroma itself is little effected beyond dissection at the junction between the normal segment and the atheroma, and that the normal segment is substantially stretched. (Reproduced with permission, Waller et al. JACC 1989;13:969.)

(31,32; Fig. 11.4). Finally, intimal hyperplasia also develops on the inner surface of isolated Dacron grafts in the first 3 months after placement, as mesenchymal cells grow through the Dacron mesh. Thus we believe that restenosis is a normal biologic response to injury, which is independent of atherosclerosis; it is driven by normal cellular elements of the vascular wall.

Wound Healing: A Three-Phase Process

The importance of this insight is that recent studies of the molecular and cell biology of wound healing can contribute greatly to our understanding of vascular intimal hyperplasia. Wound healing is a generalized biologic response that has been most extensively studied in the

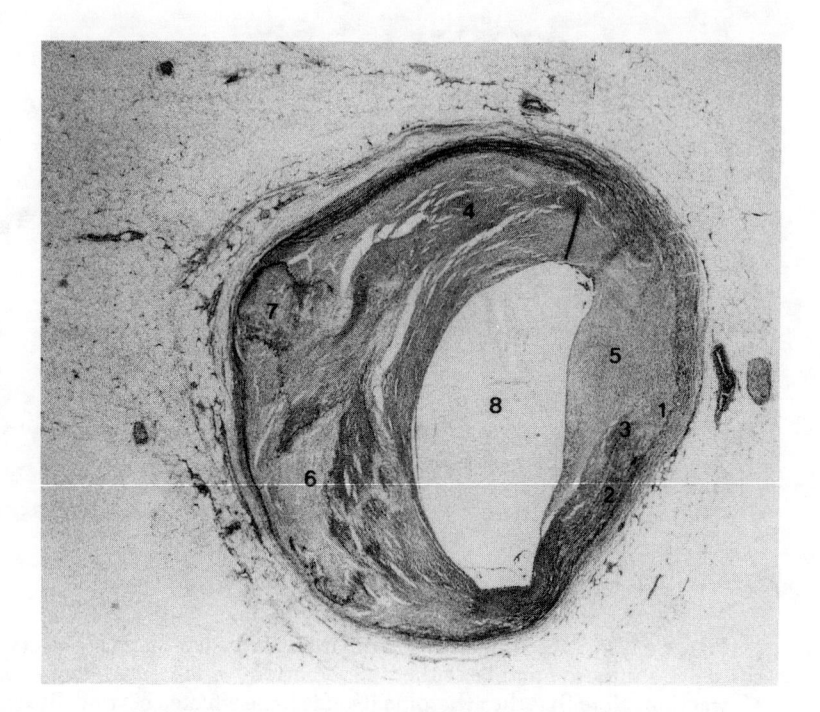

Figure 11.4. A coronary artery cross-section 2 months after PTCA. There is complete destruction of the media in the normal segment, with prominent intimal hyperplasia. *(1)* External elastica; *(2)* media; *(3)* internal elastica; *(4)* collagen; *(5)* myofibroblastic lesion; *(6)* atheroma; *(7)* calcification; *(8)* lumen.

skin and the eye. We will first describe the general wound-healing process, then apply it specifically to restenosis. Healing has been described as three overlapping phases (33).

The first phase of wound healing is the *inflammatory* phase. Blood and serum coagulate to form a primitive extracellular matrix, filling in the gap between the wound margins. An important component of this early matrix is fibronectin, which has binding domains for inflammatory cells and for many biologically active substances. Platelets also adhere to the wound surface, becoming activated as they aggregate. The activated platelets release local vasoconstrictors, expose binding sites for fibrin, and release growth factors. Within a few hours monocytes enter the wound site and also secrete growth factors.

These growth factors are thought to initiate and be maintained in the subsequent phases of wound healing (33–37) Skin healing, for instance, is markedly accelerated by direct application of growth factors (34). This area of research is new, and the number of known growth factors could double in the next decade. Further, the known factors are produced by many different cells and have more than one biologic action and overlapping functions. Some factors can either potentiate or inhibit each other's effects depending on the environment (35,36). With the caveat that our list is a simplification, we have listed in Table 11.1 the growth factors that may play an important role in wound healing and their most important potential roles in restenosis. Platelet-derived growth factor (PDGF) released from the alpha granules of platelets is a potent stimulus to smooth muscle cell migration and proliferation (38,39). The action of PDGF may not be confined to the early period of inflammation, however, since it is also secreted both by activated macrophages and by local smooth muscle cells in the area of tissue injury. Although PDGF can stimulate smooth muscle cell proliferation independently, it does not act alone. PDGF and fibroblast growth factor (FGF) make cells competent to be acted upon by a second class of growth factors that cause progression to actual DNA synthesis. The latter group includes epidermal growth factor (EGF) and insulinlike growth factor I (IGF-1) (40–43). Fibroblast growth factor (FGF) is a stimulus to endothelial cell proliferation (40); EGF and IGF-1 stimulate mesenchymal cell proliferation (41,42). Transforming growth factor (TGF) beta is the most important known growth factor in regulating the extracellular matrix and can function as a potent inhibitor of smooth muscle cell proliferation (44–47). TGF beta activates the expression of proteoglycans and collagen in the matrix, decreases the synthesis of enzymes that degrade matrix pro-

Table 11.1. Potential Role of Growth Factors in Restenosis

GROWTH FACTOR	POTENTIAL ACTION IN RESTENOSIS
PDGF	Stimulate SMC migration and proliferation
FGF	Cause endothelial cell and fibroblast proliferation
EGF	Replace heparin on cell surface, promote SMC proliferation
IGF-1	Promote SMC proliferation and extracellular matrix production
TGF	Regulate matrix remodeling, possibly regulate other growth factors

SMC = smooth muscle cell.

teins, and increases the synthesis of receptors that bind cells to matrix proteins (44,45). The magnitude of TGF beta effect on extracellular matrix synthesis can be profound: in one study TGF beta increased the synthesis of chondroitin sulfate proteoglycan, which is the dominant extracellular matrix protein early in intimal hyperplasia, by twentyfold over control (46).

The time course of appearance and disappearance of growth factors in response to injury is now being defined in several laboratories. We have defined the time course and magnitude of PDGF and IGF-1 mRNA expression after aortic denudation in the rat. There is a twofold increase in PDGF B-chain mRNA and a ninefold induction of IGF-1 mRNA expres-

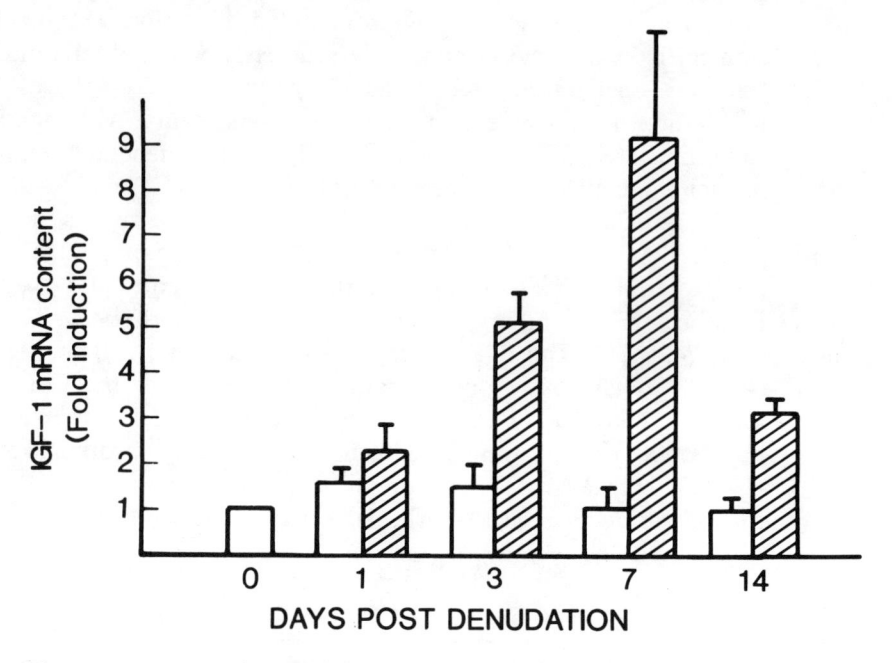

Figure 11.5. Quantification of rat aortic insulinlike growth factor (IGF-1) messenger RNA (mRNA) content after balloon denudation *(hatched bars)* or sham operation *(open bars)*. IGF-1 mRNA was estimated by densitometric scanning of autoradiographic bands in five separate solution hybridization-RNase protection assays. In each experiment, total RNA pooled from four rat aortas was blotted at each time point. All values (mean ± SEM) are expressed relative to aortic IGF-1 mRNA content of untreated rats (time zero). (Reproduced from Cercek et al., Circ Res 1990; 66:1758, with permission.)

sion beginning at day 3, peaking at day 7, and returning to baseline at 2 weeks (Fig. 11.5) (48). Cromack et al. have found a similar time course for appearance of TGF beta protein in healing nonvascular tissue (49). Thus the local tissue level of at least three growth factors is markedly increased during wound healing. We are now identifying the cellular source of these growth factors by in-situ hybridization. We believe that these and other studies will show that locally produced growth factors are the major stimulus for smooth muscle cell proliferation and extracellular matrix production after blood vessel injury.

The Phase of Cellular Proliferation

The second phase of wound healing is marked by migration of local mesenchymal cells into the wound site. Because the wound surface appears granular under a hand lens, it has been called the granulation phase. The fibronectin extracellular matrix facilitates attachment and detachment of cells as they migrate. Depending on tissue type, these migrating cells may be epithelial or endothelial cells on the wound surface, and fibroblasts or smooth muscle cells deeper in the tissue. As the epithelial or endothelial cells cover the wound surface by migration and proliferation, the fibroblast and/or smooth muscle cells below the surface proliferate and synthesize new extracellular matrix components.

Smooth muscle cell proliferation is controlled by the action of mitogens (e.g., PDGF, IGF-1) and the opposing effects of inhibitors, which include both tissue heparin and TGF beta. The smooth muscle cell has two phenotypes, one associated with the resting contractile state, the other with the proliferative-synthetic state. The contractile phenotype is a quiescent cell with numerous myofilaments, which provides both vasomotion and structural support to the normal vessel. The synthetic phenotype, which appears in abundance at wound sites, has abundant synthetic organelles (e.g., free ribosomes, Golgi apparatus, rough endoplasmic reticulum). This is the phenotype that produces extracellular matrix proteoglycan and collagen during wound healing. The contractile phenotype is unresponsive to growth factors; synthetic phenotype cells are responsive (50). When tissue is injured, quiescent contractile smooth muscle cells dedifferentrate ("modulate") to the more primitive synthetic phenotype in a matter of a few days, then migrate into the injured area and proliferate.

The mechanisms responsible for modulation of the smooth muscle phenotype are not yet known, but pieces of evidence suggest that both endothelial cells and growth factors play an important role. Quiescent endothelial cells are potent inhibitors of smooth muscle cell growth, but lose this property when they themselves are proliferating. The inhibitory effect of endothelial cells on smooth muscle cells is probably mediated by a heparinlike factor manufactured by the endothelial cell (51). Thus removal of heparin from the smooth muscle cell surface may be one mechanism by which it modulates its phenotype and becomes responsive to growth factors (52,53).

The Production of Extracellular Matrix

The third phase of wound healing is extracellular matrix deposition and remodeling. When the wound is covered by the proliferating surface cells, the mesenchymal cells beneath the surface slow their proliferation and begin to produce large amounts of proteoglycan. Proteoglycans are a diverse group of structurally related macromolecules. The common structural element is their protein backbone, to which are attached linear glycosoaminoglycans.

There are two major extracellular matrix proteoglycans: chondroitin and dermatin. Both are sulfated. Smooth muscle cells synthesize chondroitin and dermatin. During healing, these proteoglycans predominate in the extracellular matrix. Both denudation and stretching injury are now known to increase the synthesis of these proteoglycans, which, like fibronectin, promote smooth cell migration and proliferation (54). The secretion of chondroitin and dermatin is regulated by TGF beta (55,56).

The third important proteoglycan is heparin sulfate. Whereas smooth muscle cells synthesize the other two proteoglycans, endothelial cells synthesize heparin. The heparin proteoglycan in the endothelial cell basal lamina probably controls smooth muscle cell phenotype. One possible mechanism is that heparin competes with EGF for smooth muscle cell binding sites. Thus it is possible that heparin prevents growth factor access to the cell surface (53). A second possible mechanism for the striking antiproliferative effect of heparin may be its ability to potentiate the biologic activity of TGF beta. Heparin dissociates TGF beta from its carrier protein, thereby rendering it active (57). Although it is antiproliferative, heparin also markedly stimulates the synthesis of proteoglycans by smooth muscle cells, possibly by activating TGF beta (54).

The Three Phases of Restenosis: A Hypothetical Construct

Restenosis can be regarded as the unique vascular representation of the general wound healing process for several reasons. First, angioscopy and postmortem studies establish that vascular injury is extensive after angioplasty. Second, serial angiography shows that restenosis appears during the third phase of healing, when extracellular matrix formation and remodeling occur (3,4). Third, histology shows synthetic smooth muscle cells scattered in a huge mass of extracellular matrix (12,31), the typical tissue finding at 1–3 months of wound healing regardless of tissue type. Fourth, this extracellular matrix is proteoglycan. Finally, we now know that growth factors such as PDGF, IGF-1, and TGF beta are expressed at the vascular injury site, and that these factors stimulate smooth muscle cell proliferation and extracellular matrix synthesis. Thus, although the mechanism of vascular restenosis is not known, we can construct a hypothesis (Fig. 11.6) for the specific temporal sequence of restenosis.

Phase 1: The Immediate Reaction to Denudation and Stretch

The insertion and manipulation of the balloon causes circumferential denudation of endothelial cells from the blood vessel surface. The force of dilation is also transmitted to the vessel wall. The atheroma fissures and the normal wall stretches equally to the atheroma and the normal segment. When the dilating force exceeds the limit of the normal seg-

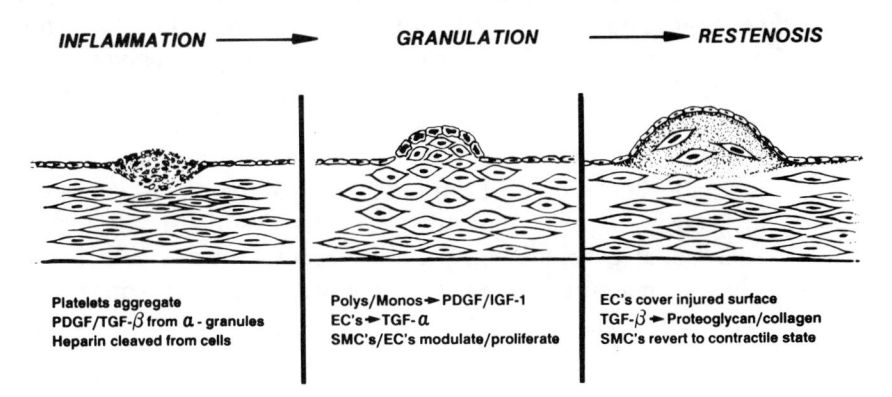

Figure 11.6. A hypothetical schema for restenosis following injury to the vascular surface. The names of the phases of wound healing have been retained to support the analogy between the two phenomena.

ment to stretch, the junction between normal and atherosclerotic tissue is most commonly the first site of rupture, causing the internal elastic lamina and media to be torn apart, and establishing dissection planes in the vessel wall (16–18). Platelets aggregate at these sites of vascular injury. The platelets release biologically active substances, the most important of which are growth factors (58), and an endoglycosidase that cleaves heparin proteoglycan from the surface of endothelial and smooth muscle cells (51,52). When heparin is cleaved, the smooth muscle cells change to the synthetic phenotype and become receptive to growth factors (50,53). The heparin released into the extracellular space also binds PDGF, EGF, and FGF locally (58), increasing the local concentration of growth factors.

Phase 2: The Tissue Reaction to Released Blood Elements

Within 48 hours of injury, some of the smooth muscle cells in the media begin to increase DNA synthesis (59) and proliferate (50). PDGF is central to this response; it also induces the cells to express their own progression factor IGF-1. By day 4, the smooth muscle cells begin to migrate to the injured area, and endothelial cells migrate from the lateral edge of the damaged blood vessel surface (53,59), traversing a fibronectin extracellular matrix that fills the fissured areas on the vessel surface (60–62). Endothelial migration is promoted by FGF (40).

By the end of the first week, many of the local smooth muscle cells have migrated from the media to the intima, although only half of these cells proliferate (63). The synthetic smooth muscle cells begin to produce chondroitin sulfate and dermatin sulfate proteoglycan (62), which gradually replace fibronectin as the dominant extracellular matrix component (62). Depending on the size of the area denuded, endothelial cells cover the injured surface by about day 7 (63,64). If the area of denudation is small (e.g., less than 1 cm long), intimal hyperplasia does not ensue (65), suggesting that below a critical time (5–7 days) or lesion diameter, endothelial coverage can prevent smooth muscle cell proliferation. Thus the magnitude of injury probably determines the magnitude of intimal hyperplasia.

Phase 3: Intimal Hyperplasia and Restenosis

When the injured blood vessel surface is covered by endothelial cells, they cease proliferating and begin synthesis of heparin proteoglycan

(54). Adjacent smooth muscle cells avidly bind the heparin (quiescent smooth muscle cells bind ten times more heparin than proliferating cells) (52). Simultaneously, TGF beta is cleaved from its protein carrier, which makes it active. Thus two potent inhibitors of smooth muscle cell proliferation are now active at the wound site, and the smooth muscle cells become less responsive to the proliferative effects of growth factors like PDGF and IGF-1 (51). Since the synthesis of proteoglycan by smooth muscle cells is independent of migration and proliferation, however, extracellular matrix production accelerates under the potent stimulus of TGF beta. Because the integrity of the blood vessel surface has been restored, the loss of proteoglycan from the injured surface is dramatically reduced (66,67), causing rapid accumulation of proteoglycan. Thus the stage for the typical appearance of intimal hyperplasia is set: proliferating smooth muscle cells in an expanding mass of extracellular matrix (31) initially dominated by proteoglycan.

The magnitude of extracellular matrix production determines whether angiographic and clinical manifestations of restenosis appear. Intimal hyperplasia reaches a peak at 4–12 weeks (Fig. 11.7; 68–71). The gradual return to contractile smooth muscle cell phenotype is paral-

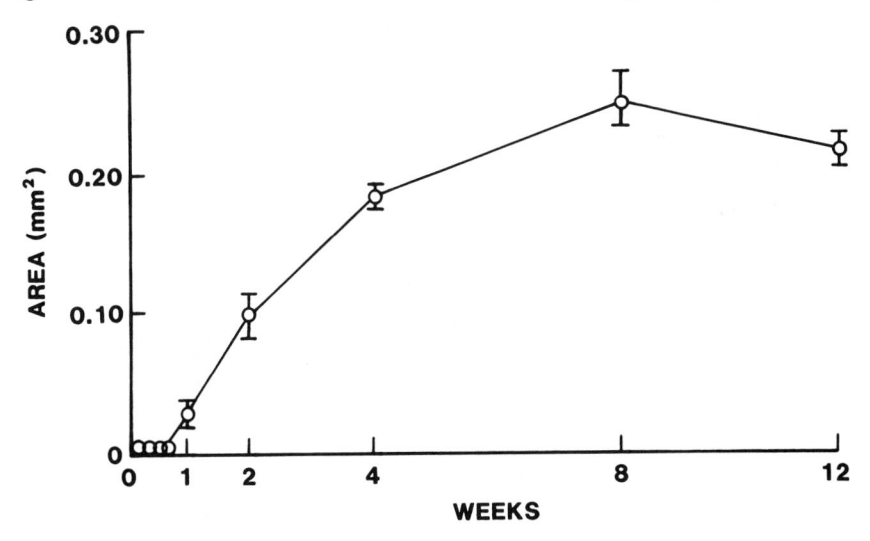

Figure 11.7. The rate of intimal hyperplasia following balloon denudation of the rat aorta. The graph expressing rate of increase of intimal thickness has the same morphologic appearance as that of the angiographic rate of restenosis reported by Nobuyoshi et al. (3). (Replotted from data published by Clowes et al. [69]).

leled by a change in the extracellular matrix: proteoglycan is gradually replaced by collagen and elastin (72). In the relatively normal segments of the vessel, reappearance of contractile smooth muscle cells is accompanied by both fibrotic remodeling and by restoration of responsiveness to vasoconstrictive stimuli (73,74). These two phenomena also cause the angiographic appearance of narrowing by angiography and may in part be responsible for the diminished diameter of normal segments proximal and distal to the atheroma itself (4).

By 6 months, the injury site has stabilized. The ratio of contractile to synthetic phenotype smooth muscle cells has returned to the resting state (53,75). The exception to this observation occurs in areas of chronic endothelial denudation. In such cases smooth muscle cells assume a characteristic flattened phenotype strikingly similar to that of endothelial cells, and their turnover continues at rates as high as 6 percent per day (vs. resting 0.1%) (59). This continued proliferation may account for the observation that between 6 and 12 months a small percentage of treated areas exhibit further narrowing (3).

The Pathogenesis of Restenosis: A Basis for Prevention

Although the pathogenesis of intimal hyperplasia suggests many methods for its inhibition or prevention, no intervention to prevent restenosis in man has so far been successful (Table 11.2). Before concluding that a potential intervention is useless, however, we need to critique the limitations of these clinical trials. First, the timing of drug administration may have been inappropriate. For instance, heparin binds growth factors at the injury site early after injury, facilitating cell migration and proliferation, but later heparin inhibits smooth muscle cell proliferation by cleaving TGF beta from its carrier protein and by inhibiting the action of growth factors. Thus it is possible that heparin might be effective in preventing restenosis if given continuously at 1 week rather than as a bolus during the PTCA procedure. Second, the dose of the agent delivered at the injury site may have been inadequate. For instance, thrombocytopenia profoundly inhibits intimal hyperplasia in animals (76), yet in man antiplatelet agents have been ineffective. The half-time for platelet aggregation after vascular injury is measured in hours (77,78), suggesting that a transient, locally effective agent would be much more effective than low-dose oral administration over several weeks. Finally, there is the remarkable irony that we cannot yet iden-

Restenosis: From Pathogenesis to Prevention

Table 11.2. Potential Therapies in Restenosis

TARGET	EXAMPLES	ACTION
I. Inflammatory Phase		
Platelets	Aspirin, dipyridamole	Inhibit adhesion and aggregation
	Sulotroban	Block thromboxane receptor
	Monoclonal antibodies	Block IIa/IIIb fibrinogen receptor
Inflammatory cells	Steroids	Inhibit accumulation and activation
	Fish oil	Inhibits activation
	Cyclosporin A	Inhibits T-lymphocytes
II. Granulation Phase		
SM cell	Vincristine/actinomycin	Destroy SMCs
SMC receptor	Heparin	Inhibit SMC modulation
	Trapidil	Antagonize PDGF action
III. Matrix Remodeling Phase		
Synthetic SMC	Colchicine, DSMO	Reduce secretory organelles
Mesenchymal cells	Retinoids	Reduce matrix synthesis

tify the desired biologic outcome of therapy. For instance, acceleration of wound healing could rapidly restore the endothelial surface but could also stimulate the proliferation of smooth muscle cells. One might speculate that to inhibit intimal hyperplasia, the first phase of healing should be accelerated and the third phase inhibited.

Interventions in Phase I: Platelet Inhibitors and Anti-inflammatory Agents

Platelet antagonists have both a biologic and a practical rationale. Platelets initiate the healing response to injury by releasing both growth factors and the heparin-cleaving endoglycosidase. In practical terms thrombocytopenia inhibits intimal hyperplasia after vascular injury in atherosclerotic animals (79). Thus the failure of carefully conducted clinical trials of aspirin and dipyridamole has been particularly disappointing. A randomized, blinded, placebo-controlled study of long-term oral aspirin-dipyridamole combination (330 mg–75 mg tid) combined with a 24-hour interval of intravenous dipyridamole in 376 patients found no difference in the angiographic rate of restenosis (38% vs. 39%)

at 4–7 months (80). Long-term oral 325-mg aspirin alone in the 126 patients resulted in a 27 percent restenosis rate, a level not different from a simultaneous coumadin-treated group (81). Beyond the dose-delivery limitations of these studies, it is possible that the negative results could reflect the combined effect of aspirin on thromboxane and prostacyclin metabolism. This latter limitation could be circumvented by use of specific thromboxane A_2 receptor antagonists.

There are also monoclonal antibodies to platelet receptors such as the IIb/IIIa receptor for fibrinogen. This receptor is exposed only when the platelet is activated. Thus it is possible to specifically attack the activated platelet at the wound site without necessarily affecting circulating nonactivated platelets. Monoclonal antibodies can effectively prevent platelet aggregation over 48 hours in a dose-dependent manner (78). The potential value of this more selective therapy has not yet been tested.

Anti-inflammatory agents also have a strong biologic rationale, since they inhibit the accumulation and activation of mesenchymal cells. These cells express the growth factors that initiate and maintain the sequence of intimal hyperplasia that begins with smooth muscle cell phenotypic modulation, migration, and proliferation and ends with formation of new extracellular matrix. In practical terms cortisol inhibits smooth muscle cell protein synthesis and proliferation in cell culture (82). In animals, the combination of steroids with heparin inhibits smooth muscle cell proliferation (83). As with other promising therapies, however, extrapolation to man has failed. Administration of steroids for 1 week post-PTCA did not reduce the restenosis rate in one incompletely reported study (84). Omega 3 fatty acids, which have both anti-inflammatory and antiplatelet actions, were reported to reduce restenosis in early clinical trials, but these results were not confirmed in others (85–89). Cyclospirin A, which inhibits T-lymphocyte activation, causes a highly significant reduction in both smooth muscle cell number and extracellular matrix production in the denuded rat endothelium (90). As yet, there are no clinical reports of its use.

Interventions in Phase II: Antagonists to Growth Factors and Smooth Muscle Cells

Since some cytotoxic agents can selectively destroy smooth muscle cells, agents effective in myosarcomas, such as the combination of actinomycin and vincristine, seem to be logical candidates for testing. We have found that this combination obliterates proliferating smooth muscle cells after balloon denudation in animals (91), but as yet there have been no trials of cytotoxic agents in man.

In principle, growth factor antagonists could inhibit modulation, migration, and proliferation of the smooth muscle cell. Synthetic smooth muscle cells produce ten times as much PDGF as nonproliferating cells (39), and the local tissue concentration of IGF-1 mRNA is equally increased after vascular injury (48). Trapidil prevents smooth muscle cell proliferation in animals through a nonspecific antagonism of PDGF action (92). There are also specific monoclonal antibodies to receptors for a variety of growth factors, which are potent in cell culture (93) but have not yet been tested in either animals or man.

The rationale for use of heparin is particularly powerful. Heparin is a natural inhibitor of smooth muscle cell proliferation. Further, it prevents smooth muscle cell proliferation in cell culture (94,95) and is very effective in preventing intimal hyperplasia in animals. In principle, the antiproliferative and anticoagulant domains of heparin are different, so it may be possible to separate these actions. If so an antiproliferative, nonanticoagulant form of heparin (95) could allow administration of the drug in a high enough concentration to inhibit intimal hyperplasia. As yet heparin has failed to prevent restenosis in man (96).

Angiotensin-converting enzyme inhibitors have recently been reported to prevent myointimal proliferation after vascular injury in rats (97). The mechanism of this action is not well defined but may involve inhibition of angiotensin II–mediated induction of PDGF-A gene expression (98). The potential utility of angiotensin converting enzyme inhibitors is now under active investigation in man.

Phase III: Inhibition of Extracellular Matrix Production

The rationale for inhibiting extracellular matrix production is strong, since it is this aspect of wound healing that is the direct physical cause of restenosis. A number of agents inhibit extracellular matrix synthesis. Colchicine (99) and DMSO (100) both reduce the number of secretory organelles in synthetic phenotype smooth muscle cells, and this effect is accompanied by significant reduction in the production of extracellular matrix. In the animal model, retinoids inhibit extracellular matrix production (101,102) and may inhibit keloid formation in man (102).

Despite their promise these antisecretory agents have not yet been formally tested for prevention of restenosis in man.

Finally, there are agents that prevent intimal hyperplasia by undefined actions. Lovastatin, prostaglandin, and calcium antagonists all inhibit smooth muscle cell proliferation, migration, or both (103–108).

Concomitant Removal or Ablation of Atheroma

Finally, let us speculate about the ultimate cure of restenosis. To do this, we must make some assumptions. First, we will assume that the mechanism of restoration of vascular patency by balloon dilation is stretching the normal wall and cracking the atheroma. We can visualize these effects quite clearly in postmortem cross-sections of coronary arteries (Plate VIII). Second, we will assume that intimal hyperplasia will consistently occur after vascular trauma because it is a normal biologic response. This is unquestionably true in animals. Third, we will assume that this response is usually self-limited. In the rabbit aorta, for instance, the thickness of the neointimal layer reaches about 0.22 mm^2 at 2 months posttrauma (59). Fourth, we will assume that the stretched segment narrows (recoils) over time. This is less well established but is supported by serial angiographic measurements of the normal vascular segment diameter in man. If these assumptions are accurate, then local inhibition of intimal hyperplasia alone, while highly desirable, may be inadequate to prevent restenosis. A significant segment of atheroma mass will also have to be removed.

The alternate methods of angioplasty, discussed in other chapters of this text, have not as yet been shown to reduce the restenosis rate, despite removal of atheroma mass. This has led some interventionists to conclude that removal of atheroma mass has no beneficial effect. There is, however, an unrecognized serious flaw in this reasoning: *no angioplasty technology has been tested with concomitant local inhibition of intimal hyperplasia.* Yet if the magnitude of intimal hyperplasia can be therapeutically reduced, one could anticipate that the vessel with the largest lumen postangioplasty will be least likely to develop restenosis. For this reason we speculate that the best results will be obtained with the combination of balloon, atheroma ablation, and local inhibition of intimal hyperplasia. Thus an understanding of the biologic process of both successful angioplasty and of restenosis suggests that ablation or extraction of atheroma in combination with local vascular stretching will ultimately become the method for restoring the vascular lumen to its original diameter and keeping it that way.

Summary

Restenosis is now the most important unsolved clinical and economic problem in the management of coronary heart disease. We have clues to the pathogenesis of restenosis that define directions for its prevention. We know that the immediate effect of angioplasty is the creation of fissures in the atheroma, stretching of the normal segment of the vessel, and extensive trauma to the intimal surface. Since the histologic appearance of the restenotic lesion is intimal hyperplasia, we can hypothesize that the specific temporal sequence of restenosis is platelet aggregation, inflammatory cell infiltration, release of growth factors, medial smooth muscle cell modulation and proliferation, proteoglycan synthesis, and extracellular matrix remodeling. Each milestone in this process can be inhibited. Although we have focused on pharmacologic methods to reduce intimal hyperplasia, we must recognize the real possibility, even likelihood, that this effect alone will not resolve the problem of restenosis. PTCA does not reduce atheroma mass. Partial or complete removal of the obstructing mass of atheroma may also be required. Rotational and directional atherectomy (109) and excimer laser angioplasty (110–112), discussed in other chapters, are all now in large-scale coronary angioplasty trials. While neither removal of atheroma mass nor inhibition of intimal hyperplasia alone may solve the problem of restenosis, it can and will be largely eliminated, we believe, by a combination of these three methods.

References

1. Holmes DR, Vlietstra R, Smith H, et al. Restenosis after percutaneous transluminal coronary angioplasty (PTCA): a report from the PTCA Registry of the National Heart, Lung and Blood Institute. *Am J Cardiol*, 1984;53:77C–81C.
2. Val PG, Bourassa MG, David PR, et al. Restenosis after successful percutaneous transluminal coronary angioplasty: the Montreal Heart Institute Experience. *Am J Cardiol* 1987; 60:50B–55B.
3. Nobuyoshi M, Kimura T, Noksaka H, et al. Restenosis after successful

percutaneous transluminal coronary angioplasty: serial angiographic follow-up of 229 patients. *J Am Coll Cardiol* 1988;12:616–623.
4. Serruys PW, Luijten HE, Beatt KJ, et al. Incidence of restenosis after successful coronary angioplasty: a time-related phenomenon. A quantitative angiographic study in 342 consecutive patients at 1, 2, and 3 months. *Circulation* 1988;77:361–372.
5. Bertrand ME, Lablanche JM, Fourrier JL, Gommeaux A, Ruel M. Relation to restenosis after percutaneous transluminal coronary angioplasty to vasomotion of the dilated coronary arterial segment. *Am J Cardiol* 1989;63:277–281.
6. King SB. Information from the Emory University PTCA Data Base, presented at the 20th Annual American College of Cardiology Conference at Snowmass, Colorado January 1989 (unpublished).
7. Brown PW. The outlook for the coronary angioplasty industry. (Industry report). Hambrect and Quist, Inc., 1986.
8. Ellis SG, Roubin GS, King SB, Douglas JS, Cox WR. Importance of stenosis morphology in the estimation of restenosis risk after elective percutaneous transluminal coronary angioplasty. *Am J Cardiol* 1989; 63:30–34.
9. Forrester JS, Litvack F, Grundfest W, Hickey A. A perspective of coronary disease seen through the arteries of living man. *Circulation* 1987; 75:505–513.
10. Uchida Y, Hasegawa K, Kawamura K, Shibuya I. Angioscopic observation of the coronary luminal changes induced by percutaneous transluminal coronary angioplasty. *Am Heart J* 1989; 117:769–776.
11. Mizuno Y, Miyamoto A, Shibuya T, et al. Changes of angioscopic macromorphology following coronary angioplasty. *Circulation* 1988; 78:II-289.
12. Austin GE, Ratliff NB, Hollman J, Tabeil S, Phillips D. Intimal proliferation of smooth muscle cells as an explanation for recurrent coronary artery stenosis after percutaneous transluminal coronary angioplasty. *J Am Coll Cardiol* 1985; 6:369–375.
13. Block P, Myler R, Stertzer S, Fallon J. Morphology after transluminal angioplasty in human beings. *N Engl J Med* 1981; 305:382–385.
14. Giraldo AA, Esposo OM, Meis JM. Intimal hyperplasia as a cause of restenosis after percutaneous transluminal coronary angioplasty. *Arch Pathol Lab Med* 1985; 109:173–175.
15. Ueda M, Becker AE, Fujimoto T. Pathologic changes induced by repeated percutaneous transluminal coronary angioplasty. *Br Heart J* 1987; 58:635–643.
16. Gravanis MB, Roubin GS. Histopathologic phenomena at the site of

percutaneous transluminal coronary angioplasty. *Human Pathol* 1989; 20:477–485.
17. Saner HE, Gobel FL, Salmonowitz E, Erlien DA, Edwards JE. The disease-free wall in coronary atherosclerosis: its relation to degree of obstruction. *J Am Coll Cardiol* 6:1096–1099.
18. Waller BF. Morphologic correlates of coronary angiographic patterns at the site of percutaneous transluminal coronary angioplasty. *Clin Cardiol* 1988;11:817–822.
19. Potkin BN, Roberts WC. Effects of percutaneous transluminal coronary angioplasty on atherosclerotic plaques and relation of plaque composition and arterial size to outcome. *Am J Cardiol* 1988; 62:41–50.
20. Kochi T, Takebayashi S, Block PC, Hiroki T, Nobuyoshi M. Arterial changes after percutaneous transluminal coronary angioplasty: results at autopsy. *J Am Coll Cardiol* 1987; 10:592–599.
21. deMorais CF, Lopes EA, Checchi H, Arie S, Poileggi F. Percutaneous transluminal coronary angioplasty—histopathological analysis of nine necropsy cases. *Virchows Arch* (A) 1986; 410:195–202.
22. Soward AL, Essed CE, Serruys PW. Coronary arterial findings after accidental death immediately after successful percutaneous transluminal coronary angioplasty. *Am J Cardiol* 1985; 56:794–795.
23. Schneider J, Gruntzig A. Percutaneous transluminal coronary angioplasty: morphological findings in 3 patients. *Pathol Res Pract* 1985; 180:348–352.
24. Mizuno K, Kurita A, Imazeki N. Pathological findings after percutaneous transluminal coronary angioplasty. *Br Heart J* 1984; 52:588–590.
25. Bruneval P, Guermonprez JL, Perrier P, Carpentier A, Camilleri JP. Coronary artery restenosis following transluminal coronary angioplasty. *Arch Pathol Lab Med* 1986;110:1186–1187.
26. Waller B. "Crackers, breakers, stretchers, drillers, scrapers, shavers, burners, welders, and melters"—the future treatment of atherosclerotic coronary artery disease? A clinical–morphologic assessment. *J Am Coll Cardiol* 1989;13:969,987.
27. Sanborn TA, Faxon DP, Haudenschild C, Gottsman SB, Ryan TJ. The mechanism of transluminal angioplasty: evidence for formation of aneurysms in experimental atherosclerosis. *Circulation* 1983; 68:1136–1140.
28. Steele PM, Chesebro JH, Stanson AW, et al. Balloon angioplasty: natural history of the pathophysiologic response to injury in a pig model. *Circ Res* 1985;57:105–112.
29. Leung DY, Glagov S, Mathews MB. Cyclic stretching stimulates synthesis of matrix components by arterial smooth muscle cells in vitro. *Science* 1976; 191:475–477.

30. Clowes AW, Clowes MM, Fingerle J, Reidy MA. Kinetics of cellular proliferation after arterial injury V. Role of acute distension in the induction of smooth muscle proliferation. *Lab Invest* 1989;60(3):360–364.
31. Simpson JB, Selmon MR, Robertson GC, et al. Transluminal atherectomy for occlusive peripheral vascular disease. *Am J Cardiol* 1988; 61:96G–101G.
32. Greisler HP, Ellinger J, Schwarcz TH, Golan J, Raymond RM, Kim DU. Arterial regeneration over polydioxanone prostheses in the rabbit. *Arch Surg* 1987;122:715–721.
33. Clark RAF. Overview and general considerations of wound repair. In: Clark RAF, Henson PM, eds. The molecular and cellular biology of wound repair. New York: Plenum Press, 1988.
34. Brown GL, Nanney LB, Griffen J, et al. Enhancement of wound healing by topical treatment with epidermal growth factor. *N Engl J Med* 1989; 321:76–79.
35. Nemeth G, Bolander M, Martin G. Growth factors and their role in wound and fracture healing. In: Barbul A, Pines E, Caldwell M, Hunt TK, eds. Growth factors and other aspects of wound healing: biological and clinical implications. Progress in clinical and biological research. New York: Alan R. Liss, 1988;266: 1–17.
36. Hjelmeland LM, Harvey AK. Growth factors: soluble mediators of wound repair and occular fibrosis. *Birth Defects* 1988; 24:87–102.
37. Knighton DR, Fiegel VD, Austin, LL, Ciresi KF, Butler EL. Classification and treatment of chronic nonhealing wounds. *Ann Surg* 1986; 204:322–330.
38. Ross R, Raines EW, Bowen-Pope DF. The biology of platelet–derived growth factor. *Cell* 1986; 46:155–169.
39. Walker LN, Bowen-Pope DF, Ross R, Reidy MA. Production of platelet–derived growth factor-like molecules by cultured arterial smooth muscle cells accompanies proliferation after arterial injury. *Proc Natl Acad Sci* 1986; 83:7311–7315.
40. Folkman J, Klagsbrun M. Angiogenic factors. *Science* 1987; 235:442–447.
41. Stiles CD, Capone GT, Scher CD, Antoniades HN, Van Wyk JJ, Pledger WJ. Dual control of cell growth by somatomedins and platelet–derived growth factor *Proc Natl Acad Sci* 1979; 76:1279–1283.
42. Waterfield MD. Epidermal growth factor and related molecules. *Lancet* 1989; June (1): 1243–1246.
43. Spencer EM, Skover G, Hunt TK. Somatomedins: do they play a pivotal

role in wound healing? Growth factors and other aspects of wound healing: biological and clinical implications New York: Alan R. Liss, 1988: 103–116.
44. Roberts AB, Flanders KC, Kondaiah P, et al. Transforming growth factor beta: biochemistry and roles in embryogenesis, tissue repair and remodeling and carcinogenesis. In: Recent progress in hormone research. Vol. 44. Academic Press, 1988.
45. Sprugel KH, McPherson JM, Clowes AW, Ross R. The effects of different growth factors in subcutaneous wound chambers. In: Growth factors and other aspects of wound healing: biological and clinical implications. New York: Alan R. Liss, 1988;266:77–91.
46. Chen JK, Hoshi H, McKeehan WL. Transforming growth factor type beta specifically stimulates synthesis of proteoglycan in human adult arterial smooth muscle cells. *Proc Natl Acad Sci* 1987; 84: 5287–5291.
47. Ignotz RA, Massague J. Transforming growth factor–beta stimulates the expression of fibronectin and collagen and their incorporation into the extracellular matrix. *J Biol Chem* 1986; 261:4337–4345.
48. Cercek B, Fishbein MC, Forrester JS, Helfant RH, Fagin JA. Induction of IGF-1 m-RNA in rat aorta after balloon denudation. *Circ Res* 1990; 66:1755–1760.
49. Cromack DT, Sporn MB, Roberts AB, Merino MJ, Dart LL, Norton JA. Transforming growth factor beta levels in rat wound chambers. *J Surg Res* 1987; 42:622–628.
50. Campbell GR, Campbell JH, Manderson JA, Horrigan S, Rennick RE. Arterial smooth muscle: a multifunctional mesenchymal cell. *Arch Pathol Lab Med* 1988; 112:977–986.
51. Castellot JJ, Wright TC, Karnovsky MJ. Regulation of vascular smooth muscle cell growth by heparin and heparin sulfates. *Seminars in Thrombosis and Hemostasis* 1987; 13:489–503.
52. Castellot JJ, Addonizio ML, Rosenberg RD, Karnovsky MJ. Cultured endothelial cells produce a heparin–like inhibitor of smooth muscle cell growth. *J Cell Biol* 1981; 90:372–379.
53. Campbell JH, Campbell GR. Endothelial cell enfluences on vascular smooth muscle phenotype. *Ann Rev Physiol* 1986; 48:295–306.
54. Wight TN. Cell biology of arterial proteoglycans. *Arteriosclerosis* 1989; 9:1–20.
55. Bassols A, Massague J. Transforming growth factor beta regulates the expression and structure of extracellular matrix chondroitin/dermatan sulfate proteoglycans. *J Biol Chem* 1988; 263:3039–3045.
56. Kinsella MG, Wight TN. Modulation of sulfated proteoglycan synthe-

sis by bovine aortic endothelial cells during migration. *J Cell Biology* 1986; 102:678–687.
57. McCaffrey TA, Falcone DJ, Brayton CF, Agarwal LA, Welt FGP, Weksler BB. Transforming growth factor–beta activity is potentiated by heparin via dissociation of the transforming growth factor beta/alpha$_2$–macroglobulin inactive complex. *J Cell Biol* 1989; 109:441–448.
58. Lobb RR. Clinical applications of heparin–binding growth factors. *Eur J Clin Invest* 1988; 18:321–336.
59. Clowes AW, Reidy MA, Clowes MM. Kinetics of cellular proliferation after arterial injury. I. Smooth muscle growth in the absence of endothelium. *Lab Invest* 1983; 49:327–333.
60. Holund B, Clemmensen K, Junker P, Lyon H. Fibronectin in experimental granulation tissue. *Acta Pathol Microbiol Immunol Scand* 1982; 90:159–165.
61. Anseth A. Glycosaminoglycans in corneal regeneration. *Exp Eye Res* 1961; 1:122–127.
62. Bently JP. Rate of chondroitin sulfate formation in wound healing. *Ann Surg* 1967; 165:186–191.
63. Clowes AW, Schwartz SM. Significance of quiescent smooth muscle migration in the injured rat carotid artery. *Circ Res* 1985; 56:139–145.
64. Fishman JA, Ryan GB, Karnovsky MJ. Endothelial regeneration in the rat carotid artery and the significance of endothelial denudation in the pathogenesis of myointimal thickening. *Lab Invest* 1975; 32:339–351.
65. Reidy MA, Schwartz SM. Endothelial regeneration III. Time course of intimal change after small defined injury to rat endothelium. *Lab Invest* 1981; 44:301.
66. Clowes AW, Clowes MM, Reidy MA. Kinetics of cellular proliferation after arterial injury. III. Endothelial and smooth muscle growth in chronically denuded vessels. *Lab Invest* 1986; 54:295–303.
67. Alvai M, Moore S. Glycosaminoglycan composition and biosynthesis in the endothelium–covered neointima and de–endothelialized rabbit aorta. *Exp Mol Pathol* 1985; 42:389–400.
68. Stemerman MB, Spaet TH, Pitlick F, Cintron J, Lejnieks I, Tiell ML. Intimal healing: the pattern of reendothelialization and intimal thickening. *Am J Pathol* 1977; 7:125–137.
69. Clowes AW, Reidy MA, Clowes MM. Mechanisms of stenosis after arterial injury. *Lab Invest* 1983; 49:208–215.
70. Schwartz SM, Campbell GR, Campbell JH. Replication of smooth muscle cells in vascular disease. *Circ Res* 1986; 58:427–444.
71. Clowes AW, Kirkman TR, Riedy MA. Mechanisms of arterial graft

healing. Rapid transmural capillary ingrowth provides a source of intimal endothelium and smooth muscle in porous PTFE prostheses. *Am J Pathol* 1986; 123;220-230.
72. Diegelmann RF, Rothkopf LC, Cohen IK. Measurement of collagen biosynthesis during wound healing. *J Surg Res* 1975; 19: 239-243.
73. Consigny PM, Tulenko TN, Nichosia RF. Immediate and long-term effects of angioplasty-balloon dilation on normal rabbit iliac artery. *Arteriosclerosis* 1986; 6:265-276.
74. Castaneda-Zuniga WR, Laerum F, Rysavy J, Rusnak B, Amplatz K. Paralysis of arteries by intraluminal balloon dilation. *Radiology* 1982; 144:75-76.
75. Manderson JA, Mosse PRL, Safstrom JA, Young SB, Campbell GR. Balloon catheter injury to rabbit carotid artery I. Changes in smooth muscle phenotype. *Arteriosclerosis* 1989; 9:289-296.
76. Minar E, Ehringer H, Ahmadi R, et al. Platelet deposition at angioplasty sites and its relation to restenosis in human iliac and femoropopliteal arteries. *Radiol* 1989; 170:767-772.
77. Wilentz JR, Sanborn TA, Haudenschild CC, Valeri CR, Ryan TJ, Faxon DP. Platelet accumulation in experimental angioplasty: time course and relation to vascular injury. *Circulation* 1989; 75:636-642.
78. Harker LA. Role of platelets and thrombosis in mechanisms of acute occlusion and restenosis after angioplasty. *Am J Cardiol* 1989; 60:20B-28B.
79. Fingerle J, Johnson R, Clowes AW, Majesky MW, Reidy MA. Role of platelets in smooth muscle cell proliferation and migration after vascular injury in rat carotid artery. *Proc Natl Acad Sci* 1986; 86:8412-8416.
80. Schwartz L, Bourassa MG, Lesperance J, et al. Aspirin and dipyridamole in the prevention of restenosis after percutaneous transluminal coronary angioplasty. *N Engl J Med* 1988; 318:1714-1719.
81. Thronton MA, Gruentzig AR, Hollman J, King SB, Douglas JS. Coumadin and aspirin in prevention of recurrence after transluminal coronary angioplasty: a randomized study. *Circulation* 1984; 69:721-727.
82. Jarvelainen H, Halme T, Ronnemaa R. Effect of cortisol on the proliferation and protein synthesis of human aortic smooth muscle cells in culture. *Acta Med Scand* 1982; 660(suppl):114-122.
83. Gordon JB, Berk BC, Bettman, Selwyn AP, Rennke H, Alexander RW. Vascular smooth muscle proliferation following balloon injury is synergistically inhibited by low molecular weight heparin and hydrocortisone. *Circulation* 1987; 76(suppl IV):IV-213.
84. Liu MW, Roubin GS, King SB. Research on coronary artery stenosis.

Restenosis after coronary angioplasty. Potential biological determinants and role of intimal hyperplasia. *Circulation* 1989; 79:1374–1387.

85. Grigg LE, Kay T, Manolas EG, Hunt D, Valentine PA. Does Max–EPA lower the risk of restenosis after PTCA: a prospective randomized trial. *Circulation* 1987; 76:IV-214.

86. Reis GJ, Boucher TM, Sipperly ME, et al. Randomised trial of fish oil for prevention of restenosis after coronary angioplasty. *Lancet* 1989; July (2):177–181.

87. Dehmer GJ, Popma JJ, Van den Berg EK, et al. Reduction in the rate of early restenosis after coronary angioplasty by a diet supplemented with n–3 fatty acids. *N Engl J Med* 1988; 391-733-740.

88. Slack JD, Pinkerton CA, Van Tassel J, et al. Can oral fish oil supplement minimize restenosis after percutaneous transluminal coronary angioplasty? *J Am Coll Cardiol* 1987; 9(suppl):64A.

89. Milner MR, Gallino RA, Leffingwell A, Pichard AD, Rosenberg J. High dose omega–3 fatty supplementation reduces clinical restenosis after coronary angioplasty. *Circulation* 1988; 78(suppl II):634.

90. Jonasson L, Holm J, Hansson GK. Cyclosporin A inhibits smooth muscle proliferation in the vascular response to injury. *Proc Natl Acad Sci* 1988; 85:2303–2306.

91. Barath P, Arakawa K, Cao J, et al. Low dose of antitumor agents prevents smooth muscle cell proliferation after endothelial injury. *J Am Coll Cardiol* 1989; 13:252A.

92. Liu MW, Roubin GS, King SB. Research on coronary artery stenosis. Restenosis after coronary angioplasty. Potential biological determinants and role of intimal hyperplasia. *Circulation* 1989; 79:1374–1387.

93. Danielpour D, Dart LL, Flanders KC, Roberts AB, Sporn MB. Immunodetection and quantitation of the two forms of transforming growth factor–beta (TGF–beta$_1$ and TGF–beta$_2$) secreted by cells in culture. *J Cell Physiol* 1989; 138:79–86.

94. Clowes AW, Clowes MM. Kinetic of cellular proliferation after arterial injury: II. Inhibition of smooth muscle growth by heparin. *Lab Invest* 1985; 52:611–616.

95. Paul R, Herbert JM, Maffrand JP, et al. Inhibition of vascular smooth muscle cell proliferation in culture by pentosan polysulphate and related compounds. *Thromb Res* 1987; 46:793–801.

96. Ellis SG, Roubin GS, Wilenz J, Lin S, Douglas JS Jr, King SB. Results of a randomized trial of heparin and aspirin vs aspirin alone for prevention of acute closure and restenosis after angioplasty (PTCA). *Circulation* 1987; 76(suppl IV):IV-213.

97. Powell JS, Clozel JP, Muller RKM, et al. Inhibitors of angiotensin–cov-

erting enzyme prevent myointimal proliferation after vascular injury. *Science* 1989; 245:186–188.
98. Naftilan AJ, Pratt RE, Dzau VJ. Induction of platelet–derived growth factor A–chain and c–myc gene expressions by angiotensin II in cultured rat vascular smooth muscle cells. *J Clin Invest* 1989; 83:1419–1424.
99. Chaldakov GN, Vankov VN. Morphological aspects of secretion in the arterial smooth muscle cell, with special reference to the golgi complex and microtubular cytoskelton. *Atherosclerosis* 1986; 61:175–192.
100. Katsuda S, Okada Y, Nakanishi I, Tanaka J. Inhibitory effect of dimethyl sulfoxide on the proliferation of cultured arterial smooth muscle cells: relationship to the cytoplasmic microtubules. *Exp Mol Pathol* 1988; 48:48–58.
101. Daly TJ, Weston WL. Retinoid effects on fibroblast proliferation and collagen synthesis of vitro and on fibrotic disease in vivo. *J Am Acad Dermatol* 1986; 15:900–902.
102. Panabiere–Castaings MH. Retinoic acid in the treatment of keloids. *J Dermatol Surg Oncology* 1988; 14:1275–1276.
103. Sahni R, Maniet AR, Voci G, Banka VS. Prevention of restenosis by lovastatin (Abstr). *Circulation* 1989;80(4):II–65.
104. Morisaki N, Kanzaki T, Motoyama N, Saito Y, Yoshida S. Cell cycle–dependent inhibition of DNA synthesis by prostaglandin I_2 in cultured rabbit aortic smooth muscle cells. *Atherosclerosis* 1988; 71:165–171.
105. Nilsson J, Olsson AG. Prostaglandin E_1 inhibits DNA synthesis in arterial smooth muscle cells stimulated with platelet–derived growth factor. *Atherosclerosis* 1984; 53:77–82.
106. Nomoto A, Hirosumi J, Sekiguchi C, Mutoh S, Yamaguchi I, Aoki H. Antiatherogenic activity of FR 34235 (Nilvadipine), a new potent calcium antagonist: effect on cuff-induced intimal thickening of rabbit carotid artery. *Atherosclerosis* 1987; 64:255–261.
107. Nilsson J, Sjolund M, Palmberg L, VonEuler AM, Jonzon, Thyberg J. The calcium antagonist nifedipine inhibits arterial smooth muscle proliferation. *Atherosclerosis* 1985; 58:109–122.
108. Betz E, Hammerle D, Viele D. Ca^{2+}-entry blockers and atherosclerosis. *Int. Angiol* 1984; 3:33.
109. Simpson JB, Robertson GC, Selmon MR, et al. Restenosis following successful directional coronary atherectomy. *Circulation* 1989; 80(4):2311A.
110. Litvack F, Grundfest WS, Goldenberg T, Laudenslager J, Forrester J. Percutaneous excimer laser angioplasty of aortocoronary saphenous vein grafts. *J Am Coll Cardiol* 1989; 14:803–808.

111. Litvack F, Grundfest W, Eigler N, et al. Percutaneous excimer laser coronary angioplasty. *Lancet* 1989; II:102–103.
112. O'Neill WW, Friedman HZ, Cragg D, et al. Initial clinical experience and early follow-up of patients undergoing mechanical rotary endarterectomy. *Circulation* 1989; 80(4):2318A.

Index

Ablation as tissue effect of lasers. *See* Laser/tissue interaction
Absorption of light, 2, 6–10, 29–34
ACC/AHA lesion classifications, 88–89
Acoustic injury zone, 36
Acoustic transients, 10, 36
Actinomycin, 257
Advanced Interventional Systems, Inc., 64, 66, 128
Albumin-heparin conjugates, 217–18
Alexandrite lasers, 182
American College of Cardiology-American Heart Association Task Force, 88
American National Standards Institute (ANSI), 223, 231
Amplatz shape catheters, 77
Amplification, process of, 5
Anastomoses of arteries, 193–94, 195
Angioscopic visualization, 66
Angiotensin-converting enzyme inhibitors, 257

ANSI. *See* American National Standards Institute
Anti-inflammatory agents, 255–56
Aorto-ostial stenoses, 92, 93, 127, 142–44
Argon lasers
  applications, 15–16, 192
  development, 2, 3, 183–84
  features, 181–82
  histologic effects, 28, 38, 195
Arterial recoil, 194, 195, 199–202
Aspirin, 79, 86, 107, 255–56
Atheroma, 243, 258, 259
Atherosclerotic tissue
  fluorescent identification of, 14
  laser ablation, 8, 30–33, 44–45
Average power, 9, 29, 172

Balloon angioplasty. *See also* Laser balloon angioplasty
  as adjunct to laser procedure, 78, 90, 102, 104
  case study, 133–35

Balloon angioplasty (cont.)
  development, 183
  histologic effects, 42
  limitations, 72, 127
  mechanisms of, 98–99
  restenosis and, 44, 111
Balloon-guided laser delivery systems, 64–65, 68
Beer-Lambert equation, 7
Bend point lesion case study, 136–37
Bending loss, 52–54, 55, 56
Bondability of fiber coatings, 54–55
Brillouin scattering, 57, 58

Calcified tissue ablation, 15, 31, 32, 33, 185
Calcium antagonists, 79, 86, 258
Canadian Cardiovascular Society, 89
Carbon dioxide lasers
  applications, 15, 16
  development, 2
  energy delivery, 178–79, 184
  features, 28, 177
  histologic effects, 55, 193, 195
Cardiovascular tissue
  laser ablation, 30–33, 35–38
  relaxation, 40–41
  thermal diffusion constants, 11
Carotenoids, 14
Catheterization laboratories, 75–76
Catheters for laser angioplasty. See also Optical fibers
  design, 60–64
  development, 202–9
  guidance systems, 64–66
  handling techniques, 77, 82
  numerical aperature, 52
  overview, 49
  selection of, 76–77
  sizing, 81, 129
  technical problems, 109
Cavity dumping, 173, 174
Cellular proliferation of wound healing, 249–50

Center for Devices and Radiological Health, 222
Chalcogenide, 179
Chondroitin, 250, 252
Chopped mode CW lasers, 27, 35–38, 173, 184
Chromophores, 10, 12
Circumflex graft case study, 162–64
Cladding materials. See Core/cladding materials
Coatings of optical fibers, 54–55
Colchicine, 257
Complete occlusions. See Total occlusions
Continuous-wave lasers
  applications, 15–18, 32
  energy delivery, 9–10, 27–28, 29, 172–73, 175
  guidance systems, 65
  histologic effects, 35–38, 43–45
  optical fibers, 58
  thrombogenicity of, 39–40
Core/cladding materials, 51, 52, 54, 55
Coronary arteries. See Dissection of vessels; Perforation of vessels
Coronary artery bypass graft (CABG)
  case study, 160–62
  incidence of, 72, 94, 95
Coupling of laser energy, 59–60, 110
CW lasers. See Continuous-wave lasers
Cyclospirin A, 256
Cytotoxic agents, 256–57

Dead space in multiple fiber systems, 63
Debris formation, 38–39
Denudation of vessel walls, 251–52
Dermatin, 250, 252
Description of device (form), 234–35
Dessication of thrombus, 194
Dielectric breakdown, 13, 14, 34
Diffraction of light, 6–10
Diffuse disease, 92, 127, 140–42, 172

Index

Dipyridamole, 255
Discrete stenosis case study, 129–30
Displacement of tissue, 63
Dissection of vessels, 68, 78–79, 152–58, 243
Distal vessel embolization, 38–39
DMSO, 257
Dotter effect, 102, 111
Dye lasers, 181, 183, 185

ELCA. See Excimer laser coronary angioplasty
Electrocautery, 192, 193
Embolism generation, 38–39
Energy coupling, 59–60
Energy fluence, 9–10, 29, 59, 109, 176
Energy loss in optical fibers, 56–57, 109
Epidermal growth factor (EGF), 247
Erbium:YAG lasers, 17, 177, 179
Excimer laser coronary angioplasty (ELCA)
  case studies, 112–25
    aorto-ostial lesion, 142–44
    bend point lesion, 136–37
    circumflex graft, 162–64
    delayed complication, 164–68
    diffuse disease, 140–42
    discrete stenosis, 129–30
    failed balloon angioplasty, 133–35
    laser dissection, 152–54
    laser perforation/emergency CABG, 160–62
    long LAD lesion, 164
    long recanalized total occlusion, 168–70
    long stenosis, 138–39
    long total occlusion, 144–47
    mechanical dissection, 155–58
    ostial LAD stenosis, 131–33
    ostial right coronary, 148–52
    RPDA graft, 158–60
  catheters, 76–77, 81, 129
  clinical procedures, 73–74, 79, 81–83, 85–88
  clinical trials/results, 85, 88–95, 99–112
  complications, 78–79, 82, 94–95, 102–6, 164–68
  guidewires, 77–78
  indications, 92–93, 127–29, 259
  laboratory design/staffing for, 75–76
  overview, 72
  patient selection, 78–79, 86
  training of practitioners, 74
Excimer lasers
  development, 2, 99
  energy delivery, 19
  features, 20–23
  guidance systems, 65
  histologic effects, 28, 36–38, 39, 42–45, 182–83
  safety/regulatory issues, 222, 225–27
  thrombogenicity of, 39–40
Excited-state dimer molecule. See Excimer lasers
Excited states, 6, 9
Expanded tip laser angioplasty catheters, 61–62, 63
Extracellular matrix production, 250, 254, 257–58

FDA. See U.S. Food and Drug Administration
Federal Laser Products Performance Standard, 223, 229, 235
Fiber core damage, 58
Fiber-optic delivery systems. See also Optical fibers
  bending loss, 52–54
  design, 20
  development, 2–4, 15–20, 26–27
  energy coupler, 59–60
  energy loss in, 109
  input/output surface damage, 57–58
  overview, 49, 66–68

Fiber-optic wave guide, 8
Fibroblast growth factor (FGF), 247
50–micron catheters, 63–64
Fissuring of vessel walls, 243, 259
Flashlamp-excited emissions, 4, 174
Fluorescence, 2, 14–15, 227
Fluoroscopic equipment, 75–76
Food and Drug Administration. *See* U.S. Food and Drug Administration
Fragmentation as tissue effect of lasers, 9
"Free-running" mode, 174

Gas chromatography, 39
Gas lasers, 20
Glass-clad silica fibers, 55–56
Growth factors and restenosis, 247–54, 256–57
Guidewires, 66, 67, 77–78
Guiding laser delivery systems, 64–68
GV Medical, 65

Halogen lasers, 2
Healing. *See* Wound healing
Heating as tissue effect of lasers, 9
Helium neon lasers, 2
Hematoporphyrin derivative, 14, 225
Heparin
  actions, 257
  bolus, 79, 87, 100, 107
  infusion, 83
  restenosis intervention and, 216–17
Heparin sulfate, 216, 250
High peak power
  features of, 172, 175, 177
  histologic effects, 34, 99
  transmission of, 110
High-torque guidewires, 77–78
Histologic analysis of irradiated tissue
  acute effects, 35–38
  chronic effects, 41–44

Holmium lasers
  energy delivery, 177–78, 179–80
  features of, 18, 28
  histologic effects, 185
"Hot tips," 17, 32, 39
Hyperflex guidewires, 77

Inflammatory phase of wound healing, 246–49
Informed consent forms, 236
Infrared (IR) lasers
  ablation and, 177
  energy delivery, 61
  optical fibers, 55, 227
  types, 177–81
Input surface damage, 57
Insulin-like growth factor (IGF), 247–48
Intermittent mode CW lasers. *See* Chopped mode CW lasers
Intimal hyperplasia, 245, 252–54, 259
Investigational device exemptions (IDE) application, 229, 231, 235, 236
Investigational plan, 231–34
Irradiation by lasers. *See* Laser/tissue interaction

Judkins shape catheters, 76, 77

Krypton lasers, 21, 192

Labeling of laser devices, 235
Laboratories, catheterization, 75–76
Laser angioplasty. *See also* Catheters for laser angioplasty; Laser balloon angioplasty (LBA)
  debris/byproduct formation, 38–39
  delivery systems for, 44–45
  development, 3–4, 26–27, 99, 172–73, 183–86
  energy delivery, 8–10
  optimal wavelengths for, 15–20, 22–23, 29–34, 177–83

Index

Laser balloon angioplasty (LBA)
  catheters, 202–9
  clinical procedures, 210–13
  clinical trials/results, 213–19
  experimental studies, 194–99
  overview, 192–94
Laser cavity, 4–6, 173, 174, 226
Laser Institute of America, 223
Laser plume, 222, 224–25
Laser regulatory issues
  description of device, 234–35
  informed consent form, 236
  investigational plan, 231–34
  labeling, 235
  manufacturing information, 235
  overview, 228–29, 238
  premarket approval applications, 237–38
  progress reports, 236–37
  reports of prior investigations, 229–31
  supplemental IDE application, 236
Laser safety issues
  laser plume, 224–25
  new technology, 225–27
  overview, 222–24, 227–28
  photosensitizers, 225
Laser/tissue interaction
  acute effects
    debris/byproduct formation, 38–39
    macroscopic/histologic analysis, 35–38
    thrombogenicity, 39–40
    vasoactivity, 40–41
  chronic effects
    macroscopic/histologic analysis, 41–44
    restenosis, 44
  energy delivery, 8, 9, 29–34
  fusion experiments, 11
  overview, 26–27
  photoacoustic ablation, 13–14
  photochemical ablation, 12–13
  safety issues, 223–24
  thermal ablation, 10–12
Laser welding, 11
Lasers
  components, 4–6
  energy delivery, 28–29
  features, 1
  histologic effects, 2
  medical applications, 2–4, 26
  observed physical phenomena, 15–20
  types, 2–3, 20–23, 27–28, 172, 177–83
Lasing medium, 4–6, 173
LBA. See Laser balloon angioplasty
Lesion morphology classification, 87–89
Light
  interaction with matter, 6–10
  physics of, 4–6
  refraction of, 49–50
Light amplification by stimulated emission of radiation. See Lasers
Long lesions, 127, 164, 242
Long-pulse mode, 22, 23
Long recanalized total occlusion case study, 168–70
Long stenosis case study, 138–39
Long total occlusion case study, 144–47
Lovastatin, 258

Macroscopic analysis of irradiated tissue
  acute effects, 35–38
  chronic effects, 41–44
Manufacturing information, 235
Matter, interaction with light, 6–10
Mesenchymal cells, 249
Metal vapor lasers, 2
Mie scattering, 7, 8
Mode-locked lasers, 27–28, 173–75
Multiple-fiber laser angioplasty catheters, 27, 62–63, 227
Myocardial infarction, 78, 79, 94, 95

Neodymium:YAG lasers
  applications, 16, 19, 211
  development, 3
  energy delivery, 28, 206–8
  features, 178, 180–81
  histologic effects, 38, 182, 183, 193, 194–95, 197–98
  peripheral vessel use, 184
Nitroglycerin, intracoronary, 81, 87, 100, 107
Noble gas lasers, 2
Nonlinear energy loss mechanisms, 57
Normal-spiking mode, 174

Omega 3 fatty acids, 256
Ophthalmologic applications of lasers, 2, 13, 192
Optical fibers. *See also* Fiber-optic delivery systems
  bending loss, 52–54
  energy loss in, 109
  fiber coating, 54–55
  fiber core damage, 58
  fiber selection, 55–56
  input surface damage, 57
  laser energy coupling, 59–60, 110–11
  numerical aperature, 52
  other energy losses, 56–57
  overview, 66–68
  physics/energy transmission, 49–52
Optical shields, 17
Ostial LAD stenosis case study, 131–33
Ostial right coronary case study, 148–52
Output surface damage, 58
"Over-the-wire" guidance systems, 64–66, 67–68

Patient report forms (PRFs), 233
Peak energy loss, 56
Peak power, 9, 29, 172, 177

Percutaneous transluminal coronary angioplasty (PTCA)
  as adjunct to laser procedure, 78
  clinical procedures, 210–16
  contraindications, 92–93, 127
  development, 98–99
  indications, 65, 259
  restenosis, 242–45, 259
  training in, 74
Perforation of vessels
  case study, 160–62
  causes, 32, 68, 105
  coronary anatomy and, 79
  incidence of, 40
  management of, 82
  manifestations of, 152
Pericardial tamponade, 82
Photoacoustic process of tissue ablation, 13–14
Photochemical process of tissue ablation, 12–13, 33–34, 99, 225
Photoexcitation, 12
Photoplasmas, 9, 10, 18
Photoplasmic process of tissue ablation, 33–34
Photosensitizers, 225
Plaque ablation, 20, 31–33, 36, 175
Plasma production, 13
Plastic-clad silica fibers, 55–56
Platelet-derived growth factor (PDGF), 216, 247, 248
Platelet inhibitors, 255–56
Plume, laser, 222, 224–25
PMA. *See* Premarket approval applications
Polymorphous lacunae, 36, 175
Population inversion, 4, 5, 6
Premarket approval applications (PMA), 231, 237–38
Progress reports, 236–37
Prostaglandins, 258
Protective clothing, 224
Proteoglycans, 250, 252
PTCA. *See* Percutaneous

Index

transluminal coronary angioplasty
Pulse duration, 19–20, 36, 38, 175, 185–86
Pulse energy, 66, 177
Pulse-stretched excimer laser, 23
Pulse width determination, 9
Pulsed lasers
  applications, 12–13, 17, 18–20, 185
  development, 99
  energy delivery, 9–10, 29, 175
  energy loss in, 57
  features, 27–28
  guidance systems, 65
  histologic effects, 36, 39–40, 42–45
  output generation, 173–75
  types, 20
Pulsed ultraviolet light, 12, 14

Q-switching, 27–28, 173, 174
Quantronix, Inc., 211

Radiation Control for Health and Safety Act, 229
Radio-frequency excited lasers, 231
Raman scattering, 57, 58
Rayleigh scattering, 7, 56
Reflection of light, 2, 6–10
Reflective energy loss, 56
Refraction of light, 2, 6–10, 32, 49–50
Regulation of lasers. *See* Laser regulation issues
Remodeling of thrombus, 194, 195
Reports of prior investigations, 229–31
Restenosis
  ablation of, 258–59
  defined, 44, 108
  incidence of, 81, 93, 111, 172, 216–19
  interventions, 255–58
  pathogenesis, 241–45, 251–55

Right posterior descending artery graft case study, 158–60
Ruby lasers, 2, 183, 192

Safety and lasers. *See* Laser safety issues
Sapphire fibers, 17, 179
Scattering of light, 2, 6–10, 29–34
Schneider Super High Flow guides, 76
Self-focusing/self-trapping effect, 58
7×200 micron catheters, 63
Shock waves, 10, 13, 18
Silica fibers, 55–56, 99
Silver halide, 179
600–micron catheters, 61, 62–63
Smoke evacuation systems, 224
Smooth muscle, 40–41, 252, 256–57
Snell's Law, 51
Solid-state lasers, 2, 172, 183
Spectranetics, Inc., 66, 75
Spectroscopic feedback, 65–66
Steroids, 256
Stretching of vessel walls, 243, 251–52, 259

Tetracycline, 14
Thallium halide, 179
Thermal fusion of tissues, 194–96
Thermal injury to tissue
  CW lasers and, 28, 175
  macroscopic/histologic analysis, 35–38
  pulsed lasers and, 17, 176, 185
Thermal process of tissue ablation, 10–12, 33–34, 175–77, 223, 224
Thermal relaxation, 11, 28, 36, 38, 175
Thermal stress crack, 58
Thermisters and thermocouples, 196
Thrombogenicity
  laser balloon angioplasty and, 194, 216
  laser type and, 39–40, 44, 45, 105, 185

Thulium:YAG lasers, 178, 180
Tissue. *See* Atherosclerotic tissue; Cardiovascular tissue; Laser/tissue interaction
Total occlusions, 92, 144–47, 168–70, 172, 242
Training of angioplasty practitioners, 74
Transforming growth factor (TGF), 247–49
Transmission of light, 2, 6–10
Trapidil, 257
12 × 200 micron catheters, 63

Ultraviolet (UV) lasers
  energy delivery, 61
  histologic effects, 32, 36, 177
  optical fibers, 55
  safety/regulatory issues, 226–27
  types, 12–13, 17, 19, 34
U.S. Food and Drug Administration, 222, 228–29, 231, 236–38
USCI, Inc., 66, 205

Vaporization as tissue effect of lasers, 9

Vascular tissue. *See* Cardiovascular tissue
Vasoactivity, 40–41, 44
Vibrational rotational state, 6
Vincristine, 257

Wavelengths of emitted light
  determination of, 5–6
  light absorption/scattering and, 29–34
  optimal types for laser angioplasty, 15–20, 175–77
White light, 1
Wound healing process
  cellular proliferation phase, 249–50
  extracellular matrix phase, 250
  inflammatory phase, 245–49
  overview, 45

Xenon lasers, 19, 21, 100

Yttrium-aluminum-garnet lasers, 2

Zirconium fluoride, 17, 179

RD 598.35 .L37 C67 1992
Coronary laser angioplasty